Big Data Analytics in HIV/AIDS Research

Ali Al Mazari
Alfaisal University, Saudi Arabia

A volume in the Advances in Healthcare Information Systems and Administration (AHISA) Book Series

IGI Global
DISSEMINATOR OF KNOWLEDGE

Published in the United States of America by
IGI Global
Medical Information Science Reference (an imprint of IGI Global)
701 E. Chocolate Avenue
Hershey PA, USA 17033
Tel: 717-533-8845
Fax: 717-533-8661
E-mail: cust@igi-global.com
Web site: http://www.igi-global.com

Library of Congress Cataloging-in-Publication Data

Names: Al Mazari, Ali, 1971- editor.
Title: Big data analytics in HIV/AIDS research / Ali Al Mazari, editor.
Description: Hershey PA : Medical Information Science Reference, [2018] I Includes bibliographical references.
Identifiers: LCCN 2017022903I ISBN 9781522532033 (hardcover) I ISBN 9781522532040 (ebook)
Subjects: I MESH: Datasets as Topic I HIV Infections--epidemiology I Data Mining
Classification: LCC RA643.8 I NLM WC 503.41 I DDC 614.5/993920072--dc23 LC record available at https://lccn.loc.gov/2017022903

This book is published in the IGI Global book series Advances in Healthcare Information Systems and Administration (AHISA) (ISSN: 2328-1243; eISSN: 2328-126X)

British Cataloguing in Publication Data
A Cataloguing in Publication record for this book is available from the British Library.

Advances in Healthcare Information Systems and Administration (AHISA) Book Series

ISSN:2328-1243
EISSN:2328-126X

Editor-in-Chief: Anastasius Moumtzoglou, Hellenic Society for Quality & Safety in Healthcare and P. & A. Kyriakou Children's Hospital, Greece

MISSION

The **Advances in Healthcare Information Systems and Administration (AHISA) Book Series** aims to provide a channel for international researchers to progress the field of study on technology and its implications on healthcare and health information systems. With the growing focus on healthcare and the importance of enhancing this industry to tend to the expanding population, the book series seeks to accelerate the awareness of technological advancements of health information systems and expand awareness and implementation.

Driven by advancing technologies and their clinical applications, the emerging field of health information systems and informatics is still searching for coherent directing frameworks to advance health care and clinical practices and research. Conducting research in these areas is both promising and challenging due to a host of factors, including rapidly evolving technologies and their application complexity. At the same time, organizational issues, including technology adoption, diffusion and acceptance as well as cost benefits and cost effectiveness of advancing health information systems and informatics applications as innovative forms of investment in healthcare are gaining attention as well. **AHISA** addresses these concepts and critical issues.

COVERAGE

- Medical informatics
- Nursing Expert Systems
- IT security and privacy issues
- IT Applications in Physical Therapeutic Treatments
- Clinical Decision Support Design, Development and Implementation
- Management of Emerging Health Care Technologies
- E-Health and M-Health
- Role of informatics specialists
- IS in Healthcare
- Telemedicine

The Advances in Healthcare Information Systems and Administration (AHISA) Book Series (ISSN 2328-1243) is published by IGI Global, 701 E. Chocolate Avenue, Hershey, PA 17033-1240, USA, www.igi-global.com. This series is composed of titles available for purchase individually; each title is edited to be contextually exclusive from any other title within the series. For pricing and ordering information please visit http://www.igi-global.com/book-series/advances-healthcare-information-systems-administration/37156. Postmaster: Send all address changes to above address.

Titles in this Series

For a list of additional titles in this series, please visit:
https://www.igi-global.com/book-series/advances-healthcare-information-systems-administration/37156

Novel Applications of Virtual Communities in Healthcare Settings
Christo El Morr (York University, Canada)
Medical Information Science Reference • ©2018 • 247pp • H/C (ISBN: 9781522529583) • US $235.00

Handbook of Research on Data Science for Effective Healthcare Practice and Administration
Elham Akhond Zadeh Noughabi (University of Calgary, Canada) Bijan Raahemi (University of Ottawa, Canada) Amir Albadvi (Tarbiat Modares University, Iran) and Behrouz H. Far (University of Calgary, Canada)
Medical Information Science Reference • ©2017 • 545pp • H/C (ISBN: 9781522525158) • US $255.00

Patent Law and Intellectual Property in the Medical Field
Rashmi Aggarwal (Institute of Management Technology Ghaziabad, India) and Rajinder Kaur (Panjab University, India)
Medical Information Science Reference • ©2017 • 257pp • H/C (ISBN: 9781522524144) • US $200.00

Design, Development, and Integration of Reliable Electronic Healthcare Platforms
Anastasius Moumtzoglou (P&A Kyriakou Children's Hospital, Greece)
Medical Information Science Reference • ©2017 • 357pp • H/C (ISBN: 9781522517245) • US $205.00

Cloud Computing Systems and Applications in Healthcare
Chintan M. Bhatt (Charotar University of Science & Technology, India) and S. K. Peddoju (Indian Institute of Technology Roorkee, India)
Medical Information Science Reference • ©2017 • 282pp • H/C (ISBN: 9781522510024) • US $205.00

For an entire list of titles in this series, please visit:
https://www.igi-global.com/book-series/advances-healthcare-information-systems-administration/37156

IGI Global
DISSEMINATOR OF KNOWLEDGE

701 East Chocolate Avenue, Hershey, PA 17033, USA
Tel: 717-533-8845 x100 • Fax: 717-533-8661
E-Mail: cust@igi-global.com • www.igi-global.com

This work is dedicated to my father, Adnan, and mother, Farhah, and family, who at all times enable and inspire me with their bravery, faith, hope, and love to fly toward my imaginations and dreams!!!

Always yours,
Ali Al Mazari

Editorial Advisory Board

List of Reviewers

Table of Contents

Detailed Table of Contents

Reverse transcriptase (RT) is a vital enzyme in the process of transcription of HIV-1. The nucleoside analogues of RT inhibitors (NRTIs) act by substrate competition and chain termination as they resemble a nucleotide. To understand the basis of RT resistance in HIV-1, in this chapter, one of the clinically essential mutants Q151M of RT which exhibits multi-resistance to many NRTIs was modeled and docked with NRTIs in comparison to wild type (WT). The results of docking indicate that the WT showed high affinity with all inhibitors compared to the mutant (MT). It can be suggested that the high affinity in WT could be attributed to the favorable interactions with all inhibitors that lacks in MT due to amino acid substitution that leads to structural changes in MT protein, which alters the favorable network of interaction and eventually imparts resistance to all inhibitors.

The traditional way of formatting information from transactional systems to make them available for "statistical processing" does not work in a situation where data is arriving in huge volumes from diverse sources, and where even the formats could be changing. Faced with this volume and diversification, it is essential to develop techniques to make best use of all of these stocks in order to extract the maximum amount of information and knowledge. Traditional analysis methods have been based largely on the assumption that statisticians can work with data within the confines of their own computing environment. But the growth of the amounts of data is changing that paradigm, especially which ride of the progress in computational data analysis. This chapter builds upon sources but also goes further in the examination to answer this question: What needs to be done in this area to deal with big data challenges?

The term big data refers to the data that exceeds the processing or analyzing capacity of existing database management systems. The inability of existing DBMS to handle big data is due to its large volume, high velocity, pertaining veracity, heterogeneous variety, and on-atomic values. Nowadays, healthcare plays a vital role in everyone's life. It becomes a very large and open platform for everyone to do all kinds of research work without affecting human life. When it comes to disease, there are so many types found all over the world. But among them, AIDS (acquired immunodeficiency syndrome) is a disease that spreads so quickly and can easily turn life to death. There are many studies going on to create drugs to cure this deadly disease, but until now, there has been no success. In cases such as this, big data is implemented for better a result, which will have a good impact on society.

HIV/AIDS big data analytics evolved as a potential initiative enabling the connection between three major scientific disciplines: (1) the HIV biology emergence and evolution; (2) the clinical and medical complex problems and practices associated

Protease (PR) is an important enzyme required for the posttranslational processing of the viral gene products of type-1 human immunodeficiency virus (HIV-1). Protease inhibitors (PI) act as competitive inhibitors that bind to the active site of PR. The I84V mutation contributes resistance to multiple PIs, and structurally, this mutation affects both sides of the enzyme active site. In order to get insights about this major resistance site to PR inhibitors using in silico approaches, in this chapter, the wild-type (WT) and mutant (MT) I84V of PR were modeled and docked with all PR inhibitors: Atazanavir, Darunavir, Indinavir, Lopinavir, Nelfinavir, Saquinavir, and Tipranavir. Docking results revealed that in comparison to the WT, the binding score was higher for the MT-I84V. Thus, it can be suggested that the high affinity towards inhibitors in the MT could be due to the presence of energetically favorable interactions, which may lead to tight binding of inhibitors with the MT protein, leading to the development of PR resistance against PIs in HIV-1 eventually.

In the last two decades, several advancement studies have increased the care of HIV-infected individuals. Specifically, the development for preparation of combination antiretroviral therapy has resulted in a dramatic decline in the rate of deaths from AIDS. The term “HIV-associated neurocognitive disorder” (HAND) has been used to distinguish the spectrum of neurocognitive dysfunction associated with HIV infection. HIV can pass to the CNS during the early stages of infection and last in the CNS. CNS inflammation and infection lead to the development of HAND. The brain can serve as a sanctuary for ongoing HIV replication, even when the systemic viral suppression has been achieved. HAND can remain in patients treated with combination antiretroviral therapy, and its effect on survival, quality of life, and everyday functioning make it a significant unresolved problem. This chapter discusses details of the computational modeling studies on mechanisms and structures of human dopamine transporter (hDAT) and its interaction with HIV-1 trans activator of transcription (Tat).

Foreword

The increasingly sophisticated technologies granted and contributed to the humanity further insights and understanding of our needs and problems. This book takes the advantages of technological developments and advancements through investigating the use of Big Data Analytics in the intersection area of three dominant sciences or disciplines: biology, medical and computing. The mission of constructing this book as a new domain for Big Data Analytics was not easy, mainly when applied in the area of a disastrous infection and disease, HIV/AIDS. The term "Big Data" is novel, despite data is mature. The term "Analytics" is also innovative, despite computer processing and analysis is well known since ages. The application of the combination of those two terms, i.e., Big Data Analytics, in medical and healthcare domains to serve clinicians is also a pioneering task, despite their application in other sciences such as security, business, finance, etc. To some, *Data* may mean easy to find, analyze and convert into information; yet, the skills requirements, tools and engines necessary to identify, access, collect, organize, manage, secure, manipulate and process large data sets remains a real scientific and practical challenge. Data sets can be structured, semi-structured or unstructured; data can also be numerical, textual, or in multimedia format; data also be public, private or sensitive; and so on. Dealing with medical issues with biological background is also another challenge, as HIV/ADS infection. Since years, the progress toward understanding and controlling HIV virus and AIDS disease is slow, despite scientists have made an acceptable management of this tough infectious disease. In response, this book comes in time to try uncovering significant aspects of HIV/AIDS with biological perspective. The book therefore, constructs a new scientific and research domain in the area of infectious diseases with particular focus on HIV/AIDS using a novel tool known as Big Data Analytics. The integration between computational, biology, medicine, pharmacology and clinical domains created by this book derives the scientific synergy and collaborative interests among scientists from those domains to understand and tackle HIV/AIDS problem using new approach and tools. The book then initiates a new trend of thinking and decision making in a novel, yet critical area of interest, i.e., HIV/AIDS and infectious diseases; this may help solving this challenging problem.

Preface

With the advent of the new technologies, Big Data science in particular, scientists made a significant progress in the study of medical problems from biological perspective. This book, HIV/AIDS Big Data Analytics in HIV/AIDS Research, evolved as a potential initiative enabling the connection between three major scientific disciplines: (1) the HIV biology emergence and evolution; (2) the clinical and medical complex problems and practices associated with the infections and diseases; and (3) the computational methods for the mining of HIV/AIDS biological, medical and clinical Big Data. The aim of this initiative is to underline and respond to the Big Data problems at the intersection and multidisciplinary science of these three disciplines. The first objective in this work is to highlight the problems associated with HIV/AIDS Big Data Management from different perspectives including: Management Software, Applications and Approaches; Big Data Architect and Warehouses; Big Data Governance; HIV/AIDS Big Data Security and Privacy, etc. This will address the emergence and evolution of HIV/AIDS Big Data Management Domain to understand how such massive data can be collected, stored, managed, secured, handled, governed, used, etc. It is believed that these key issues are crucial for the development and implementation of Big Data Analytics in the HIV/AIDS industry.

The second objective is to provide the development and implementation of different computational techniques and analytics for HIV/AIDS Big Data Analysis with focus on the key big biological and complex clinical variables of HIV/AIDS to be considered by practitioners and scientists. This will involve the development, implementation and testing of Computational HIV/AIDS Big Data Analytics, Techniques, Models and Algorithms for the Prediction, Classification, Visualization, Clustering, Optimization and Distributed Processing problems. These will extend the understanding of HIV/AIDS Big Data for clinical decision making and the design of Combination Antiretroviral Therapy (CART), known also as or Highly Active Antiretroviral Therapy (HAART) agents.

The third objective is to provide Big Data Analytics for knowledge discovery in specific domains of the HIV/AIDS infection and disease. This will introduce several Big Data Analytics to improve the current knowledge in key domains including HIV/AIDS Epidemiology and Pathology, Evolutionary Patterns, Genotypes and Phenotypes, Immune System Evolution, Viral Dynamics, Drug Resistance Dynamics, Antiretroviral Interactions, Transmission and Adherence. These efforts will generate and improve key and new types of knowledge needed for the management of HIV/AIDS infection and disease.

Due to the lack of a comprehensive and complete reference book that integrates biological and clinical understanding of HIV/AIDS with focus on Big Data Analytics, it can be seen that this book could be unique in its contribution, value, nature, scope and tools. To the best of available knowledge, there is no such book that provides a complete coverage and discussion of HIV biological and clinical problems together with the Big Data Analytics problems and solutions. Therefore, the main objective of this work is expected to supply the description of these problems and solutions using Big Data Analytics with the support of real examples and case studies from biology, medical and computational sciences. The lack of such publication is clearly due to the difficulty of obtaining the complete knowledge from Big Data located at the intersection of the three disciplines at the same time. The most important challenge here is due to the HIV/AIDS Big Data complexity and variability belongs to this multidisciplinary with three big faces that can be attributed by many features. The challenge to establish skills for solving such complexity starts at the entry gate to this multidisciplinary by understanding its Big Data, and then at the decision making to what read, understand and think about. This book attempted to fill all of these gaps and serve as an entry gate to the multidisciplinary of biology, clinical and computing of a particular infectious disease using a new approach used by other disciplines, i.e., Big Data Analytics.

As practitioners, clinicians will be able to obtain clinical view of HIV/AIDS Big clinical Data and problems or solutions, and biologists will also be able to obtain biological view of HIV/AIDS Big biological data problems and solutions. Moreover, computational scientists will be able to obtain technical, computational and analytical view of HIV Big Data Analytics with an area of application to model problems and solutions. Most scientists feel more comfortable when using one individual source at the intersection of several disciplines. For example, PhD students in the area of bioinformatics, medical informatics and biomedical informatics struggle largely to pick up the right reference to read; mainly for the development and application of the new area of Big Data Analytics in the domains of medicine, biomedical and healthcare. Clinicians and biologist also struggle to understand and explore the contributions made by the ICT integration and Big Data Analytics within their industries. Computational scientists also struggle to identify the gaps and challenges within the area of big biological and clinical data that they can examine and get advantage of it using their ICT tools, techniques, algorithms and Analytics. The key value therefore is in providing a reference enabling translating HIV/AIDS Big Data sets into meaningful public health interventions.

The HIV/AIDS Big Data Analytics in HIV/AIDS Research book covers key issues in the area of HIV/AIDS Big Data. In the introduction, the author introduces the advances and new trends in the area of HIV/AIDS Big Data Analytics. The chapter discusses the emergence and evolution of Big Data Analytics, with focus on Medical and Biomedicine domains, and particularly HIV/AIDS Big Data Computational Analysis Techniques including Prediction, Classification, Visualization, Clustering, Optimisation and Big Data Distributed Processing Techniques. The chapter also discusses the HIV/AIDS Big and Complex Data Management from different perspectives and provides an HIV/AIDS Big Data Analytics Taxonomy.

The first chapter investigates the reason of multi resistance mediated by the substitution Q151M of RT which exhibits multiple resistances to many NRTIs such as ABC, AZT, DDI, D4T, FTC, TDF and 3TC in comparison to wild type (WT). The findings of this chapter show the effect of binding affinity of WT and MT- Q151M of RT with both thymine (AZT D4T, FTC and 3TC) and guanine (ABC, DDI and TDF) analogues of NRTIs. The second chapter focuses on the challenges around the era of "data revolution" through the description and review big data, and then knowledge discovery from data using analytics methods. The chapter then explains and presents how the most basic of statistical methodologies has developed to create very flexible tools, and how statistics and computational tools should act together to better analyze big data in order to extract valuable information.

The third chapter describes the types of predicative measures to understand HIV/AIDS including Medical, Environmental and Operational, despite the operational remains with no clear vision. The Medical Predicative Measures are invented for fighting with HIV/AIDS, and the Environmental Predicative Measures focus on many environmental factors such as poverty, culture, religion and traditions, appear to play an essential role in the rapid and global development of AIDS epidemic. The fourth chapter provides a review on the computational and data mining Perspectives on HIV/AIDS in Big Data Era. The chapter focuses on the research opportunities in this domain, identifies the challenges facing the development of big data analytics in HIV/AIDS domain, and then highlights the future research directions of big data in the healthcare and clinical sectors.

The fifth chapter discusses the overview of various legal frameworks governing health information, dispels misconceptions about privacy regulations, and highlights how these legal frameworks provide privacy, confidentiality, and security to this sensitive information, in precise, the contribution may maximize the utility of big data to improve HIV/AIDS prevention and treatment. The sixth chapter provides the development of a stochastic model to demonstrate that in men who have sex with men (MSM) populations that practice unprotected anal intercourse (UAI), the prevalence of the HIV-1 infection decays when there is a transition from role versatility to role segregation without assuming that the long-term probability of acquisition from UIA sex with receptive infected partners is negligible. The chapter demonstrates that the high prevalence of the HIV-1 infection in MSM populations can still theoretically be attributed to role versatility.

The seventh chapter provides the development and application of molecular model to understand drug resistance to protease inhibitors. The chapter introduces the model to understand the differences in the binding affinity between the clinically essential mutant (MT- I84V) and the wild-type (WT) of HIV-1 protease protein which eventually lead to PR resistance. The eighth chapter provides a review on the computational modeling research on mechanism and structures of Human dopamine transporter (hDAT) as well as its interaction with HIV-1 trans-activator of transcription (Tat).

With the above contribution, this book is expected to serve as a significant reference for Computational Scientists, Statisticians, Computational Biologists, Bioinformaticians, Biomedical Scientists, Clinical Practitioners, Pharmacologists and other researchers in the areas of Computing, Big Data Analytics, Machine Learning, Data Mining, Pharmacology, Infectious Diseases and Evolution Biology. The book can also serve as a complementary textbook for advanced courses in the area of data mining, machine learning, medical sciences of infectious diseases, computational biology and biomedical informatics multidisciplinary courses designed for undergraduate, postgraduates and doctorate research students.

As potential titles of courses associated with this book, 'HIV Big Data Computation', 'Big Data Analytics in Bioinformatics', 'Big Data Mining and Modeling in HIV/AIDS', 'Computational Methods for Big Data Analysis', 'Computing Methods in Biomedical Informatics', Big Data Analytics for HIV Dynamics', and so forth, can be considered in this context. As target audience for this book, research centers and researchers in the areas of Big Data Analytics, data mining, machine learning, algorithmic design in life sciences, bioinformatics, biomedical informatics, medical informatics, pharmacology, drug discovery and design, and evolution biology, all can be considered as primary target. This book can also be used by postgraduate students as a complementary or a secondary textbook for advanced courses in the area of Big Data Analytics, data mining, machine learning, and medical sciences of infectious diseases, biostatistics, computational biology and biomedical informatics.

Practitioners from computing and clinical industries can also get advantage of this book; it will be useful for computer applications developers in the area of Big Data Analytics, and may enable them to easily investigate and identify major requirements of computational infrastructure, application and platforms. For clinicians, this book will be useful for clinical practices in the area of infectious diseases and immunology; it may enable them to easily identify and analytically understand the different aspects of infection of the disease they manage or investigate which is similar to HIV/AIDS

In due course, this book is expected to help understanding the different aspects of HIV/AIDS Big Data Management. This will derive and represent the understanding of the HIV/AIDS Big Data construction, architect and its intersection with the computational, biomedical, pharmacological and other domains. The book is also expected to make it possible to understand and identify the key Big Data variables and Big Databases aspects for HIV/AIDS evolution, treatment and management using computational techniques and algorithms. This will represent the application of HIV/AIDS Big Data Analytics as an interest of research communities from different disciplines. In addition, this work is aimed to understand HIV/AIDS Big Data mining and modeling for issue-specific knowledge discovery in the area of medicine. This may provide the robust ICT integration explaining the use of these Big Data Analytics technologies within biology and therapy of HIV. This will accelerate and influence the bioinformatics and biomedical informatics paradigm.

Acknowledgment

With all my hearty wishes, I would like to thank all of those who helped in making this book. Special thanks go to my beloved friends Dr. Ahmed Bani-Mustafa, Dr. Qusai Shambour, Prof. Emmanuel Nyakwende, Dr. Hashem Al Adarous, and all others I knew. Many thanks with appreciation to the Development Editor, Ms. Jordan Tepper, in particular, and Melissa Wagner, Assistant Marketing Manager, at the IGI Global. Thanks also to my beloved sister, Safa Al Mazari, for her assistance in wrapping up and organizing this book. A very special thank to all those living at my home, wife, boys and daughters for giving the space and time to make this book a reality.

Ali Al Mazari
Alfaisal University, Saudi Arabia

Introduction

ADVANCES IN HIV/AIDS BIG DATA ANALYTICS: INTRODUCTION

Understanding the different aspects of HIV/AIDS Big Data Management, and identifying the key Big Data variables and Big Databases aspects for HIV/AIDS evolution, treatment and management, remain of research interest. Understanding HIV/AIDS Big Data mining and modelling for knowledge discovery in the area of medicine is also a key area of research. The applications of Big Data Analytics in the area of HIV/AIDS represent an evolved initiative enabling the connection between three major scientific disciplines: medicine, biology and computing. This connection integrates the scientific insights provided through HIV biology emergence and evolution, clinical and medical complex problems and practices associated with the infections and diseases, and the computational methods for the mining of HIV/AIDS biological, medical and clinical Big Data. Therefore, this chapter introduces the advances and new trends in the area of HIV/AIDS Big Data Analytics. In this chapter, the focus will be on the emergence and evolution of Big Data Analytics, and on the applications of such initiative in medicine, biology and biomedicine domains. The chapter develop a novel HIV/AIDS Big Data Taxonomies with focus on HIV/AIDS Big Data Management, Computational Analytics and HIV/AIDS research issues of interest.

HIV/AIDS BIG DATA CHALLENGE

The recent revolutionary developments, advancements and applications of DNA sequencing tools and technologies increased the availability of genome sequences and data of humans and other millions of species; the available data is most likely doubling every year. Many advantages have been reported and seen through the use and processing of such genomic data in different domains including biology for understanding evolutionary behaviours, in medicine for understanding and managing infections and diseases, in pharmacology for drug design and manufacturing, etc. However, many challenges remain residual when dealing with big data, mainly when datasets are structured, semi-structured and/or unstructured. Datasets can also be challenging with different types including numerical, textual, or in different multimedia formats; and datasets can be public, private, sensitive or under other security category.

Moreover, a remaining challenge for HIV/AIDS Big Data is when dealing with the integration of such datasets located within spread databases including hospital databases, national or private medical centres, molecular labs, and even research centres and other repositories. Regardless of whether it's locally or internationally, there is a huge amount of data located everywhere and it needs to be consolidated for more significance, mainly with the advent and availability of modern data warehousing tools and technologies. In earlier research and studies, scientists used to have a small, but acceptable, amount of data to investigate problems, however, this may not be the case anymore considering the availability of big data. Figure 1 illustrates a taxonomy that covers various aspects and categories of HIV/AIDS Big Data problems and challenges.

Figure 1. Taxonomy of HIV/AIDS big data problems and challenges

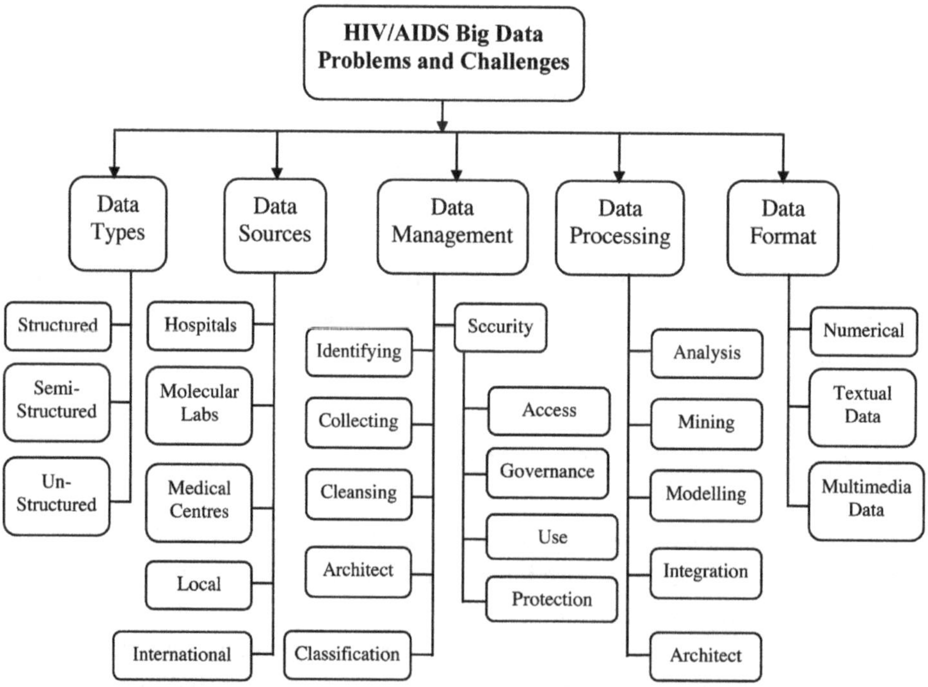

HIV/AIDS CLINICAL AND MEDICAL CHALLENGES

Worldwide, HIV infection and its consequential AIDS are ranked at the top of the list of most disastrous health problems. There have been substantial efforts over the past two decades to address the threats posed by HIV infection and AIDS; these include the development of potent Antiretroviral (ARV), effective clinical tests, genotypic databases and using these programs for the effective treatment and prevention of HIV/AIDS. However, the numbers of people living with HIV and deaths due to AIDS continue to grow. An estimated 39.5 million people worldwide were living with HIV in 2006, of whom 4.3 million were newly infected and an estimated 2.9 million lost their lives to AIDS.

The capacity of HIV to mutate and produce genetic variations, so-called viral quasispecies, remains the most critical factor behind the failure of the approved Combination Antiretroviral Therapy (CART), formerly Highly Active Antiretroviral Therapy (HAART). The existence of these variations has enabled HIV to acquire resistance to the available ARVs; this can significantly reduce the benefits of the therapies. Understanding the ways in which these genetic variations emerge and evolve may enable the determination of which drugs are most effective for each infected individual. HIV targets a type of the white blood cell known as a CD4 T-cell, a fundamental component of the immune system. Because CD4 T-cells enable the body to fight off certain types of infectious attack, an individual becomes more vulnerable immunologically with the depletion of these cells. In a variable period of time—from one to twenty years or more—HIV-infection exhausts the CD4 T-cells, resulting in AIDS and, typically, death then follows within several years of AIDS onset.

ARV agents are designed to inhibit HIV replication. The start of an effective treatment regimen enables the continuity of CD4 T-cell production. However, complicating factors usually emerge, limiting the production of these cells. The rapid development of genetic variations that confer drug resistance associated with one or more ARV agents is ranked at the top of these factors. Genotypic testing has been introduced to identify the mutations associated with drug resistance. These tests determine the new mutations within the PR and RT nucleotide sequences. A genotypic assay compares PR and RT sequences with the analogous data from previous tests of the same individual, and/or with a wild-type reference sequence, to identify the precise mutations associated with resistance to individual ARVs and classes of ARVs. The HIV viral load (VL) and leukocyte subset analysis assays are used to determine the number of HIV copies and the counts of CD4 T-cell in a blood sample, respectively. These assays together give information related to the impact of resistance mutations on viral replication and on immunological damage, respectively. Despite the ability to monitor these parameters, the earliest pathways in the development of resistance-associated mutations and the impact of these on the vulnerability of the immunological and virological responses are not yet clearly defined. Analysis of HIV variability alone, even when determined directly by sequence analysis is problematic, because of the complex interdependencies between the high genetic variability of HIV mutations and mutational patterns, individual ARV agent(s) and classes of ARVs and the responses of the immune system and the capacity of the virus to mutate to also escape immunological attack. Figure 2 illustrates a taxonomy that covers various aspects and categories of HIV/AIDS research topics of interest.

HIV/AIDS BIG DATA COMPUTATIONAL ANALYTICS

Computational methods for the analysis of the genomic and proteomic structures of viruses have the potential to provide major insights into biology, medicine and pharmacy. These methods can be used for the analysis of the genotypic, phenotypic, evolutionary and treatment profiles of viral infections and diseases, to accelerate the discovery of potent therapeutic agents, to improve knowledge of the biology of these microbes, to advance the management of infectious diseases, and, ultimately, to enhance health care, saving lives, time and costs, and improving the quality of life. Many computational methods, including algorithms and models, have been used in the development of repositories of gene and protein molecular sequences, and of computer-based genotyping applications. In the area of HIV/AIDS Big Data Computational Analysis, different techniques can be considered for the advances in this new domain. Figure 1.3 illustrates a taxonomy that covers various techniques for the development of algorithms and models servicing as HIV/AIDS Big Data Computational Analytics.

Figure 2. Taxonomy of HIV/AIDS research topics of interest

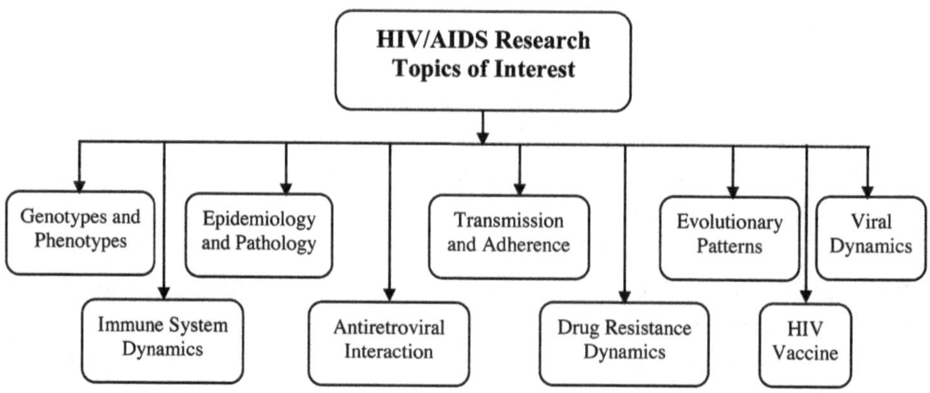

Figure 3. Taxonomy of HIV/AIDS big data computational analytics

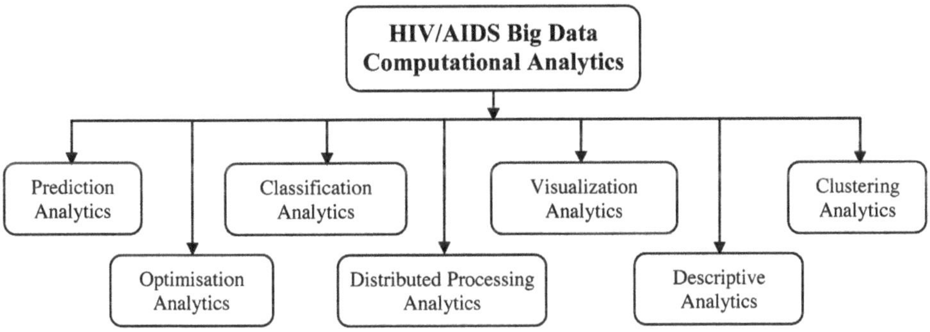

HIV/AIDS BIG DATA ANALYTICS MOTIVATION

HIV/AIDS Big Data Analytics evolved as a potential initiative enabling the connection between three major scientific disciplines: (1) the HIV biology emergence and evolution; (2) the clinical and medical complex problems and practices associated with the infections and diseases; and (3) the computational methods for the mining of HIV/AIDS biological, medical and clinical Big Data. The book aims to underline and respond to the Big Data problems at the intersection and multidisciplinary science of these three disciplines. The first objective in this book is to highlight the problems associated with HIV/AIDS Big Data Management from different perspectives including: Management Software, Applications and Approaches; Big Data Architect and Warehouses; Big Data Governance; HIV/AIDS Big Data Security and Privacy, etc. As in Part A, this will address the emergence and evolution of HIV/AIDS Big Data Management Domain to understand how such massive data can be collected, stored, managed, secured, handled, governed, used, etc. It is believed that these key issues are crucial for the development and implementation of Big Data Analytics in the HIV/AIDS industry.

The second objective is to provide the development and implementation of different computational techniques for HIV/AIDS Big Data Analysis with focus on the key big biological and complex clinical variables of HIV/AIDS to be considered by practitioners and scientists. As in Part B, this will involve the development, implementation and testing of Computational HIV/AIDS Big Data Analytics, Techniques, Models and Algorithms for the Prediction, Classification, Visualization, Clustering, Optimisation and Distributed Processing problems. These will extend the understanding of HIV/AIDS Big Data for clinical decision making and antiretroviral design. The third objective is to provide Big Data Analytics for knowledge discovery in specific domains of the HIV/AIDS infection and disease. As in Part C, the book will introduce several Big Data Analytics to improve the current knowledge in key domains including HIV/AIDS Epidemiology and Pathology, Evolutionary Patterns, Genotypes and Phenotypes, Immune System Evolution, Viral Dynamics, Drug Resistance Dynamics, Antiretroviral Interactions, Transmission and Adherence. These efforts will generate and improve key and new types of knowledge needed for the management of HIV/AIDS infection and disease. In summary, focal aspects of this book include:

- Understanding the different aspects of HIV/AIDS Big Data Management. This will derive and represent the understanding of the HIV/AIDS Big Data construction, architect and its intersection with the computational, biomedical, pharmacological and other domains.
- Understanding and identification of the key Big Data variables and Big Databases aspects for HIV/AIDS evolution, treatment and management using computational techniques and algorithms. This will represent the application of HIV/AIDS Big Data Analytics as an interest of research communities from different disciplines.
- Understanding HIV/AIDS Big Data mining and modelling for issue-specific knowledge discovery in the area of medicine. This will provide the robust ICT integration explaining the use of these Big Data Analytics technologies within biology and therapy of HIV. This will accelerate and influence the bioinformatics and biomedical informatics paradigm.

THE NEED FOR HIV/AIDS BIG DATA ANALYTICS

Due to the lack of a comprehensive and complete reference book that integrates biological and clinical understanding of HIV/AIDS with focus on Big Data Analytics, it can be seen that this book will be unique in its contribution, value, nature, scope and tools. To the best of available knowledge, there is no such book that provides a complete coverage and discussion of HIV biological and clinical problems together with the Big Data Analytics problems and solutions. Therefore, the main objective of this book is to supply the description of these problems and solutions using Big Data Analytics with the support of real examples and cases studies from biology, medical and computational sciences. The lack of such publication is clearly due to the difficulty of obtaining the complete knowledge from Big Data located at the intersection of the three disciplines at the same time. The most important challenge here is due to the HIV/AIDS Big Data complexity and variability belongs to this multidisciplinary with three big faces that can be attributed by many features. The challenge to establish skills for solving such complexity starts at the entry gate to this multidisciplinary by understanding its Big Data, and then at the decision making to what read, understand and think about. This book attempts to fill all of these gaps and serve as entry gate to the multidisciplinary of biology, clinical and computing of a particular infectious disease using a new approach used by other disciplines, i.e., Big Data Analytics.

Clinicians will be able to obtain clinical view of HIV/AIDS Big clinical Data and problems or solutions, biologists will be able to obtain biological view of HIV/AIDS Big biological data problems and solutions, and computational scientists will be able to obtain technical, computational and analytical view of HIV Big Data Analytics with an area of application to model problems and solutions. Most scientists feel more comfortable when using one individual source at the intersection of several disciplines. For example, PhD students in the area of bioinformatics, medical informatics and biomedical informatics struggle largely to pick up the right reference to read; mainly for the development and application of the new area of Big Data Analytics in the domains of medicine, biomedical and healthcare. Clinicians and biologist also struggle to understand and explore the contributions made by the ICT integration and Big Data Analytics within their industries. Computational scientists also struggle to identify the gaps and challenges within the area of big biological and clinical Data that they can examine and get advantage of it using their ICT tools, techniques, algorithms and Analytics. The key value therefore is in providing a reference enabling translating HIV/AIDS Big Data sets into meaningful public health interventions.

THE TARGET AUDIENCE AND USE

This book will serve as a significant reference for Computational Scientists, Statisticians, Computational Biologists, Bioinformaticians, Biomedical Scientists, Clinical Practitioners, Pharmacologists and other researchers in the areas of Computing, Big Data Analytics, Machine Learning, Data Mining, Pharmacology, Infectious Diseases and Evolution Biology. The book can also serve as a complementary textbook for advanced courses in the area of data mining, machine learning, medical sciences of infectious diseases, computational biology and biomedical informatics multidisciplinary courses designed for undergraduate, postgraduates and doctorate and post-doctorate research students.

Potential titles of courses associated with this book may include: 'HIV Big Data Computation', 'Big Data Analytics in Bioinformatics', 'Big Data Mining and Modeling in HIV/AIDS', 'Computational Methods for Big Data Analysis', 'Computing Methods in Biomedical Informatics', Big Data Analytics for HIV Dynamics', and so forth. This book can be used as complementary reading for courses in bioinformatics, biomedical informatics, statistics and life sciences where these specialisations are offered. The target audience for this book will include:

- **Research Centres and Researchers:** Specifically, in the areas of Big Data Analytics, data mining, machine learning, algorithmic design in life sciences, bioinformatics, biomedical informatics, medical informatics, pharmacology, drug discovery and design, and evolution biology, as a primary target audience.
- **Postgraduate Students:** This book can be used as a complementary textbook for advanced courses in the area of Big Data Analytics, data mining, machine learning, medical sciences of infectious diseases, Biostatistics, computational biology and biomedical informatics, as a secondary target audience.
- **Computing Industry Practitioners:** This book will be useful for computer applications developers in the area of Big Data Analytics, data mining, machine learning and life sciences. The book will enable them to easily investigate and identify major requirements of computational infrastructure, application and platforms, as a secondary target audience.
- **Clinical Industry Practitioners:** This book will be useful for clinical practices in the area of infectious diseases and immunology. The book will enable them to easily identify and analytically understand the different aspects of infection of the disease they manage or investigate which is similar to HIV/AIDS, as a secondary target audience.

ORGANIZATION OF THE WORK

This work involves eight chapters. In the introduction chapter, this chapter, the author introduces the advances and new trends in the area of HIV/AIDS Big Data Analytics. The chapter discusses the emergence and evolution of Big Data Analytics, with focus on Medical and Biomedicine domains, and particularly HIV/AIDS Big Data Computational Analysis Techniques including Prediction, Classification, Visualization, Clustering, Optimisation and Big Data Distributed Processing Techniques. The chapter also discusses the HIV/AIDS Big and Complex Data Management from different perspectives and provides an HIV/AIDS Big Data Analytics Taxonomy.

The first chapter investigates the reason of multi resistance mediated by the substitution Q151M of RT which exhibits multiple resistances to many NRTIs such as ABC, AZT, DDI, D4T, FTC, TDF and 3TC in comparison to wild type (WT). The findings of this chapter show the effect of binding affinity of WT and MT- Q151M of RT with both thymine (AZT D4T, FTC and 3TC) and guanine (ABC, DDI and TDF) analogues of NRTIs.

The second chapter focuses on the challenges around the era of "data revolution" through the description and review big data, and then knowledge discovery from data using analytics methods. The chapter then explains and presents how the most basic of statistical methodologies has developed to create very flexible tools, and how statistics and computational tools should act together to better analyse big data in order to extract valuable information.

The third chapter describes the types of predicative measures to understand HIV/AIDS including Medical, Environmental and Operational, despite the operational remains with no clear vision. The Medical Predicative Measures are invented for fighting with HIV/AIDS, and the Environmental Predicative Measures focus on many environmental factors such as poverty, culture, religion and traditions, appear to play an essential role in the rapid and global development of AIDS epidemic.

The fourth chapter provides a review on the computational and data mining Perspectives on HIV/AIDS in Big Data Era. The chapter focuses on the research opportunities in this domain, identifies the challenges facing the development of big data analytics in HIV/AIDS domain, and then highlights the future research directions of big data in the healthcare and clinical sectors.

The fifth chapter discusses the overview of various legal frameworks governing health information, dispels misconceptions about privacy regulations, and highlights how these legal frameworks provide privacy, confidentiality, and security to this sensitive information, in precise, the contribution may maximize the utility of big data to improve HIV/AIDS prevention and treatment.

The sixth chapter provides the development of a stochastic model to demonstrate that in men who have sex with men (MSM) populations that practice unprotected anal intercourse (UAI), the prevalence of the HIV-1 infection decays when there is a transition from role versatility to role segregation without assuming that the long-term probability of acquisition from UIA sex with receptive infected partners is negligible. The chapter demonstrates that the high prevalence of the HIV-1 infection in MSM populations can still theoretically be attributed to role versatility.

The seventh chapter provides the development and application of molecular model to understand drug resistance to protease inhibitors. The chapter introduces the model to understand the differences in the binding affinity between the clinically essential mutant (MT- I84V) and the wild-type (WT) of HIV-1 protease protein which eventually lead to PR resistance.

The eighth chapter provides a review on the computational modelling research on mechanism and structures of Human dopamine transporter (hDAT) as well as its interaction with HIV-1 trans-activator of transcription (Tat).

Chapter 1
Computational Analysis of Reverse Transcriptase Resistance to Inhibitors in HIV-1

Ameeruddin Nusrath Unissa
National Institute for Research in Tuberculosis (NIRT), India

Luke Elizabeth Hanna
National Institute for Research in Tuberculosis (NIRT), India

ABSTRACT

Reverse transcriptase (RT) is a vital enzyme in the process of transcription of HIV-1. The nucleoside analogues of RT inhibitors (NRTIs) act by substrate competition and chain termination as they resemble a nucleotide. To understand the basis of RT resistance in HIV-1, in this chapter, one of the clinically essential mutants Q151M of RT which exhibits multi-resistance to many NRTIs was modeled and docked with NRTIs in comparison to wild type (WT). The results of docking indicate that the WT showed high affinity with all inhibitors compared to the mutant (MT). It can be suggested that the high affinity in WT could be attributed to the favorable interactions with all inhibitors that lacks in MT due to amino acid substitution that leads to structural changes in MT protein, which alters the favorable network of interaction and eventually imparts resistance to all inhibitors.

DOI: 10.4018/978-1-5225-3203-3.ch001

INTRODUCTION

Human immunodeficiency virus (HIV) continues to be a major global public health issue. In 2015, globally 1.1 million people died, 36.7 million people living with HIV and 2.1 million people newly infected from HIV-related diseases. Sub-Saharan Africa is the most affected region, which accounts for two-thirds of the global total of new HIV infections. HIV infection is often diagnosed through rapid diagnostic tests, which detect the presence or absence of HIV antibodies. Although, there is no cure for HIV infection, however, effective antiretroviral (ARV) drugs can control the virus and help prevent transmission so that people with HIV, and those at substantial risk, can live healthy, long and productive lives. Expanding ART prevention choices to all people living with HIV can help avert 21 million AIDS-related deaths and 28 million new infections by 2030 (World Health Organization, 2016).

Reverse transcriptase (RT) is an important enzyme in the transcription process of the type-1 HIV (HIV-1). The RT enzyme functions as RNA-dependent DNA polymerization and DNA-dependent DNA polymerization. The enzyme RT is a heterodimer comprises of p66 and p51 subunits. The first 440 amino acids of p66 and p51 are identical, and both subunits appear to contain a polymerase function. The C-terminal portion of p66 contains the RNase H domain. The p66 subunit contains the DNA-binding groove and the active site; the p51 subunit displays no enzymatic activity and functions as a scaffold for the enzymatically active p66 subunit. The p66 subunit has five subdomains namely fingers, palm, thumb, connection and RNase H subdomains (Shafer et al., 2001; Erickson & Burt, 1996).

The nucleoside RT inhibitors (NRTIs) are prodrugs that are triphosphorylated by host cellular enzymes. The triphosphorylated NRTIs then compete with natural deoxynucleoside triphosphates (dNTPs) for incorporation into the newly synthesized DNA chains where they cause chain termination. There are two biochemical mechanisms of NRTI drug resistance. The first mechanism is mediated by mutations that allow the RT enzyme to discriminate against NRTI during synthesis, thereby preventing their addition to the growing DNA chain relative to the natural dNTP substrates (Larder & Stammers, 1999; Sarafianos et al., 1999; Huang et al., 1998). The second mechanism is mediated by mutations in RT that increase the rate of hydrolytic removal of the chain terminating NRTI and thus enable continued DNA synthesis (Arion et al., 1998; Boyer et al., 2001; Meyer et al., 1998). This mechanism of resistance has also been referred to as pyrophosphorolysis, nucleotide excision, and primer unblocking. The hydrolytic removal requires a pyrophosphate donor, which in most cells is usually ATP (Meyer et al, 1999).

The NRTI resistance mutations include i. M184V, ii. thymidine analog mutations (TAM), iii. mutations selected by non- thymidine analogs, iv. multi-nucleoside resistance mutations. M184V is the most commonly occurring NRTI resistance mutation. The phenotypic and clinical significance of M184V is influenced by the presence or absence of other NRTI resistance mutations. For example, the presence of K65R or L74V in combination with M184V is sufficient for high-level resistance to both ABC and DDI. In contrast, three or more TAM plus M184V are required for high-level abacavir (ABC) and didanosine (DDI) resistance (Whitcomb et al., 2003; Guha & Halder, 2012). Mutations in thymidine analogs *viz* zidovudine (AZT or ZDV) and stavudine (D4T) decrease susceptibility to these NRTI and to a lesser extent to ABC, DDI, and tenofovir (TDF) (Whitcomb et al., 2003; Guha & Halder, 2012). TAM accumulates in two distinct but overlapping patterns. The Type I pattern includes the mutations M41L, L210W, and T215Y. The Type II pattern includes D67N, K70R, T215F, and K219Q/E. Mutation D67N also occurs commonly with type I TAM (Cozzi-Lepri et al., 2005). However, K70R and L210W rarely occur together. Type I TAM causes higher levels of phenotypic and clinical resistance to the thymidine analogs and cross-resistance to ABC, DDI, and TDF than do the type II TAM. Indeed, the presence of all three Type I TAMs markedly reduces the clinical response to ABC, DDI, and TDF (Cozzi-Lepri et al., 2005; Miller et al., 2004). Another important substitution K65R causes intermediate resistance to TDF, ABC, DDI, lamivudine (3TC), and emtricitabine (FTC), low-level resistance to D4T, and increased susceptibility to AZT/ZDV. L74V causes intermediate resistance to DDI and ABC, and a slight increase in susceptibility to ZDV and TDF6 (Cozzi-Lepri et al., 2005). Amino acid insertions at codon 69 generally occur in the presence of multiple TAM, and in this setting are associated with intermediate resistance to 3TC and FTC and high-level resistance to each of the remaining NRTI (Rhee et al., 2006).

Q151M is a 2-bp mutation (CAG→ATG) that is usually accompanied by two or more of the following mutations: A62V, V75I, F77L, and F116Y. The Q151M complex causes high-level resistance to AZT, D4T, DDI, and ABC, and intermediate resistance to TDF, 3TC, and FTC (Zaccarelli et al., 2004). This complex developed in 5% of patients who received DDI in combination with AZT or D4T, but is rarely selected by 3TC or FTC containing regimens. Thus, in the light of above we were interested to find the reason of multi resistance mediated by the substitution Q151M of RT which exhibits multiple resistance to many NRTIs such as ABC, AZT, DDI, D4T, FTC, TDF and 3TC in comparison to wild type (WT).

MATERIALS AND METHODS

Homology Modeling of Mutant RT

The target RT protein sequence (P04585) was obtained from the Uniprot database (see http://www.uniprot.org/) and was submitted to protein alignment program (BLASTp) (Altschul et al., 1997). The protein sequence was searched against protein database (PDB) (see http://www.rcsb.org/pdb/home/home.do), in the program. From the analysis, the crystal structure of RT protein 3MEC of HIV-1 was taken as template and WT (Lansdon et al., 2010).

Model Building

The MT-RT was created from WT template sequence (3MEC) of RT from HIV-1 by substitution of methionine at position 151 instead of glutamine. Additionally, in the template protein 3MEC, A chain was retained and the heteroatoms such as water and others were removed. The MT-model was built by providing command line options for sequence alignment between WT and MT, and then a series of commands were provided for model building using the software MODELLER9v14 (Sali, 1995).

Model Evaluation

The generated model was validated by Ramachandran plot (Lovell et al., 2003). Besides, the deviation was analyzed using PDBeFOLD between the WT and the model upon structural superimposition (Krissinel & Henrick, 2003).

Ligands

In this study, the ligands (ABC, AZT, DDI, D4T, FTC, TDF and 3TC) used were obtained from ncbi database (see https://www.ncbi.nlm.nih.gov/). Chemsketch software was used to obtain the structure of the ligand in Mol format and structural conversion was performed using version 2 of a software called Discovery studio.

Discovery Studio (DS)

The software was used for visualization purpose of modeled protein and docking data.

Docking Protocol

Docking was carried out with the help of software-GOLD (Jones et al., 1995). Dockings were performed under 'Standard default settings' mode. The cavity atom file containing the atom number of binding residues of HIV-1 RT such as Gly112, Asp113, Tyr115, Gln151, and Asp185 in WT and Met151 in MT was prepared for all ligands (ABC, AZT, DDI, D4T, FTC, TDF and 3TC). The binding residues were selected based on comparison between the binding regions of 3MEC and MT model (Lansdon et al., 2010).

BIOVIA-2016

This software was used to determine the interactions between the ligands and proteins.

RESULTS

Template Selection and Homology Modeling of MT of RT

Using BLASTp search against PDB, 3MEC was identified as the template as it displayed maximum identity with the RT protein (Figure 1). Mutant model of RT was built based on substitution at codon 151 in the WT- protein sequence (P04585) of RT of HIV-1, using MODELLER 9v14 (Figure 2). The generated model was validated by structural superimposition (Figure 3). The root mean square deviation (RMSD) between the WT and MT was 0.9 Å, indicating the reliability of the model. This was also supported by Ramachandran plot analysis showing 98% of residues in the allowed region (Figure 4).

Docking Between WT and MT-RTs With NRTIs

The generated model was used for docking studies and the docked complexes (Figures 5 -11) were visualized using DS. Docking of NRTIs (ABC, AZT, DDI, D4T, FTC, TDF, 3TC) with RTs resulted in ten poses. Of the ten poses, the best ligand pose was selected based on top GOLD score (Figure 12). The WT-RT showed high score with all inhibitors compared to the MT-Q151M which displayed lower score.

Figure 1. BLASTp result showing 99% identity between template (3MEC) and the target WT-RT sequence (P04585) of HIV-1

NCBI Blast:Protein Sequence (550 letters)

Chain A, Hiv-1 Reverse Transcriptase In Complex With Tmc125
Sequence ID: 3MEC_A **Length:** 560 **Number of Matches:** 1

Range 1: 1 to 552 GenPept Graphics Next Match Previous Match

Score	Expect	Method	Identities	Positives	Gaps
1108 bits(2867)	0.0	Compositional matrix adjust.	549/552(99%)	549/552(99%)	2/552(0%)

```
Query  1    PISPIETVPVKLKPGMDGPKVKQWPLTEEKIKALVEICTEMEKEGKISKIGPENPYNTPV  60
            PISPIETVPVKLKPGMDGPKVKQWPLTEEKIKALVEICTEMEKEGKISKIGPENPYNTPV
Sbjct  1    PISPIETVPVKLKPGMDGPKVKQWPLTEEKIKALVEICTEMEKEGKISKIGPENPYNTPV  60

Query  61   FAIKKKDSTKWRKLVDFRELNKRTQDFWEVQLGIPHPAGLKKKKSVTVLDVGDAYFSVPL  120
            FAIKKKDSTKWRKLVDFRELNKRTQDFWEVQLGIPHPAGLKKKKSVTVLDVGDAYFSVPL
Sbjct  61   FAIKKKDSTKWRKLVDFRELNKRTQDFWEVQLGIPHPAGLKKKKSVTVLDVGDAYFSVPL  120

Query  121  DEDFRKYTAFTIPSINNETPGIRYQYNVLPQGWKGSPAIFQSSMTKILEPFRKQNPDIVI  180
            DEDFRKYTAFTIPSINNETPGIRYQYNVLPQGWKGSPAIFQSSMTKILEPFRKQNPDIVI
Sbjct  121  DEDFRKYTAFTIPSINNETPGIRYQYNVLPQGWKGSPAIFQSSMTKILEPFRKQNPDIVI  180

Query  181  YQYMDDLYVASDLEIGQHRTKIEELRQHLLRWGLTTPDKK--KEPPFLWMGYELHPDKWT  238
            YQYMDDLYV SDLEIGQHRTKIEELRQHLLRWGLTTPDKK  KEPPFLWMGYELHPDKWT
Sbjct  181  YQYMDDLYVGSDLEIGQHRTKIEELRQHLLRWGLTTPDKKHQKEPPFLWMGYELHPDKWT  240

Query  239  VQPIVLPEKDSWTVNDIQKLVGKLNWASQIYPGIKVRQLCKLLRGTKALTEVIPLTEEAE  298
            VQPIVLPEKDSWTVNDIQKLVGKLNWASQIYPGIKVRQLCKLLRGTKALTEVIPLTEEAE
Sbjct  241  VQPIVLPEKDSWTVNDIQKLVGKLNWASQIYPGIKVRQLCKLLRGTKALTEVIPLTEEAE  300

Query  299  LELAENREILKEPVHGVYYDPSKDLIAEIQKQGQGQWTYQIYQEPFKNLKTGKYARMRGA  358
            LELAENREILKEPVHGVYYDPSKDLIAEIQKQGQGQWTYQIYQEPFKNLKTGKYARMRGA
Sbjct  301  LELAENREILKEPVHGVYYDPSKDLIAEIQKQGQGQWTYQIYQEPFKNLKTGKYARMRGA  360

Query  359  HTNDVKQLTEAVQKITTESIVIWGKTPKFKLPIQKETWETWWTEYWQATWIPEWEFVNTP  418
            HTNDVKQLTEAVQKITTESIVIWGKTPKFKLPIQKETWETWWTEYWQATWIPEWEFVNTP
Sbjct  361  HTNDVKQLTEAVQKITTESIVIWGKTPKFKLPIQKETWETWWTEYWQATWIPEWEFVNTP  420

Query  419  PLVKLWYQLEKEPIVGAETFYVDGAANRETKLGKAGYVTNRGRQKVVTLTDTTNQKTELQ  478
            PLVKLWYQLEKEPIVGAETFYVDGAANRETKLGKAGYVTNRGRQKVVTLTDTTNQKTELQ
Sbjct  421  PLVKLWYQLEKEPIVGAETFYVDGAANRETKLGKAGYVTNRGRQKVVTLTDTTNQKTELQ  480

Query  479  AIYLALQDSGLEVNIVTDSQYALGIIQAQPDQSESELVNQIIEQLIKKEKVYLAWVPAHK  538
            AIYLALQDSGLEVNIVTDSQYALGIIQAQPDQSESELVNQIIEQLIKKEKVYLAWVPAHK
Sbjct  481  AIYLALQDSGLEVNIVTDSQYALGIIQAQPDQSESELVNQIIEQLIKKEKVYLAWVPAHK  540

Query  539  GIGGNEQVDKLV  550
            GIGGNEQVDKLV
Sbjct  541  GIGGNEQVDKLV  552
```

Figure 2. Structure of RT -WT (green) and 3-D model of MT-Q151M (yellow)

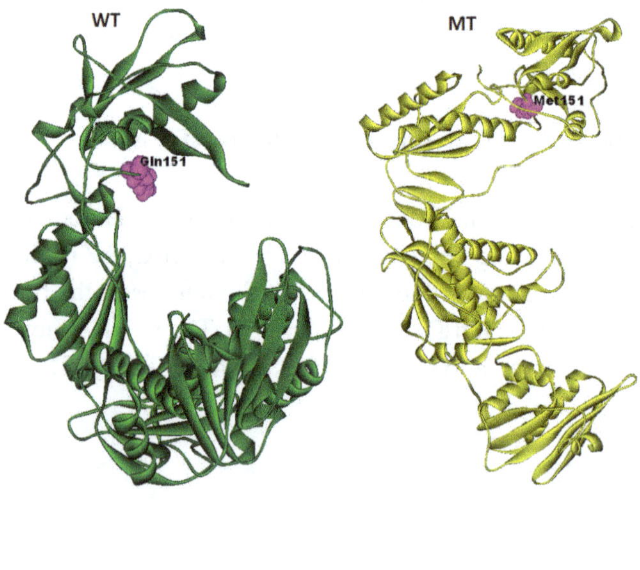

Figure 3. Superimposition of template-3MEC (green) and MT (yellow) showing an RMSD of 0.9 Å

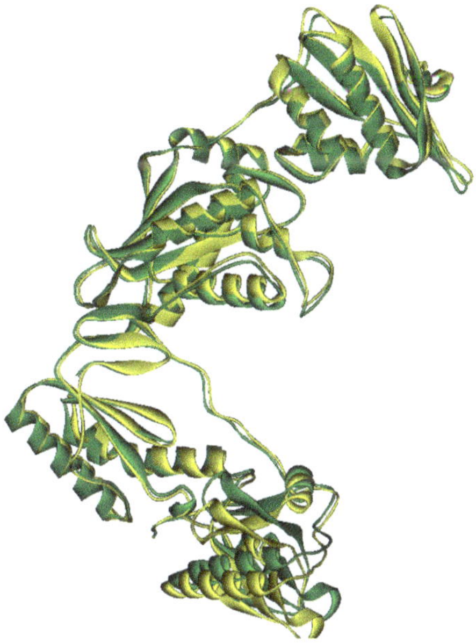

Figure 4. Ramachandran plot
Number of residues in favoured region (~98.0% expected): 541 (98.4%)
Number of residues in allowed region (~2.0% expected): 7 (1.3%)
Number of residues in outlier region: 2 (0.4%)

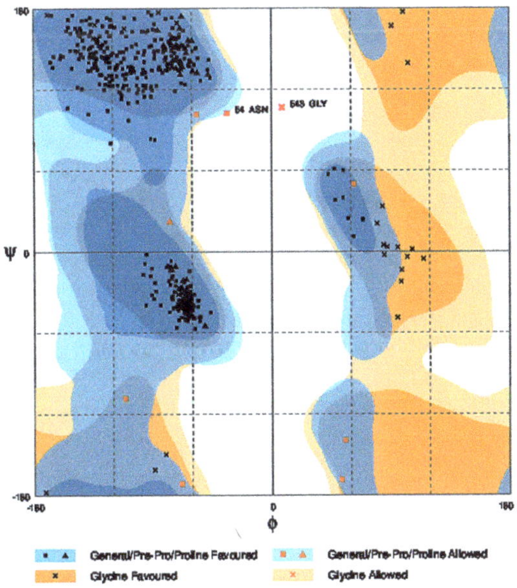

Figure 5. Docking complex WT and MT of RT with ABC (dark blue)

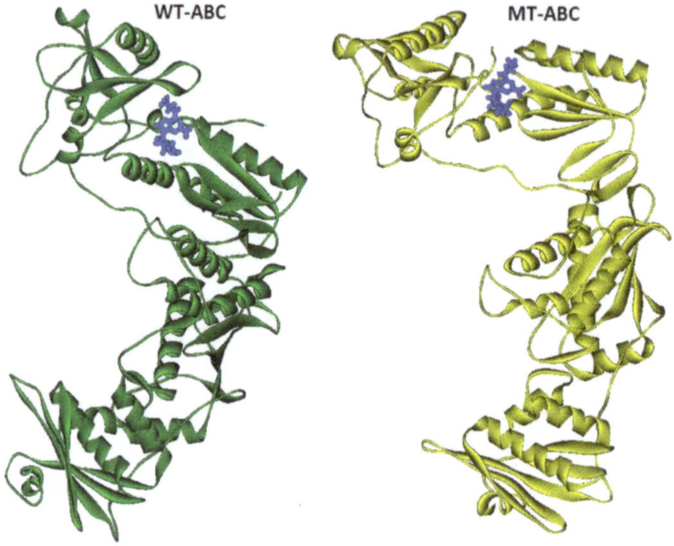

Figure 6. Docking complex of WT and MT with AZT (mustard)

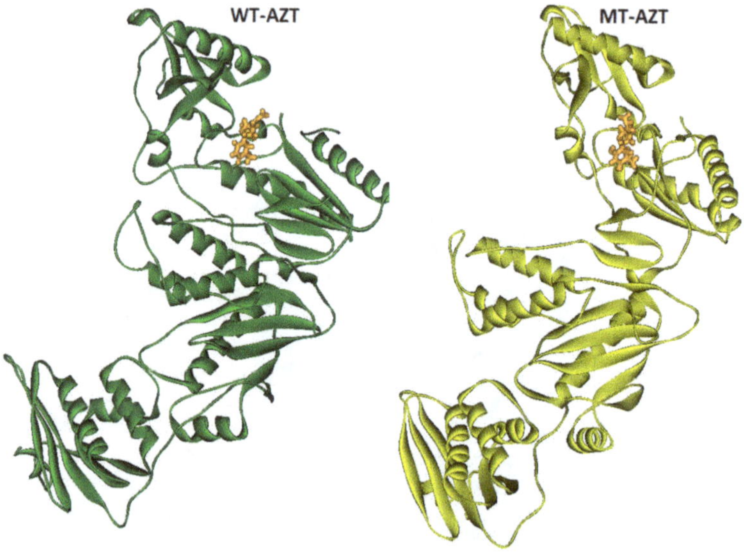

Figure 7. Docking complex of WT and MT with D4T (red)

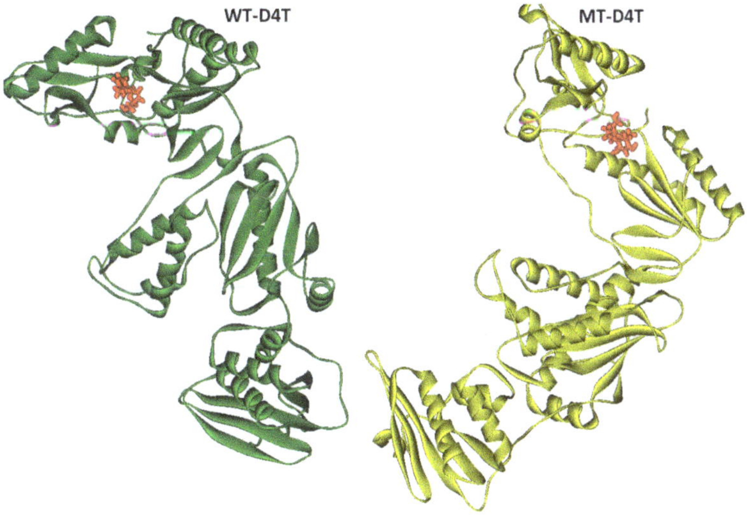

Figure 8. Docking complex of WT and MT with DDI (light blue)

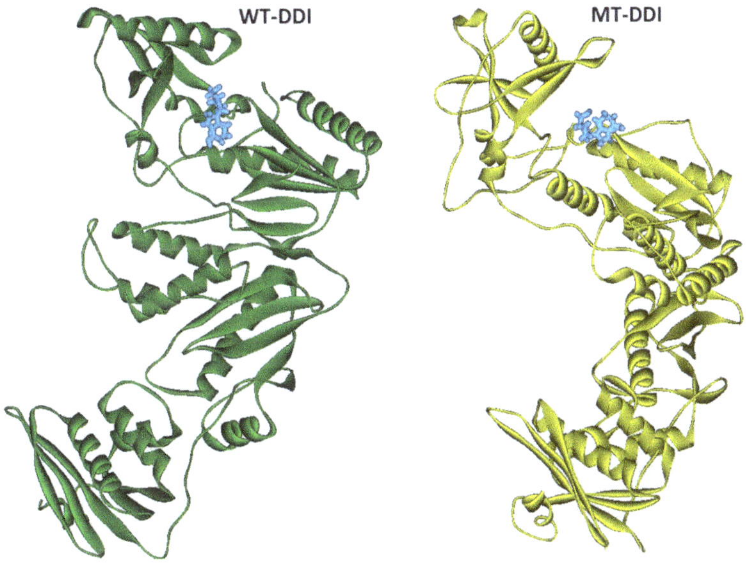

Figure 9. Docking complex of WT and MT with FTC (pink)

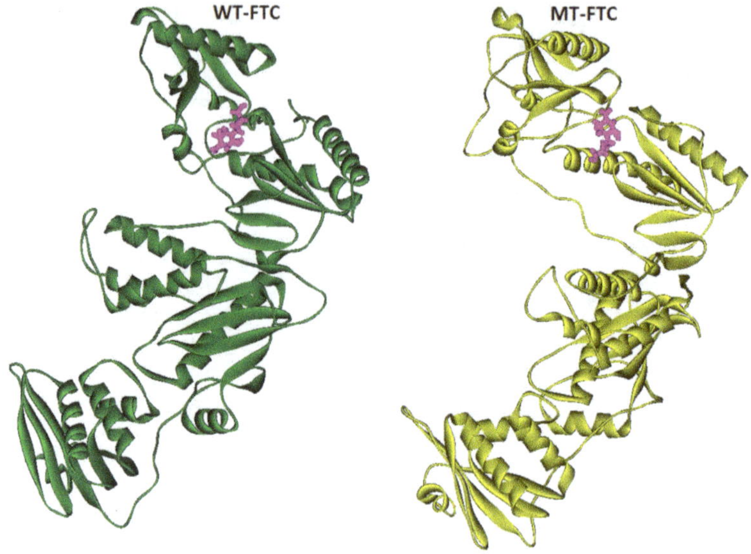

Figure 10. Docking complex of WT and MT with TDF (brown)

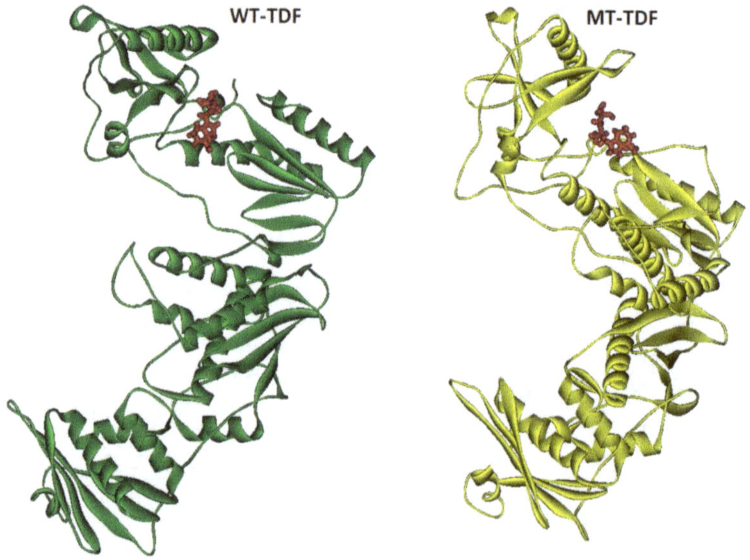

Figure 11. Docking complex of WT and MT with 3TC (cyan)

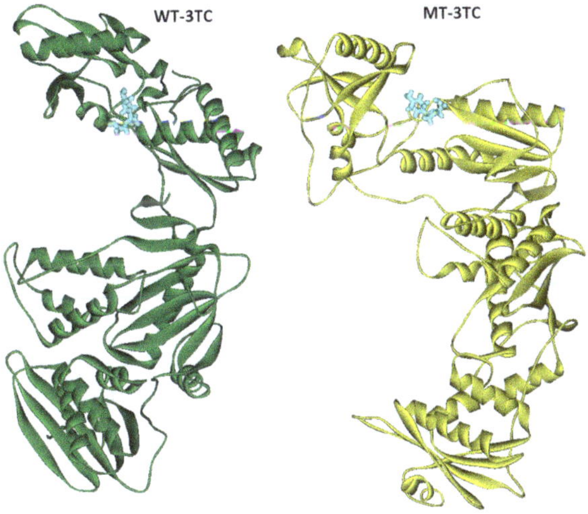

Figure 12. Docking score of WT and MT of RT with NRTIs

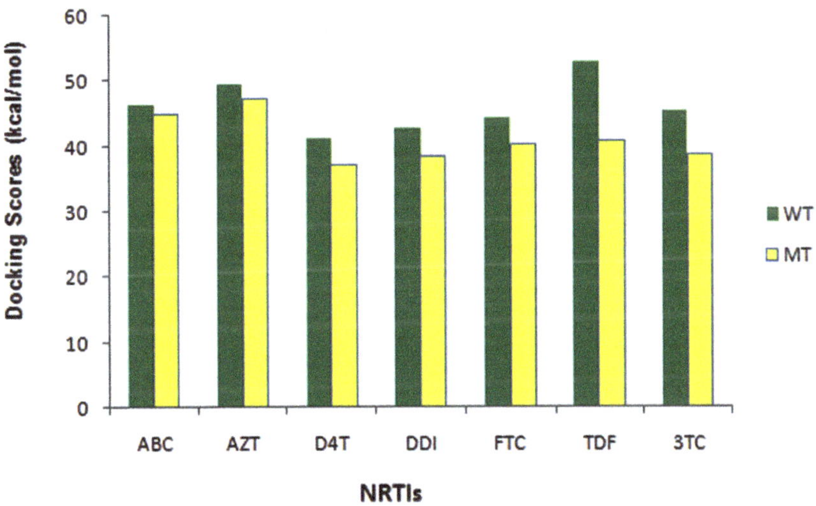

Interactions of RT Enzymes With the NRTIs

Of all other types of protein-ligand interactions such as hydrophobic (alkyl, pi-alkyl) electrostatic (charge), van der Waals, the significance of Hydrogen (H) bonds is very important, as they contribute towards structural integrity and functionality of protein-ligand complex.

In WT-RT complexed with ABC, followed by van der Waals interactions, 2 Hydrogen (H) bonds (conventional H) between ABC and residues Asp113 and Asp185 were formed, respectively. Further, two carbon H bonds between ABC and Tyr115 and Gln151 were formed. It is interesting to note the presence of Gln151 (mutation site) in direct contact with the drug through H bonding. In case of MT complexed with ABC, three conventional H bonds were observed between the drug and one with Val111 and two with Asp185 residues. In addition, the pi –alkyl and alkyl interactions in WT and MT are shown in Figure 13.

In case of WT complexed with AZT, 2 conventional H bonds were formed between the drug molecule and Tyr115 and Gln151 (mutation site), respectively. The residue Tyr115 was also involved in Pi- sigma interaction with the drug. Of note, an unfavorable positive-positive interaction was formed between AZT and the residue Arg72. Further, an attractive charge was observed between AZT and Asp113. In MT complex, similar to WT a conventional H bond was formed between the drug molecule and the residue Tyr115. Also, two carbon H bonds were observed between the AZT and the residues Tyr115 and Asp113. More importantly, two unfavorable donor-donor interactions were also observed between the drug and residues Asp113 and Phe116. Besides the residue Asp113 was also involved in salt bridge formation. Other interactions (van der Waals interactions, alkyl and Pi-alkyl) in WT and MT were found as evident in Figure 14.

In D4T complexed with WT-RT, 2 conventional H bonds were formed between the D4T and Phe116 and Gln151 (mutation site), respectively, while in case of MT complex with D4T more number of H bond interactions were found. Of which 3 were conventional H bonds between the drug and residues Asp113, Tyr115 and

Figure 13. Interactions of WT and MT of RT with ABC at its binding site

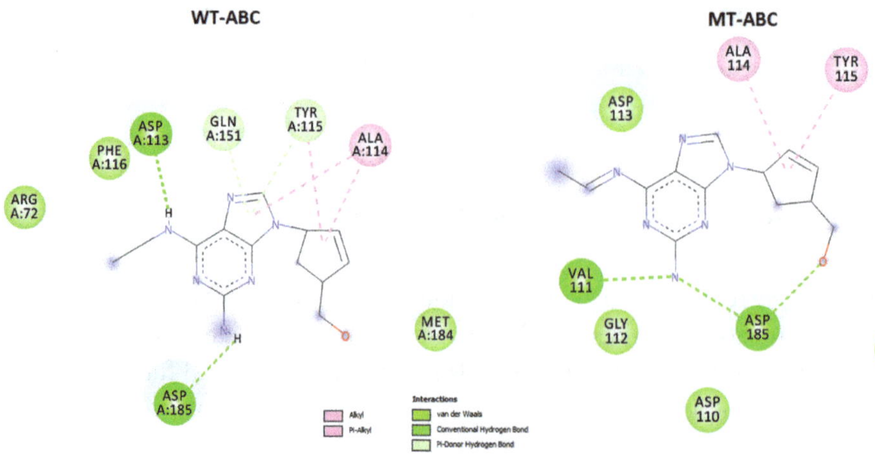

Figure 14. Interactions of WT and MT with AZT at its binding site

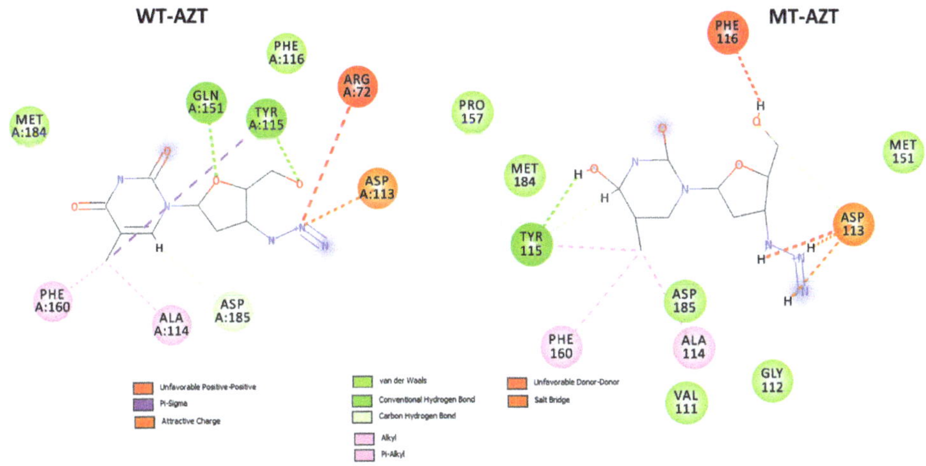

Asp185, 4 were carbon H bonds between D4T and Val111, Asp113, Phe116 and Asp185 were formed, respectively. This is followed by of van der Waals, alkyl, Pi-alkyl interactions as shown in Figure 15.

In WT combined with DDI, a conventional H and carbon H bonds were formed between DDI and the residue Asp113. On the other hand in case of MT-complex, a conventional H bond between DDI and the residue Val111 was found, further 4 H bonds were formed, and of these two were carbon H bonds and another two were conventional H bonds between DDI and the residue Asp113, similar to WT. Other types of interactions are shown in Figure 16.

In WT complexed with FTC, it is important to note that no other types of interactions were found apart from van der Waals interactions and two conventional H bonds, which were formed between FTC and the residue Tyr115 and Asp185, respectively. In case of MT, two conventional H bonds were formed between the drug and residues Tyr115 and Asp113, respectively. Although the compound FTC contains fluorine and sulphur atoms, but they were not involved in any bonding with the WT or MT-RT (Figure 17).

In TDF complexed with WT, two conventional H bonds were formed between the phosphate group of TDF and Asp113 and Gln151 (mutation site), respectively. A carbon H bond was found between the phosphate group of TDF and Asp113. Further, an unfavorable positive-positive interaction was formed between TDF and the residue Arg72, similar to the interaction with the drug AZT. In addition, an attractive charge was observed between the phosphate group of TDF and Asp113, again similar to the interactions with the drug AZT. While in case of MT complex, many H bonds (5 conventional and 4 carbon H) interactions were found with residues Val111 Asp113 and Asp185 as shown in Figure 18.

Figure 15. Interactions of WT and MT with D4T at its binding site

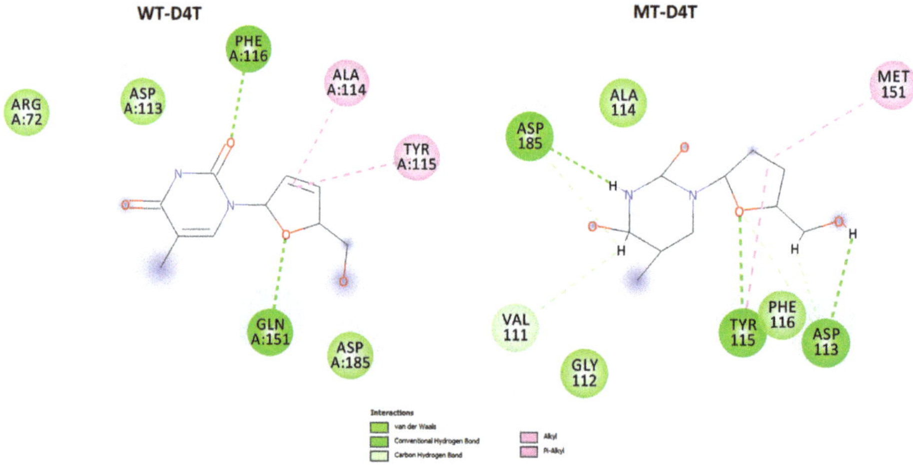

Figure 16. Interactions of WT and MT with DDI at its binding site

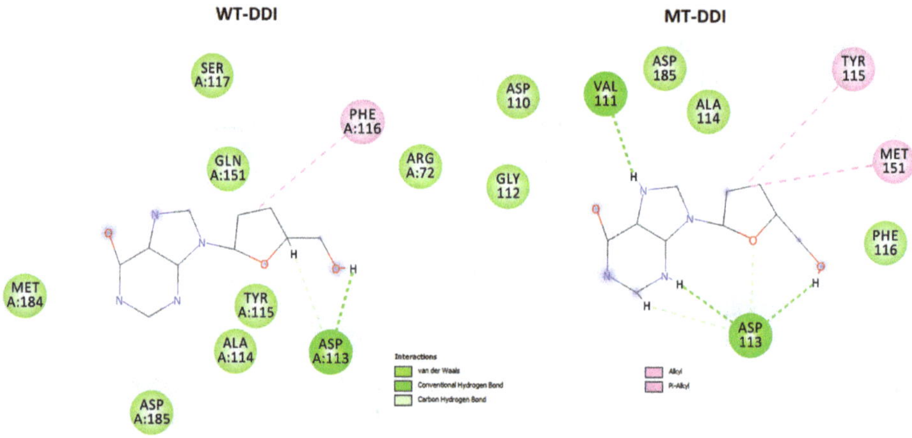

In case of WT complexed with 3TC, three conventional H bonds were formed between the drug and two with Asp113 and one with Gln151 (mutation site), respectively. Two carbon H bonds were found between 3TC and Asp185. Further, a pi-sulphur bond was formed between the drug molecule and the residue Tyr115. In MT-complex, similar to WT three conventional H bonds were formed but all with the residue Asp113. Four carbon H bonds were formed between the drug molecule and two with Val111, and other two with Asp113 and Asp185, respectively as shown in Figure 19.

Figure 17. Interactions of WT and MT with FTC at its binding site

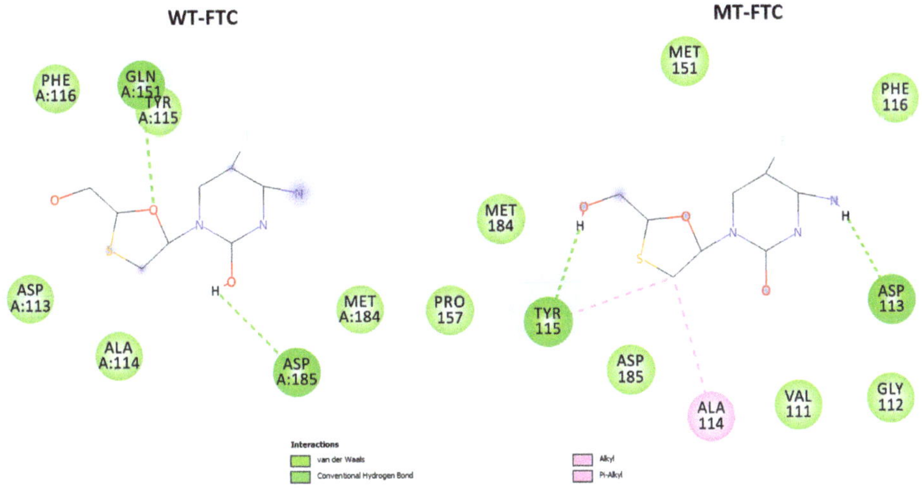

Figure 18. Interactions of WT and MT with TDF at its binding site

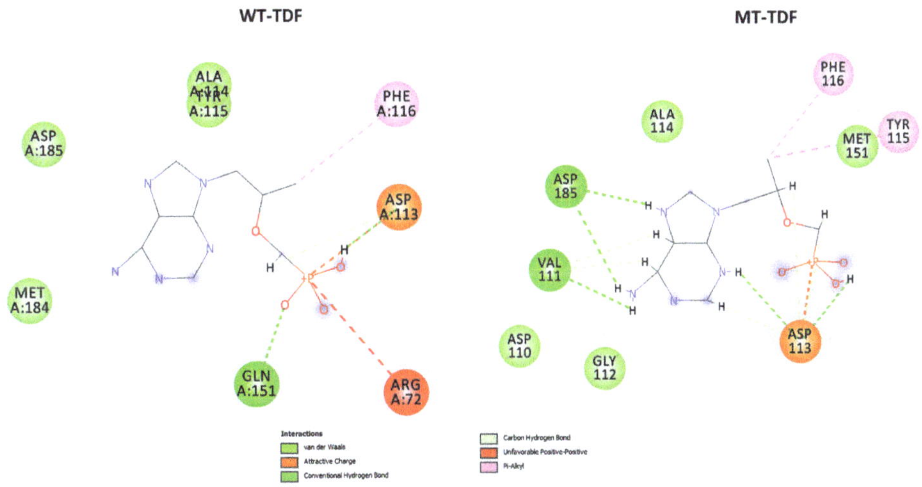

DISCUSSION

There are two mechanisms through which resistance to NRTIs occurs, in the first and primary mechanisms of mutations (M184V, K65R and Q151M) appear at or near the NRTIs binding site of the RT gene. In the second mechanism, the mutations inhibit the functions of NRTIs even if they bind to the RT gene correctly, by enhancing the process of pyrophosphorolysis through removal of chain terminating

Figure 19. Interactions of WT and MT with 3TC at its binding site

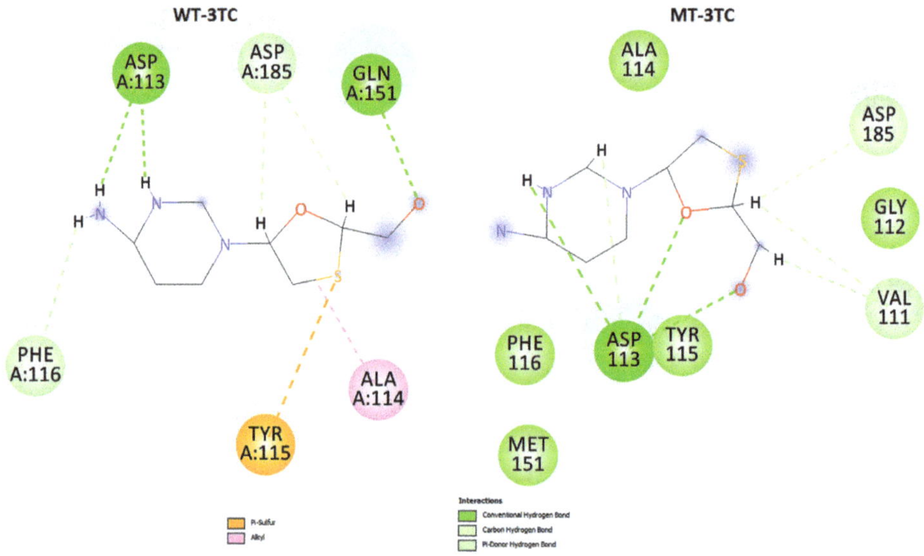

residue and reinstate an extendable primer (resumes RNA and DNA synthesis). Of the primary mutations, the Q151M mutation was less studied in comparison to the other two. In connection to which, in this study, the modeled MT-Q151M of HIV-1 RT was docked with seven NRTIs (ABC, AZT, DDI, D4T, FTC, TDF and 3TC) to understand the binding differences in comparison to WT and the eventual cause for RT resistance to these NRTIs. Based on docking results it can be suggested that the reason for the high score in WT could be probably due to favorable interactions with all inhibitors. In contrast, the low score represents less affinity in MT- Q151M towards the inhibitors could be attributed to absence of such interactions and could be a cause for its resistance against all inhibitors. Of significance, the presence of residue Gln151 (mutation site) in direct contact with the 5 NRTIs such as ABC, AZT, D4T, TDF and 3TC through H bonding (Figures 13, 14, 15, 18, 19) at the active site suggests it catalytic role in WT-RT enzyme, in addition to its clinical relevance. Although, the mutated residue Met151 was not in direct contact through hydrogen bonding, however, the residue was in van der waals contact distance or involved in alkyl and pi-alkyl interactions at the active site. Besides, the probable reason for the favorable interactions could in turn be due to the substitution of Met in the MT protein in place of Gln in WT, as Met contains a extra sulphur and a methyl group instead of Gln which contains a amide group, might have induced much structural changes in the protein's side chain, which was evident by showing less score owing to the changes in the profile of interactions in the MT-Q151M.

Alternatively, the effect of docking could be better understood in conjunction with more powerful tool such as molecular dynamics, although, the insights provided in this study can be meaningful to know the impact of such substitution and its consequent changes in binding ability. To our knowledge, this is the first study of such kind to show the effect of binding affinity of WT and MT- Q151M of RT with both thymine (AZT D4T, FTC and 3TC) and guanine (ABC, DDI and TDF) analogues of NRTIs. In addition, this analysis suggests that further structural studies more particularly based on MD are needed to enlighten our knowledge on the fundamental molecular mechanism of mutation-acquired RT resistance to NRTIs.

REFERENCES

Altschul, S. F., Madden, T. L., Schäffer, A. A., Zhang, J., Zhang, Z., Miller, W., & Lipman, D. J. (1997). Gapped BLAST and PSI-BLAST: A new generation of protein database search programs. *Nucleic Acids Research*, *25*(17), 3389–3402. doi:10.1093/nar/25.17.3389 PMID:9254694

Arion, D., Kaushik, N., McCormick, S., Borkow, G., & Parniak, M. A. (1998). Phenotypic mechanism of HIV-1 resistance to 3 '-azido-3 '-deoxythymidine (AZT): Increased polymerization processivity and enhanced sensitivity to pyrophosphate of the mutant viral reverse transcriptase. *Biochemistry*, *37*(45), 15908–15917. doi:10.1021/bi981200e PMID:9843396

Boyer, P. L., Sarafianos, S. G., Arnold, E., & Hughes, S. H. (2001). Selective excision of aztmp by drug-resistant human immunodeficiency virus reverse transcriptase. *Journal of Virology*, *75*(10), 4832–4842. doi:10.1128/JVI.75.10.4832-4842.2001 PMID:11312355

Cozzi-Lepri, A., Ruiz, L., Loveday, C., Phillips, A. N., Clotet, B., Reiss, P., …, , & Lundgren, J.D. (2005). Thymidine analogue mutation profiles: Factors associated with acquiring specific profiles and their impact on the virological response to therapy. *Antiviral Therapy*, *10*(7), 791. PMID:16312176

Erickson, J. W., & Burt, S. K. (1996). Structural mechanisms of HIV drug resistance. *Annual Review of Pharmacology and Toxicology*, *36*(1), 545–571. doi:10.1146/annurev.pa.36.040196.002553 PMID:8725401

Guha, S. K., & Haldar, S. N. (2012). Drug Resistance in HIV. Medicine Update, 84–88.

Huang, H., Chopra, R., Verdine, G. L., & Harrison, S. C. (1998). Structure of a covalently trapped catalytic complex of HIV-1 reverse transcriptase: Implications for drug resistance. *Science*, *282*(5394), 1669–1675. doi:10.1126/science.282.5394.1669 PMID:9831551

Jones, G., Willett, P., & Glen, R. C. (1995). Molecular recognition of receptor sites using a genetic algorithm with a description of desolvation. *Journal of Molecular Biology*, *245*(1), 43–53. doi:10.1016/S0022-2836(95)80037-9 PMID:7823319

Krissinel, E., & Henrick, K. (2003). Protein structure comparison in 3D based on secondary structure matching (PDBeFold) followed by Cα alignment, scored by a new structural similarity function. *Proceedings of the 5th International Conference on Molecular Structural Biology*, 88.

Lansdon, E. B., Brendza, K. M., Hung, M., Wang, R., Mukund, S., Jin, D., ... Liu, X. (2010). Crystal structures of HIV-1 reverse transcriptase with etravirine (TMC125) and rilpivirine (TMC278): Implications for drug design. *Journal of Medicinal Chemistry*, *53*(10), 4295–4299. doi:10.1021/jm1002233 PMID:20438081

Larder, B. A., & Stammers, D. K. (1999). Closing in on HIV drug resistance. *Nature Structural Biology*, *6*(2), 103–106. doi:10.1038/5787 PMID:10048915

Lovell, S. C., Davis, I. W., Arendall, W. B. III, de Bakker, P. I., Word, J. M., Prisant, M. G., ... Richardson, D. C. (2003). Structure validation by Cα geometry: Φ, ψ and Cβ deviation. *Proteins*, *50*(3), 437–450. doi:10.1002/prot.10286 PMID:12557186

Meyer, P. R., Matsuura, S. E., Mian, A. M., So, A. G., & Scott, W. A. (1999). A mechanism of AZT resistance: An increase in nucleotide-dependent primer unblocking by mutant HIV-1 reverse transcriptase. *Molecular Cell*, *4*(1), 35–43. doi:10.1016/S1097-2765(00)80185-9 PMID:10445025

Meyer, P. R., Matsuura, S. E., So, A. G., & Scott, W. A. (1998). Unblocking of chain terminated primer by HIV-1 reverse transcriptase through a nucleotide-dependent mechanism. *Proceedings of the National Academy of Sciences of the United States of America*, *95*(23), 13471–13476. doi:10.1073/pnas.95.23.13471 PMID:9811824

Miller, M. D., Margot, N., Lu, B., Zhong, L., Chen, S. S., Cheng, A., & Wulfsohn, M. (2004). Genotypic and phenotypic predictors of the magnitude of response to tenofovir disoproxil fumarate treatment in antiretroviral-experienced patients. *The Journal of Infectious Diseases*, *189*(5), 837–846. doi:10.1086/381784 PMID:14976601

Rhee, S. Y., Taylor, J., Wadhera, G., Ben-Hur, A., Brutlag, D. L., & Shafer, R. W. (2006). Genotypic predictors of human immunodeficiency virus type 1 drug resistance. *Proceedings of the National Academy of Sciences of the United States of America*, *103*(46), 17355–17360. doi:10.1073/pnas.0607274103 PMID:17065321

Sali MODELLER. (1995). *Implementing 3D Protein Modeling, mc2, vol. 2:5.* Molecular Simulations Inc.

Sarafianos, S. G., Dasi, K., Dingi, J., Boyer, P. L., Hughes, S. H., & Arnold, E. (1999). Touching the heart of HIV-1 drug resistance: The fingers close down on the dNTP at the polymerase active site. *Chemistry & Biology*, *6*(5), R137–R146. doi:10.1016/S1074-5521(99)80071-4 PMID:10322129

Shafer, R. W., Dupnik, K., Winters, M. A., & Eshleman, S. H. (2001). A guide to HIV-1 reverse transcriptase and protease sequencing for drug resistance studies. *HIV Sequence Compendium*, *2001*, 1. PMID:22324021

Whitcomb, J. M., Parkin, N. T., Chappey, C., Hellmann, N. S., & Petropoulos, C. J. (2003). Broad nucleoside reverse-transcriptase inhibitor cross-resistance in human immunodeficiency virus type 1 clinical isolates. *The Journal of Infectious Diseases*, *188*(7), 992–1000. doi:10.1086/378281 PMID:14513419

World Health Organization, HIV/AIDS, Media Centre-Fact Sheet. (n.d.). Retrieved from http://www.who.int/mediacentre/factsheets/fs360/en/

Zaccarelli, M., Perno, C. F., Forbici, F., Soldani, F., Bonfigli, S., Gori, C., ... De Longis, P. (2004). Q151M-mediated multinucleoside resistance: Prevalence, risk factors, and response to salvage therapy. *Clinical Infectious Diseases*, *38*(3), 433–437. doi:10.1086/381097 PMID:14727218

Chapter 2
Statistical and Computational Needs for Big Data Challenges

Soraya Sedkaoui
Khemis Miliana University, Algeria & Montpellier University, France

ABSTRACT

The traditional way of formatting information from transactional systems to make them available for "statistical processing" does not work in a situation where data is arriving in huge volumes from diverse sources, and where even the formats could be changing. Faced with this volume and diversification, it is essential to develop techniques to make best use of all of these stocks in order to extract the maximum amount of information and knowledge. Traditional analysis methods have been based largely on the assumption that statisticians can work with data within the confines of their own computing environment. But the growth of the amounts of data is changing that paradigm, especially which ride of the progress in computational data analysis. This chapter builds upon sources but also goes further in the examination to answer this question: What needs to be done in this area to deal with big data challenges?

DOI: 10.4018/978-1-5225-3203-3.ch002

INTRODUCTION

With the advent of digital technology and smart devices, a large amount of digital data is being generated every day. Individuals are putting more and more publicly available data on the web. Many companies collect information on their clients and their respective behavior. As such, many industrial and commercial processes are being controlled by computers. The results of medical tests are also being retained for analysis. Financial institutions, companies, and health service providers, administrations generate large quantities of data through their interactions with suppliers, patients, customers, and employees. Beyond those interactions, large volumes of data are created through Internet searches, social networks, GPS systems, and stock market transactions.

This brings us to think about the legend of the wise 'Sissa' in India. When King 'Belkib' asked about the reward he desired, after his invention, he asked to receive a grain of rice for the first square, two grains for the second, four grains for the third and so on. The king agreed, but he didn't know that on the last square of the board he should drop 2^{63} grains, or more than 700 billion tons. In their book "Race Against the Machine," Brynjolfsson and Mcaffee (2011) referenced the fable of the chess and rice grains to make the point that "exponential increases initially look a lot like linear, but they are not. As time goes by – as the world move into the second half of the chessboard – exponential growth confounds our intuition and expectation".

Thus currently, not only is the quantity of digitally stored data much larger, but the type of data is also very varied, thanks to the various new technologies (Sedkaoui & Monino, 2016). Data volume will continue to grow and in a very real way, the data produced, as well as other data accumulated, constitutes a constant source of knowledge. This widespread production of data has resulted in the 'data revolution' or the age of 'big data'. Big data gets global attention and can be best described using the three Vs: volume, variety and velocity. These three dimensions often are employed to describe the phenomenon. Each dimension presents both challenges for data management and opportunities to advance decision-making. In another way, every data tells a story and data analytics, in particular the statistical methods coupled with the development of IT tools, piece together that story's reveal the underlying message.

This 3 V's provide a challenge associated with working with big data. The volume put the accent on the storage, memory and computes capacity of a computing system and requires access to a computing cloud. Velocity stresses the rate at which data can be absorbed and meaningful answers produced. The variety makes it difficult to develop algorithms and tools that can address that large variety of input data. So, there are still many difficulties and challenges in the use of big data technologies. And, if decision-makers can't understand the power of data processing and analytics, they may be, in some ways, the “Belkibs” of big data value. The key is applying proper analytics and statistics methods to the data. Thus, from this data companies derive information and then producing knowledge, or which it called the target paradigm of “knowledge discovery”, described as a “knowledge pyramid” where data lays at the base. To advance successfully the paradigm effectiveness data analysis is needed.

The analysis of big data involves multiple distinct phases which include data acquisition and recording, information extraction and cleaning, data integration, aggregation and representation, query processing, data modeling and analysis and interpretation. These all are the methods of modern statistical analysis necessary for dealing with big data challenges. But, each of these phases introduces other challenges: Heterogeneity, scale, timeliness, complexity, quality, security...

Modern data analysis is very different from other methods which existed prior. Also, data is very different from data which existed before. In another word, the nature of modern data (greatest dimension, diverse types, mass of data) does not authorize the use of most conventional statistical methods (tests, regression, classification). Indeed, these methods are not adapted to these specific conditions of application and in particular suffer from the scourge of dimension. These issues should be seriously considered in big data analytics and in the development of statistical procedures.

Consider a simple example to explain a quantitative variable Y through a set $\{X1, \ldots Xp\}$ of quantitative variables: $Y = f(X1, \ldots Xp) + \varepsilon, [(yi, xi), i = 1, \ldots, n]$

If the function is assumed to be linear and p is small, on the order of ten; the problem is well known and widely discussed in the literature. In the case where the function f is not exactly linear and n is large, it is possible to accurately estimate a larger number of parameters and therefore to envisage more sophisticated models. Keeping to the usual Gaussian model, even the simplest case of a polynomial model quickly becomes problematic. Indeed, when the function is linear, take $p = 10$, the model selection procedure is facing a group of 2^{10} possible models and shrewd algorithms allow to cope.

However, consider to estimate f, a simple polynomial of second or third degree, with all its interactions, leads us to consider a large number of parameters and thus, by combinatorial explosion, an astronomical number of possible models. Other methods must then be considered taking into account necessarily the algorithmic computational complexity. This explains the involvement of another discipline, computing. The concern of computability outweighs the mathematical definition of the problem comes down to optimizing a criterion adjustment of the function f over a set of more or less rich solutions.

These methods have often been developed in another disciplinary environment: computers, artificial intelligence, K-means, neural networks, decision trees… support vector machines become credible alternatives since the number of observations is sufficient or the number of variables is very important.

Development of new statistical methods is an interdisciplinary field that draws on computer sciences, artificial intelligence, machine learning, and visualization models etc. So, two technical entities have come together. First, there is big data for massive amounts of data. Second, there is advanced analytics, which is actually a collection of different tool types, including those based on predictive analytics, data mining, statistics, clustering, data visualization, text analytics, artificial intelligence, and so on (Shroff, 2013; Siegel, 2016).

Current technologies software tries to overcome the challenges that "V's" raises. One of these is Apache Hadoop, which is open source software that its main goal is to handle large amounts of data in a reasonable time. While one major aspect of big data is the computational handling of network induced data, another is the proper application of data analytic and statistical tools for large scale use in business and commercial contexts. Cukier and Mayer-Schoenberger (2013a; 2013b, p.29) see a paradigmatic change in the statistical handling of large data:

Using great volumes of information ... require three profound changes in how we approach data. The first is to collect and use a lot of data rather than settle for small amounts or samples as statisticians have done for well over a century. The second is to shed our preference for highly curated and pristine data and accept messiness: in an increasing number of situations, a bit of inaccuracy can be tolerated, because the benefits of using vastly more data of variable quality outweigh the costs of using smaller amounts of very exact data. Third, in many instances, we will need to give up our quest to discover the cause of things, in return for accepting correlations. With big data, instead of trying to understand precisely why an engine breaks down or why a drug's side effect disappears, researchers can instead collect and analyze massive quantities of information about such events and everything that is associated with them, looking for patterns that might help predict future occurrences. Big data helps answer what, not why, and often that's good enough.

Big data deals with unconventional, unstructured databases, which can reach petabytes, exabytes or zetabytes, and require specific treatments for their needs, either in terms of storage or processing/display (Vermesan and al, 2014). The challenges include not just the obvious issues of scale, but also heterogeneity, lack of structure, error-handling, timeliness, provenance, and visualization, at all stages of the analysis driving from data acquisition to result interpretation. The ultimate goal is not only to collect, combine, or process all data, but also to increase its value and efficiency. This means that it must evolve from big data to 'smart data', since the effectiveness of companies' strategies now depends on the quality of data. Which should be kept in mind as the analysis unfolds.

It would require tailored statistical methods and data quality control to superimpose on large data streams to make sense of the data and use them for statistical inference and decisions. More frequently than not also good theoretic insights and models of the subject discipline would be helpful to identify the 'payoff relevance' of data for predictive purposes (Harford, 2014). This explains the formation of handling data through scalable tools as developed in econometrics, psychometrics, technometrics etc.

The goal of this chapter is to show what is specifically the power of 'data'? And why it is so important for companies? And how big data can benefit from the mixture of two fields: 'computer science' and 'statistics' in order to make the inquiry from data a more successful endeavor, rather than dwelling on theoretical issues of dubious value. This chapter presents the main statistical computing issues and challenges in the age of data deluge, and examines whether traditional statistical approach and methods substantially differ from the new trend of big data analytics. In another word, the objective writing this chapter is to present and explain the important role of computing statistical methods in data analysis and knowledge extraction, and the necessity of developing such methods.

To show that the challenges around the era of "data revolution" focus on data uses, Author will firstlyl describe, review, and reflect on big data, by defining what is it meant in order to consolidate the divergent discourse on it and presenting its various dimensions and challenges. Also, in this chapter one section will be dedicate for introducing knowledge discovery from data and the interest of searching new analytics methods for efficiently obtain the potential value from the massive data. Then, author will explain and present how the most basic of statistical methodologies has developed to create very flexible tools, and how statistics and computational tools should act together to better analyze big data in order to extract value.

BIG DATA: THE BIGGEST GAME-CHANGING OPPORTUNITY

Nowadays, an increasing number of data silos are created across the world, which means that this growth will never stop. This data is not only voluminous; it is also continuous, streaming, real time, dynamic and volatile. This is generally described by what it called the phenomenon of "3 Vs", or "big data". Businesses can exploit big data to extract valuable information. Such information can help decision makers to enhance their strategies and optimize their plans. But, what really is subsumed under big data?

Big data qualifies under a few main characteristics: (i) It is primarily network generated on a large scale volume, by variety and velocity and comprises large amounts of information at the enterprise and public level, in the categories of terabytes (10^{13} bytes), petabytes (10^{15}) and beyond of online data. (ii) It consists of a variety and diversity of data types and formats, many of them dynamic, unstructured or semi-structured and hard to handle by conventional statistical methods. (iii) Big data is generated by disparate sources as in interactive application through IoT from wireless devices, sensors, streaming communication generated by machine-to-machine interactions (Sedkaoui, 2017).

Big data nowadays has become one of the biggest concepts in the world of IT especially with the rapid development of IoT driving the increase of data. It also brings new opportunities for the discovery of new values that are temporarily hidden. The success of large companies such as Amazon, Google, Facebook, Twitter etc. proves the emergence of a factor in the development of today's hyper-connected world. The companies, increasingly aware of the importance of data and information, which represents the result of data processing and it is in the heart of decision-making (see next section), throng to reflect on the way to "manage" to enrich and benefit. Henceforth, this gives new properties to data, as they are Meta tagged piecemeal, produced in real time, and arrive in continuous streams from multiple sources.

In addition, data is now abundant resources in many circumstances, thus data can pile-up or "many managers find themselves drowning in data" (Mann, 2004). Companies are leveraging these and many other sources of data to achieve a better understanding of their customers, employees, partners and operations, with an eye towards improving every aspect of business. But it must first of all understand the rich ecosystem and extended big data. Inside this ecosystem some phases and processes can be identified, such as: (i) Data Collection: which implies the proper use of Networks, Infrastructure, and data centers in order to access and analyze a particular set of dynamic data. (ii) Data Processing: this is influenced directly by the technologies used for the storage and database management. (iii) Data Analysis: data analytics is gaining increasing attention in business and consequently also Data-Driven Decision-making (DDD), which refers to the practice of basing decisions on the analysis of data.

Big data applications are numerous and constitute a factor in strengthening the capacity for innovation within companies. Innovation certainly comes from crosses and treatments that have not been thought originally. But nothing better than good examples to understand how big data transformed the business.

An extremely popular example is Hadoop, an Open Source framework in this field that allows applications to work with huge repositories of data and thousands of nodes. These have been inspired by Google tools such as the MapReduce and

Google File system, or NoSQL systems, which in many cases do not comply with the ACID (atomicity, consistency, isolation, durability) characteristics of conventional databases.

Spotify, an on-demand music service, uses Hadoop big data analytics, to collect data from its millions of users worldwide and then uses the analyzed data to give informed music recommendations to individual users.

The American company 'Harrah's' has made progress in sales of 8 to 10 percent by analyzing customer segmentation data, while Amazon stated that 30 percent of its turnover came from its engine analytical recommendations (McKinsey, 2011, 2013). With massive production of online data Google, in 2009, was able to predict the timely spread of influenza through simple correlation (Foster et al., 2017, Chap. 1). In the same spirit, the United Nations has developed a program anticipating epidemics and reversals of economic conditions through keywords exchanged on Twitter.

Such examples, and many others, share common principles: extreme digitalization of their process leads to extensive use of data to experiment with new business models, beyond their original boundaries. IDC (2011) describes big data technologies as a new generation of technologies and architectures, designed to economically extract value from very large volumes of a wide variety of data, by enabling high-velocity capture, discovery, and/or analysis. Technologies for big data harvesting from multiple resources have been fast growing in the forms of data mining systems; search engines; query languages; filtering systems; cloud services, etc.

Big data will fundamentally change the way businesses compete and operate. Companies that invest in and successfully derive value from their data will have a distinct advantage over their competitors (McKinsey Global Institute, 2011). It is difficult to identify the all issues brought about by big data, but there is now increasing opportunity to capitalize on the approach. The question continues as to how companies can maintain and improve our knowledge store over time.

TURN DATA INTO KNOWLEDGE FOR SUPPORTING DECISION

The explosion of data volumes will gradually increase as the Internet of Things (IoT) develops. Data volume will continue to grow and in a very real way constitutes a constant source of knowledge. The difficulty of transforming big data into value or knowledge is related to its complexity, the essence of which is broadly captured by the three Vs. Volume, Variety and Velocity are used to define the term big data. Each of these dimensions presents both challenges for data management and opportunities to advance decision-making.

Traditionally, the decision-making process is shaped on the model of limited rationality by Herbert Simon (1977): Intelligence, modelling, choice and control. The intelligence phase is all about finding the occasions over which a decision should be made (Simon, 1997). "The major role of the intelligence stage is to identify the problem and collect relevant information" (Turban et al., 2011) which would be used later in the next stages of the decision-making process.

However, with the exploitation of big data this process is being complicated and has to improve. Organizations need to use a structured view of data to improve their decision-making process. Big data has the potential to aid in identifying opportunities related to decision in the intelligence phase of Simon's model, where the term of "intelligence" refers to knowledge discovery. To achieve this structured view, they have to collect and store data, perform an analysis, and transform the results into useful and valuable information, and then it's essentially about discovering new knowledge.

In relating these three concepts: "Data, Information and Knowledge", a hierarchy can be suggested, which suggest in turn that one can be changed into other. This model is often used in the literature relating to the information and knowledge management. Several studies claim that the first appearance of knowledge hierarchy is in T.S Elliot's poem "The Rock" in 1934. In recent literature, many authors refer to the publication "From data to wisdom" of R.L Ackoff published in 1989 as a source of knowledge hierarchy.

Many other authors (Zeleny, 1987; Cleveland, 1982) have also proposed extensions of the hierarchy; Ackoff includes understanding (and some use intelligence) as its own level before attaining wisdom.

The relationship between these three words can be represented as a pyramid where knowledge occupies the highest place to highlight the fact that many data are necessary for the acquisition of knowledge.

The knowledge pyramid is by nature a multidisciplinary endeavor (Piegorsch, 2015): computer scientists construct algorithms to manipulate and organize the data, aided by statisticians and mathematicians who instruct on development and application of quantitative methodology. Then, database expert collect and warehouse the data, software designers write programs that apply the analytics algorithms to the data, engineers build electronics and hardware to implement the programming, and subject-matter/domain experts – that is, biologists, chemists, economists, and social scientists – interpret the finding.

The most important asset of large volumes of data has to do with the fact that they make it possible to apply knowledge and create considerable value. Combined with advanced analysis methods, new explanations can be provided for several phenomena. There are two ways to transforms data into a valuable contribution to a company (Sedkaoui, 2016):

- Transforming data into information is one of the stages of data value production, which is exploited in order to obtain useful information and to successfully carry out company strategies. This automatically involves database information in company decision making processes;
- Transforming data into products or processes adds value to companies. This is produced when data analysis must be implemented in the physical world.

Before one attempts to extract useful knowledge from data, it is important to understand the overall approach or the process that leads to finding new knowledge. The process defines a sequence of steps (with eventual feedback) that should be followed to discover knowledge in data. To advance successfully each step, effective data collection must be applied, description, analysis and interpretation (Walter, 2015, Chapter 1). Each step is usually realized with the help of available software tools. Data mining is a particular step in this process – application of specific algorithms for extracting models from data. The additional steps in the process, such as data preparation, data selection, data cleaning, incorporation of appropriate prior knowledge, and proper interpretation of the results of mining ensure that useful knowledge is derived from the data.

There is, however, a serious challenge in making good use of such massive datasets and trying to learn new knowledge of the system or phenomenon that created these data. Knowledge extraction from data volumes of ever increasing size requires ever more flexible tools to facilitate interactive query. Today's applications are therefore required to extract knowledge from large, often distributed, repositories of text, multimedia or hybrid content. A new generation of computational techniques and tools is required to support the extraction of useful knowledge from the rapidly growing volumes of data. The nature of this quest makes it impossible to use traditional computing techniques. Instead, various soft computing techniques are employed to meet the challenge for more sophisticated solutions in knowledge discovery.

Knowledge discovery process is an automatic, exploratory analysis and modeling of large data for understandable patterns from large and complex datasets. It's focused on the development of methodologies and techniques that 'make sense' out of data, i.e. for extracting relevant and non-trivial information from data. So, data are a set of facts i.e. cases in a database, while a pattern is an expression in some language describing a subset of the data or a model applicable to the subset. Knowledge discovery process is thus a sequence of steps that, starting from rough data, leads to the discovery of knowledge. This is particularly so where the use of data for decision-making and knowledge discovery is novel.

It may be observed that the knowledge discovery process is reminiscent of the real beginnings of statistics. However, it's not only using statistics, but also contributing to statistics. The need for effective tools for knowledge discovery and mining is large especially as a crucial component of data-warehouses. Indeed, harnessing data may also require the complete overhaul of the businesses to create structures and processes that can respond to any information gleaned in a short timeframe, potentially even in real-time.

The value of a given piece of data increases in time and depends on the variety of uses it is given. In this sense, companies must possess the capacity to absorb the entirety of data available, which allows them to assimilate and reproduce knowledge. This capacity requires specific skills familiar with statistical data analytics which becomes a fundamental skill for any scientist dealing with big data. Since statistical methods are applied at the base of the pyramid (data), the data process guided knowledge discovery will entail an integrated plan of descriptive analysis and predictive modeling.

But, examining the current state of big data use in business, as well as the main opportunities many challenges are presented. Typically, a variety of some major challenges will be discussed in the next section. These challenges are regarded mostly as internal and reflect procedural problems in collecting, archiving and handling data.

BIG DATA CHALLENGES BEYOND 3Vs

Some analysts suggest that the world is entering the 'Industrial Revolution of Data' where the amount of data will be generated not only by people and companies but also by machines and interactive devices. The dimension related to the variety involves several different issues. First of all, data – especially in an industrial environment – can be presented in several different ways, such as texts, functions, curves, images, and graphs, or a combination of these elements. On the other hand, this data shows great variety, which often reflects the complexity of the studicd phenomenon.

So data complexity is growing with the increase of its quantity its velocity and diversification of its types and sources. Variety usually means heterogeneity of data types, representation, and semantic interpretation. However, velocity means both the rate at which data arrive and the time in which it must be acted upon. There are also wider challenges relating to the use of big data within society-at-large, which have been widely discussed in the literature (Boyd & Crawford, 2012; Ekbia et al., 2015).

As previously stated, big data analytics involves multiple distinct and each of them introduces challenges. The problems start right away during data acquisition, when the data deluge requires us to make decisions, currently in an ad hoc manner, about what data to keep and what to discard, and how to store what is keeping reliably with the right data. In this section author gives a broad overview of the challenges that need to be addressed in order to build capabilities in big data analytics.

The 3 V's provide a challenge associated with working with big data. The volume put the accent on the storage, memory and computes capacity of a computing system and requires access to a computing cloud. Velocity stresses the rate at which data can be absorbed and meaningful answers produced. The variety makes it difficult to develop algorithms and tools that can address that large variety of input data.

However, many technical challenges must be addressed before this potential can be realized fully. The challenges include not just the obvious issues of scale, but also heterogeneity, quality, timeliness …, at all stages of the analysis driving from data acquisition to result interpretation. Security and privacy are also a big concern, especially when considering that the linking of databases can disclose information that was meant to remain anonymous (Sedkaoui, 2017).

Heterogeneity

Data can be both structured and unstructured. They are highly dynamic and does not have particular format. It may exists in the form of email attachments, images, pdf documents, medical records, graphics, video, audio etc. and they cannot be stored in row/column format as structured data. Transforming this data to structured format for later analysis is a major challenge in big data analytics. However, machine analysis algorithms expect homogeneous data, and cannot understand nuance. In consequence, data must be carefully structured as a first step in data analysis.

- **Scale:** Managing large and rapidly increasing volumes of data has been a challenging issue for many decades. In the past, this challenge was mitigated by processors getting faster, following Moore's law, to provide us with the resources needed to cope with increasing volumes of data. The difficulties of BD analysis derive from its large scale as well as the presence of mixed data based on different patterns or rules (heterogeneous mixture data) in the collected and stored data (heterogeneous mixture data issue). Especially, in the case of complicated heterogeneous mixture data, the data has not only several patterns and rules but characteristically, the properties of the patterns vary greatly (Fujimaki & Morinaga, 2012).

Timeliness

As the size of the data sets to be processed increases, it will take more time to analyse. In some situations results of the analysis is required immediately. So businesses need to develop partial results in advance so that a small amount of incremental computation with new data can be used to arrive at a quick determination. In BD the realization time to information is critical to extract value from various data sources, including mobile devices, radio frequency identification, the web and a growing list of automated sensory technologies.

Complexity

Complexity measures the degree of interconnectedness and interdependence in big data structures such that a small change in one or a few elements can yield very large changes or a small change that ripple across or cascade through the system and substantially affect its behavior, or no change at all (Katal and al 2013). Traditional software tools are not enough for managing the increasing volumes of data. Data analysis, organization, retrieval and modeling are also challenges due to scalability and complexity of data that needs to be analyzed.

Quality

Big data processing requires an investment in computing architecture to store, manage, analyze, and visualize an enormous amount of data. It is the indispensable raw material of one of the new century's most important activities. But it is important to be prudent in our analysis and predictions because a lot of data is not yet "the right data". There is, therefore, underlying difficulty behind big data, since more data is not necessarily better data.

Security

The vast majority of data comes from the many devices and machines reporting to each other and to those running them. From the assembly line at the manufacturing plant to the passenger jet in flight, millions of bytes of data are generated and then analyzed. Some of captured data is personal information, and as such, both cutting-edge security and responsible stewardship models must be used to make sure this information is safe and correctly used.

Privacy

The advance in big data analytics brought us tools extract and correlates this data which would make data violation much easier. That makes developing the big data applications a must without forgetting the needs of privacy principles and recommendations. The lawsuit following the Netflix Challenge is a striking example of that where linking the provided data to the IMDB movie reviews allowed to identify some users.

To make the most out of big data, the issue is not limited to the "simple" technical issues of collection, storage and processing speed. The use of big data requires rethinking the process of collecting, processing and the management of data. It's the "analysis" that will be applied to data which will justify big data, not the collection of data itself. What is truly necessary are excellent analytic skills, a capacity to understand and manipulate large sets of data, and the capacity to interpret and apply the results. The need to analyze and use enormous amounts of data more efficiently drives companies towards "data science" in the hope of unlocking the power of big data analytics.

THE NEED FOR NEW ANALYTICS METHODS

The rise of big data reflects the growing awareness of the "power" behind data, and of the need to enhance gathering, exploitation, sharing and processing. The process of gathering, processing, and interpreting data is not limited to defining ideas, but also consists of materializing them in order to ensure improved knowledge production that leads to innovation. It is the use of data that empowers decision-making. In another word, it's the "analysis" that will be applied to data which will justify big data, not the collection of data itself.

Data analysis came in in the 20th century when the information age really began. Zhang have mentioned in his book "data analytics" published in 2017, that the first real data processing machine came during the Second World War. But, the advent of the internet was sparked the true revolution in data analysis. The importance of data analysis started in the late 1960 when researchers begin to speak about databases as repositories of data. E.F. Codd (Codd, 1970) and his research group at IBM labs applied some mathematical principles and predicate logic to the field of data modelling.

Since then, data bases and their evolutions have been used as a source of information to query and manipulate data. In 1974, still at IBM labs, the first language for database was developed. SEQUEL (Structured English Query Language) (Chamberlin and Boyce, 1974), later called SQL for copyright issues, was the forerunner of all the query languages becoming the standard for relational database. In the 1970s and 1980s, computers could process information, but they were too large and too costly. Only large firms could hope to analyze data with them. Edgar F. Codd was the first to work on data organization by designing database management systems (DBMSs), in particular of relational databases.

In recent years, with the advent of Web 2.0 and the semantic Web era, data analysis have become very important, replacing the traditional storing systems in many applications. They represent now the new technology for knowledge representation, data storage and information sharing. Even with big data, data collection and analysis will become more and more important. Then, it's then necessary to adapt new approaches, new methods, new knowledge and new ways of working, resulting in new properties and new challenges, as logic referencing must be created and implemented. But, before breaking down the process of data analytics and in order to understand this process, author will define what data analytics is?

Data analytics is a process of inspecting, cleansing, transforming, and modeling data with the goal of discovering useful information, suggesting conclusions, and supporting decision-making. It focuses on knowledge discovery for predictive ad descriptive purposes, to discover new ideas or to confirm existing ideas.

It can be seen from the above definition that data analysis is a primordial step in the process of knowledge discovery in databases (KDD). This step involves the application of specific algorithms for extracting patterns (models) from data. The additional steps are data preparation, data selection, data cleaning, incorporation of appropriate prior knowledge, and proper interpretation of the results of mining (Mitra and al, 2002).

Data processing and analysis, in the present day, are brought together under the notion of "Business Intelligence" (BI), due especially to computers' increased processing capabilities. Powerful analytics tools can then be used to process the information gathered in large sets of structured and unstructured data. However, there are many technical challenges that must be addressed to realize the full potential of big data. Jagadish and al (2012) provide a comprehensive discussion of such challenges based on the notion of data analysis pipeline:

- **Data Acquisition and Recording:** It is critical to capture the context into which data has been generated, to be able to filter out non-relevant data and to compress data, to automatically generate metadata supporting rich data description and to track and record provenance.
- **Information Extraction and Cleaning:** Data may have to be transformed in order to extract information from it and express this information in a form that is suitable for analysis. Data may also be of poor quality and/or uncertain. Data cleaning and data quality verification are thus critical.
- **Data Integration, Aggregation, and Representation:** Data can be very heterogeneous and may have different metadata. Data integration, even in more conventional cases, requires huge human efforts. Novel approaches that can improve the automation of data integration are critical as manual approaches will not scale to what is required for big data. Also different data aggregation and representation strategies may be needed for different data analysis tasks.
- **Query Processing, and Analysis:** Methods suitable for big data need to be able to deal with noisy, dynamic, heterogeneous, untrustworthy data and data characterized by complex relations. However despite these difficulties, big data even if noisy and uncertain can be more valuable for identifying more reliable hidden patterns and knowledge compared to tiny samples of good data. Also the (often redundant) relationships existing among data can represent an opportunity for cross-checking data and thus improve data trustworthiness. Supporting query processing and data analysis requires scalable mining algorithms and powerful computing infrastructures.
- **Interpretation:** Analysis results extracted from big data needs to be interpreted by decision makers and this may require the users to be able to analyze the assumptions at each stage of data processing and possibly re-tracing the analysis. Rich provenance is critical in this respect.

Big data analysis are essential when organizations want to engage in predictive analysis, natural language processing, image analysis or advanced statistical techniques such as discrete choice modeling and mathematical optimization, or even if they want to mash up unstructured content and analyze it with their BI. Companies will be able to suggest data management for decision-making. The new analytical power is seen as an opportunity to invent and explore new methods which are able to detect correlations between the quantities of available data.

For example, the e-commerce giant Amazon recommends products to customers based on their browsing and purchasing habits. The "ad-tech" companies such as RocketFuel apply statistical and optimization techniques to determine which banner ads to display. Thus, devices such as "Fitbit" that the recording and monitoring of our physical activities, and their integration with other applications, allows individuals to obtain information on calories burned and food consumed. This allows a creation of new models which sell this information to insurance companies to better calculate risks.

The case of these companies in various fields illustrates the power that brings analytics for management of the proposed services and applications available. To capitalize on its potential, companies must put data analytics at the center of their strategy. That is truly necessary are excellent analytic skills, a capacity to understand and manipulate large sets of data, and the capacity to interpret and apply the results.

But, they need also to establish clear guidelines for data integrity and security, as digital ecosystems can only function efficiently if all parties involved can trust in the security of their data and communication. The analysis of big data is not only a matter of solving computational problems, even if those working on big data come from the natural sciences or computational fields. Rather, expertly analyzing big data also requires thoughtful measurement (Patty & Penn 2015), careful research design, and the creative deployment of statistical techniques.

Indeed, massive datasets will require the full range of statistical methodology to be brought to bear in order for assertions of knowledge on the basis of massive data analysis to be reliable. Following a period when the main issue is how to organize and structure databases? The question now is what to do? What analyzes developed to value and support decision-making? In another term, how should statistical procedures be designed so as to be scalable computationally to the massive datasets? These issues should be seriously considered in big data analysis and in the development of statistical procedures.

HOW ARE COMPUTATIONAL TOOLS SUPPORTING STATISTICAL METHOD TO DEAL WITH BIG DATA?

During the time of applying methods of statistical inference and statistical decisions some 70 years ago, information derived from data collection was considered costly. Models were built where information was linked to payoff relevance of a decision-making criterion (utility or payoff function), therefore statistical information was handled to satisfy these criteria. Now as masses of data are produced at relatively low costs all these data could be quickly aggregated. Statisticians have coined a term, 'value of perfect information', which is set up to integrate data points, collection and analysis through statistical inferential models i.e., exploratory data analysis (EDA) or through statistical decision models (Piegorsch, 2015). For example, achieving this goal is quite challenging to gather all the data for perfect information.

In traditional statistics, there are limited amounts of data, and it must get as much information as possible out of it. In the big data age, there is a limited amount of computational power, and companies need to make the best decision. Big data pose new challenges to statisticians both in terms of theory and application. Some of the challenges include: Size, scalability of statistical computation methods, non-random data, assessing uncertainty, sampling, modelling relationships, mixture data, real-time analysis on streaming data, statistical analysis with multiple kinds of data, data quality and complexity, protecting, privacy and confidentiality, high dimensional data …

There are several methods that are recently developed and feasible for statistical inference of big data and workable on parallel machines, including the bag of little bootstraps, aggregated estimation equation, and so on. Each method was being developed to find and design tools that explicitly reveal tradeoffs relating complexity, risk, and time.

Statistics is the traditional field that deals with the quantification, collection, analysis, interpretation, and drawing conclusions from data. Development of new statistical methods is an interdisciplinary field that draws on computer sciences, artificial intelligence, machine learning, and visualization models and so on.

Concerning statistical methods literature summarizes the change in two points (Sedkaoui, 2017):

- *The new approaches are on the crossroads of IT tools and statistics.* it's concerning Machine Learning, where algorithms generate alone, more or less models on large amounts of data;
- *These methods are not new because machine learning dated from 1960s.* this return to the center stage is due to the fact that these techniques work especially well on high amounts of information.

The applied statistics and machine learning community have been quite concerned with identifying ways to cross-validate predictions produced by these techniques, and avoid simply capitalizing on chance by overfitting their data (James and al, 2014). But, it's necessary to point that there are two computational barriers for big data analysis: the first concerns the data that can be too big to hold in a computer's memory; while the second is related to the computing task that can take too long to wait for the results. These barriers can be approached either with newly developed statistical methodologies and/or computational methodologies (Wang and al, 2015).

From an IT point of view, knowledge of Hadoop is highly desirable. It allows the creation of distributed applications and "scalable" on thousands of nodes to manage petabytes of data. The principle is to split and parallelize (distribution) data batch task to linearly reduce the computation time (scalable) depending on the number of nodes. Hadoop becomes the mining web reference tool and e-commerce.

From a statistical point of view the new challenge is both the functional representation of bases of construction and relevant models to address and take into account the complex data structures: geolocation on graphs, real-time signal, 3D images, sequences... Every problem, especially industrial, requires a specific approach after a search that a conventional engineering development. In the case of data streams, the decision support becomes adaptive or sequential. The computational tools that often are associated with the analysis of big data also can help scholars who are designing experiments or making causal inferences from observational data.

Besides the aforementioned advantages, the heterogeneity of big data also poses significant challenges to statistical inference. The model is also changing; reason why data were collected to feed statistical models but now models reinventing or adapting to best exploit available data. Processing big data, in turn, puts demand on computational frameworks and models that need to be fault tolerant, flexible and light weight; example by supporting iterative and stream computing, as well as local processing of data.

Computing and storage solutions form basis for advanced data analysis, including machine learning and statistical modeling. For example, Imai and Ratkovic (2013) extended variable selection methods to estimate treatment-effect heterogeneity, whereas Green and Kern (2012) used Bayesian additive regression trees to capture systematic heterogeneity in treatment effects.

The scalability of statistical methods also poses a major challenge. When data becomes big, the possible number of simultaneous hypotheses, as well as data points, can be on the order of millions (American Statistical Association, 2015). Data sets derived from big data sources are not necessarily random samples of the target population.

The big data introduce unique computational and statistical challenges, including scalability and storage bottleneck, noise accumulation, spurious correlation and measurement errors. These challenges are distinguished and require new computational and statistical paradigm. In order to confront the challenges mentioned above statistical methods will need to be modernized. More application is needed to overcome the methodological difficulties impeding the exploitation of big data sources.

Big data are characterized by high dimensionality and large sample size. These two features raise three unique challenges:

- High dimensionality brings noise accumulation, spurious correlations and incidental homogeneity;
- High dimensionality combined with large sample size creates issues such as heavy computational cost and algorithmic instability;
- The massive samples in big data are typically aggregated from multiple sources at different time points using different technologies (Fan and al, 2014).

Another important point, which represents an often issue in data mining and analytics, is the need for sufficiently high quality in the database. Once the implementation of the first data warehouse in the 1990s the question of the quality of the data was a major issue. In the US, the theorem 'garbage in, garbage out', or the "GIGO" principal, was immediately widespread. So there is nothing new about this description: only data quality will help produce an event, a forecast or strategic information and define an action lever. Therefore, the volume of data is of little importance, since internal data must be combined with external data in order for a company to obtain the most out of its data. The reconciliation of internal and external data has always been a challenge.

It is possible to obtain better results by making better use of available data. When researchers encounter a set of data, they need to understand not only the limits of the available set of data, but also the limits of the questions that it can respond to, as well as the range of possible appropriate interpretations. Data analysis, when it is not preceded by the word 'Big', refers to the development and sharing of useful and effective models.

Currently, one of the innovations that make it possible to share and store large volumes of data is Cloud Computing. The 'Cloud' allows access to shared computing resources through an on-demand telecommunication network or self-service modules. The cloud transforms storage infrastructure and computing power into services through the intermediary of companies that possess servers and rent out their capacities. This approach makes it possible to share costs and to provide greater data storage and processing flexibility for users. The volume of data generated and stored by enterprises made a new step. As already indicated in previous sections, this new step creates new approaches for both architectures databases, the parallelization of computations as for algorithms and methods used.

While the parallel and distributed architectures present new capabilities for storage and manipulation of data, from an inferential point of view, it is unclear how the current statistical methodology can be transported to the paradigm of big data. Cutting-edge data management, querying, and analysis techniques in computer science must be linked with fundamental approaches in statistics and machine learning to create data systems that are flexible, responsive, and predictive. Computer-science techniques need to incorporate more statistical approaches, while statistical techniques need to develop approaches for trading off statistical power and computational complexity (it will be discussed in the next section). The need to analyze and use enormous amounts of data more efficiently drives companies towards "data science" in the hope of unlocking the power of big data.

SOME NEW METHODS DEVELOPED (ALGORITHMS) FOR MASSIVE DATASETS ANALYSIS

The transformation of big data into knowledge is by no means an easy task. Therefore, it is challenging for businesses to analyze and extract knowledge from a universe due to lack of computing resources available. This section is about methods which ride of the progress in computational data analysis. Sound statistical methods that are scalable computationally to massive datasets have been proposed. From a computational perspective, much effort has been put into the most active, open source statistical environment. Software review focuses on the open source R and R packages, covering recent tools that help break the barriers of computer memory and computing power. Statistician R developers are relentless in their drive to extend the reach of R into big data. The statistical methodologies for big data can be grouped as follow:

Subsampling-Based

This means that a subsample from the original dataset is taking with respect to a carefully designed probability distribution, and uses this sample as a surrogate for the original dataset to do model estimation, prediction as well as statistical inference.

1. **The Big Data Bootstrap:** Traditionally, subsampling has been used to refer to "m-out-of-n" bootstrap, whose primary motivation is to make approximate inference owing to the difficulty or intractability in deriving analytical expressions (Efron, 1979; Jackknife, 1989). In the massive data setting, there is a serious problem: each bootstrap resample is itself massive. However, in

settings involving large datasets, the computation of bootstrap-based quantities can be prohibitively demanding. A new procedure which incorporates features of both the bootstrap and subsampling is known as the Bag of Little Bootstraps (BLB), to obtain a robust, computationally efficient means of assessing estimator quality. This method, proposed by Kleiner and al. (2014), is a combination of subsampling (Politis and al., 1999), the m-out-of-n bootstrap (Bickel and al., 1997), and the bootstrap to achieve computational efficiency. The development of BLB was motivated by the computational imperative; it can be viewed as a novel statistical procedure to be compared to the bootstrap and subsampling according to more classical criteria.

2. **Leveraging:** Leveraging methods are designed under a subsampling framework, in which one samples a small proportion of the data (subsample) from the full sample, and then performs intended computations for the full sample using the small subsample as a surrogate. Ma and Sun (2014) proposed to use leveraging to facilitate scientific discoveries from big data using limited computing resources. The key to success of the leveraging methods is to construct the weights, the nonuniform sampling probabilities, so that influential data points are sampled with high probabilities.
3. **Mean Log-Likelihood:** Liang and al. (2013) proposed a new parameter estimator, maximum mean log-likelihood estimator, for big data problems, and a resampling-based stochastic approximation method for obtaining such an estimator. The method uses Monte Carlo averages calculated from subsamples to approximate the quantities needed for the full data. Motivated from minimizing the Kullback–Leibler (KL) divergence, they approximate the KL divergence by averages calculated from subsamples. The solution to the mean score equation is obtained from a stochastic approximation procedure, where at each iteration; the current estimate is updated based on a subsample of size m drawn from the full data. As m is much smaller than n, the method is scalable to big data. Liang and al. (2013) established the consistency and asymptotic normality of the resulting estimator under mild conditions.

Divide and Conquer Method

The divide and conquer method solves big data problems in the following manner. First, the original massive dataset is divided into *K* small blocks that are manageable to the current computing facility unit. Then, the intended statistical analysis is performed on each small block. Finally, an appropriate strategy will be used to combine the results from these *K* blocks. As a result, the computation for the divide and conquer method can easily be done in parallel.

This is trivial for some models, like linear models or generalized linear models, for which the estimation procedures are linear by construction. More specifically, the estimating equations for the full data themselves can be written as a summation of all smaller blocks. The readers are referred to for more detailed discussion and theoretical properties for resulting estimators for a single parameter case.

1. **Aggregated Estimating Equations:** In recent years, there have been active researches on developing compression and aggregation schemes to support fast online analytical processing (OLAP) of various statistical analyses, such as linear regression, general multiple linear regression, logistic regression analysis… However, many advanced statistical analyses are nonlinear and thus most of the current OLAP tools cannot be used to support these advanced analyses. Aggregated estimating equations develop a computation and storage efficient algorithm for estimating equation (EE) estimation in massive data sets using a divide and conquer strategy. In each partition of the data set, the raw data is compressing into some low dimensional statistics and then discard the raw data. Results an approximation to the EE estimator, the AEE estimator, by solving an equation aggregated from the saved low dimensional statistics in all partitions. Such low dimensional statistics are taken as the EE estimates and first-order derivatives of the estimating equations in each partition. For general nonlinear assessment equations were offered a linear approximation of the estimating equations with the Taylor expansion at the solution in each block. Lin & Xi (2011) showed that the aggregated estimator has the same limit as the estimator from the full data.
2. **Parallel MCMC:** Computational intensity and sequential nature of estimation techniques for Bayesian methods in statistics and machine learning, combined with their increasing applications for big data analytics, necessitate both the identification of potential opportunities to parallelize techniques such as Monte Carlo Markov Chain (MCMC) sampling. In the Bayesian framework, it is natural to partition the data into k subsets and run parallel MCMC on each one of them. The prior distribution for each subset is often obtained by taking a power 1/k of the prior distribution for whole data in order to preserve the total amount of prior information. Neiswanger and al. (2013) proposed to use kernel density estimators of the posterior density for each data subset, and estimate the full data posterior by multiplying the subset posterior densities together. This method is asymptotically exact in the sense of being converging in the number of MCMC iterations. Wang and al (2015) replaced the kernel estimator of Neiswanger and al. (2013) with a random partition tree histogram, which uses the same block partition across all terms in the product representation of the posterior to control the number of terms in the approximation such that it

does not explode with m. Scott and al. (2013) proposed a consensus Monte Carlo algorithm, which produces the approximated full data posterior using weighted averages over the subset MCMC samples.

Divide-and-conquer is a natural computational paradigm for approaching big data problems, particularly given recent developments in distributed and parallel computing, but some interesting challenges arise when applying divide-and-conquer algorithms to statistical inference problems. One interesting issue is that of obtaining confidence intervals in massive datasets.

Massive Time-Series Datasets

The detection and analysis of events within massive collections of time-series has become an extremely important task. In particular, many scientific investigations (e.g. the analysis of microlensing and other transients) begin with the detection of events in irregularly-sampled series with both non-linear trends and non-Gaussian noise. This approach harnesses the power of Bayesian modeling while maintaining much of the speed and scalability of more ad-hoc machine learning approaches.

Coarse-to-Fine Method

Another surprising yet proved to be effective idea proposed much recently is the coarse-to-fine method. In order to make intended algorithms for the massive dataset scalable, statisticians introduced a simple solution: rounding parameters. Hence the continuous real numbers of data are simply rounded from higher decimal places to lower decimal places. A substantial number of observations are degenerated to be identical. This idea was successfully applied to the functional data analysis using smoothing spline ANOVA models (Helwig and Ma, 2016). Indeed, in recent years slanted plane methods that jointly reason about stereo/flow and super pixels have been proposed (Yamaguchi and al, 2013). While they perform very well in challenging scenarios they are however computationally very expensive, limiting their applicability to real-wold applications such as autonomous driving.

Algorithm Weakening

In the case of BLB the flexibility inheres in the choice of m (the subsample size) and in the case of Divide-Factor-Combine (DFC) it is the choice of l (the submatrix dimension). Chandrasekaran and Jordan (2013) define a notion of "algorithmic weakening," in which a hierarchy of algorithms is ordered by both computational efficiency and statistical efficiency.

The problem that they address is to develop a quantitative relationship among three quantities: the number of data points, the runtime and the statistical risk. Chandrasekaran and Jordan (2013) focus on the denoising problem, an important theoretical testbed in the study of high-dimensional inference. General framework for algorithm weakening based on relaxations of convex sets.

Convex optimization methods offer a powerful framework for statistical inference due to the broad class of estimators that can be effectively modeled as convex programs. Further the theory of convex analysis is useful both for characterizing the statistical properties of convex programming based estimators as well as for developing methods to compute such estimators efficiently.

Online Updating Approaches

Motivated from a Bayesian inference perspective, Schifano and al. (2015) extends the work of Lin and Xi (2011) in a few important ways. First, they introduce divide-and-conquer-type variance estimates of regression parameters in the linear model and estimating equation settings. Then, they develop iterative estimating algorithms and statistical inferences for linear models and estimating equations that update as new data arrive. After that, they address the issue of possible rank deficiencies when dealing with blocks of data, and the uniqueness properties of the combined and cumulative estimators when using a generalized inverse.

Instead, they propose outlier tests relying on predictive residuals, which are based on the predictive values computed from the cumulative estimate of the regression coefficients attained at the previous accumulation point. In addition, a new online-updated estimator of the regression coefficients corresponding estimator of the standard error in the estimating equation setting which takes advantage of information from the previous data are introduced by authors.

CONCLUSION

With the developing of the IoT and the coming the semantic web, new methods for representing, storing and sharing information are going to replace the traditional systems. Offering to businesses and decision-makers, unprecedented opportunities to tackle much larger and more complex big data challenges. This chapter has dealt with the issue of extraction of knowledge from data driven by statistics and computing in order to deal big data challenges. Such as: (i) the complexity of data (collected from different sources and different formats). (ii) Noisy data challenge: big data generally include different kinds of measurement errors, outliers and missing values.

(iii) Dependent data challenge: in varied types of current data, such as financial time series and so on.

To handle the challenges of big data, new statistical thinking and computational methods are needed. Because, classical statistical methods are often unsuited for big data purposes, which can be linked to a lack of flexibility in existing methods, but also to the assumptions that are typically made for mathematical convenience, and the particular way of drawing inference from data.

For example, many traditional methods that perform well for moderate sample size do not scale to massive data. Similarly, many statistical methods that perform well for low-dimensional data are facing significant challenges in analyzing high-dimensional data. In terms of statistical methods, dimension reduction and variable selection play pivotal roles in analyzing high-dimensional data. New statistical procedures with these issues in mind are crucially needed.

With the challenges and opportunities of big data and necessity of turning data into knowledge, statistics is an essential scientific discipline because of its sophisticated methods for statistical inference, prediction, quantification of uncertainty, and experimental design. Statistics is closely related to machine-learning and knowledge discovery, and depends heavily on data-visualization techniques. And knowledge discovery is on the interface of computing and statistics, and the main issues faced were to find a point of contact between the two disciplines already explored, statistics and computing science.

The collaboration between statistics and computer science is needed to control runtimes that will maintain the statistical procedures usable on large-scale data while ensuring good statistical properties. Then, analysis of the data is application oriented and driven by computation. In case of data analytics, companies analyzed requirements regarding (i) Data: types, structure, format and sources and (ii) data Processing: operations, performance and conditions.

Obviously, more can be done, following either the undertaken direction or exploring new solutions. This include the ever-changing landscape of data and their associated characteristics, evolving data analysis paradigms, challenges of computational infrastructure, data sharing and data access, and – crucially – our ability to integrate data sets and their analysis toward an improved understanding. Moreover the type of analysis which is needed to be done on the data depends highly on the results to be obtained through decision making. This can be done to (i) incorporate massive data volumes in analysis or (ii) determine upfront which big data is relevant (quality). So, the biggest challenge of the zetabytes age will not be storing all that data, it will be figuring out how to make sense of it.

ACKNOWLEDGMENT

I would like to gratefully and sincerely thank Professor H.W Gottinger for his guidance, understanding, in the planning and preparation of this chapter, and most importantly, his friendship. I must express my very profound gratitude to my mother and to my sisters and brother for providing me with unfailing support and continuous encouragement throughout my years of study and through the process of researching and writing this chapter. This accomplishment would not have been possible without them. Thank you.

REFERENCES

Ackoff, R. L. (1989). From data to wisdom. *Journal of Applied Systems Analysis, 15*, 3–9.

American Statistical Association. (2015). *Discovery with Data: Leveraging Statistics with Computer Science to Transform Science and Society, Web. 3.0*. Retrieved from http://www.amstat.org/policy/pdfs/BigDataStatisticsJune2014.pdf

Bickel, P., Gotze, F., & Van Zwet, W. (1997). Resampling fewer than n observations: Gains, losses and remedies for losses. *Statistica Sinica, 7*, 1–31.

Boyd, D., & Crawford, K. (2012). Critical questions for big data: Provocations for a cultural, technological, and scholarly phenomenon. *Information Communication and Society, 15*(5), 662–679. doi:10.1080/1369118X.2012.678878

Brynjolfsson, E., & McAfee, A. (2011). *Race Against the Machine: How the Digital Revolution is Accelerating Innovation, Driving Productivity, and Irreversibly Transforming Employment and the Economy*. Lexington, MA: Digital Frontier Press.

Chamberlin, D. D., & Boyce, R. F. (1974, April). SEQUEL: A structured English query language. *Proc. 1974 ACM SIGFIDET Workshop*, 249-264.

Chandrasekaran, V., & Jordan, M. (2013). Computational and statistical tradeoffs via convex relaxation. *Proceedings of the National Academy of Sciences of the United States of America, 13*(13), 1181–1190. doi:10.1073/pnas.1302293110 PMID:23479655

Cleveland, H. (1982, December). Information as Resource. *The Futurist*, 34–39.

Codd, E. F. (1970, June). A relational model of data for large shared data banks. *Communications of the ACM, 13*(6), 377–387.

Cukier, K., & Mayer-Schoenberger, V. (2013b). The Rise of Big Data. *Foreign Affairs, 92*(3), 28–40.

Cukier, K., & Mayer-Schonberger, V. (2013a). *Big Data: A Revolution That Will Transform How We Live, Work and Think*. Boston, MA: Houghton Mifflin Harcourt.

Efron, B. (1979). Bootstrap methods: Another look at the jackknife. *Annals of Statistics, 7*(1), 1–26. doi:10.1214/aos/1176344552

Ekbia, H., Mattioli, M., Kouper, I., Arave, G., Ghazinejad, A., Bowman, T., ... Sugimoto, C. R. (2015). Big data, bigger dilemmas: A critical review. *Journal of the Association for Information Science and Technology, 66*(8), 1523–1545. doi:10.1002/asi.23294

Eliot, T. S. (1934). *The rock*. Faber & Faber. Available at: http://www.wisdomportal.com/Technology/TSEliot-TheRock.html

Fan, J., Han, F., & Liu, H. (2014). Challenges of Big Data analysis. *National Science Review, 1*(2), 293–314. doi:10.1093/nsr/nwt032 PMID:25419469

Foster, I., Ghani, R., Jarmin, R. S., Kreuer, F., & Lane, J. (2017). *Big Data and Social Science*. Boca Raton, FL: CRC Press.

Fujimaki, R., & Morinaga, S. (2012). The Most Advanced Data Mining of the Big Data Era. *Advanced Technologies to Support Big Data Processing, 7*(2).

Green, D. P., & Holger, L. K. (2012). Modeling Heterogeneous Treatment Effects in Survey Experiments with Bayesian Additive Regression Trees. *Public Opinion Quarterly, 76*(3), 491–511. doi:10.1093/poq/nfs036

Harford, T. (2014). Big Data: A Big Mistake. *Significance, 11*(5), 14–19. doi:10.1111/j.1740-9713.2014.00778.x

Helwig, N. E., & Ma, P. (2016). Smoothing spline ANOVA for super-large samples: Scalable computation via rounding parameters. *Statistics and Its Interface, 9*(4), 433–444. doi:10.4310/SII.2016.v9.n4.a3

IDC. (2011). *World's data will grow by 50X in next decade*. IDC Study.

Imai, K., & Ratkovic, M. (2013). Estimating Treatment Effect Heterogeneity, *Randomized Program Evaluation. The Annals of Applied Statistics, 7*(1), 443–470. doi:10.1214/12-AOAS593

Jagadish, S. V. K., Septiningsih, E. M., Kohli, A., Thomson, M. J., Ye, C., Redoña, E., ... Singh, R. K. (2012). Genetic advances in adapting rice to a rapidly changing climate. *Journal Agronomy & Crop Science, 198*(5), 360–373. doi:10.1111/j.1439-037X.2012.00525.x

James, G., Witten, D., Hastie, T., & Tibshirani, R. (2014). *An introduction to statistical learning with applications in R*. New York: Springer.

Katal, A., Wazid, M., & Goudar, R. H. (2013). Big Data: Issues, Challenges, Tools and Good Practices. *IEEE Spectrum*, 404–409.

Kleiner, A., Talwalkar, A., Sarkar, P., & Jordan, M. I. (2014). A scalable bootstrap for massive data. *Journal of the Royal Statistical Society. Series B, Statistical Methodology, 76*(4), 795–816. doi:10.1111/rssb.12050

Liang, F., Cheng, Y., Song, Q., Park, J., & Yang, P. (2013). A resampling-based stochastic approximation method for analysis of large geostatistical data. *Journal of the American Statistical Association, 108*(501), 325–339. doi:10.1080/01621459.2012.746061

Liang, F., & Kim J., (2013). *A bootstrap Metropolis–Hastings algorithm for Bayesian analysis of big data*. Tech. rep., Department of Statistics, Texas A & M University.

Lin, N., & Xi, R. (2011). Aggregated estimating equation estimation. *Statistics and Its Interface, 4*(1), 73–83. doi:10.4310/SII.2011.v4.n1.a8

Ma, P., & Sun, X. (2014). *Leveraging for big data regression*. WIREs Computational Statistics.

Mann, D. (2004). *Hands-on Systematic Innovation for Business*. CREAX Press.

McKinsey. (2011). *Internet matters: The Net's sweeping impact on growth, jobs, and prosperity*. Author.

McKinsey. (2013). *Big Data, Analytics and the Future of Marketing and Sales*. New York: McKinsey.

Mitra, S., Pal, S. K., & Mitra, P. (2002). Data mining in soft computing framework: A survey. *IEEE Transactions on Neural Networks, 13*(1), 3–14. doi:10.1109/72.977258 PMID:18244404

Neiswanger, W., Wang, C., & Xing, E. (2013). *Asymptotically exact, embarrassingly parallel MCMC*. arXiv preprint arXiv: 1311-4780

Patty, J., & Penn, E. M. (2015). Analyzing Big Data: Social Choice and Measurement. *PS, Political Science & Politics, 48*(1), 95–101. doi:10.1017/S1049096514001814

Piegorsch, W. W. (2015). *Statistical Data Analytics*. New York: Wiley.

Politis, D. N., Romano, J. P., & Wolf, M. (1999). Subsampling. New York: Springer.

Schifano, E. D., Wu, J., Wang, C., Yan, J., & Chen, M.-H. (2015). Online Updating of Statistical Inference in the Big Data Setting. *Technometrics*. PMID:28018007

Scott, S.L., Blocker, A.W., Bonassi, F.V., Chipman, H., George, E., & McCulloch, R. (2013). Bayes and Big Data: The Consensus Monte Carlo Algorithm. *EFaBBayes 250 Conference*, 16.

Sedkaoui, S. (2017). The Internet, Data Analytics and Big Data. In Internet Economics: Models, Mechanisms and Management (pp. 185-210). Bentham Science.

Sedkaoui, S., & Monino, J. L. (2016). *Big data, Open Data and Data Development*. New York: ISTE-Wiley.

Shroff, G. (2013). *The Intelligent Web, Search, Smart Algorithms and Big Data*. Oxford, UK: Oxford Univ. Press.

Siegel, E. (2016). *Predictive Analytics*. New York: Wiley.

Turban, E. (2011). *Business Intelligence: A Managerial Approach* (2nd ed.). Upper Saddle River, NJ: Prentice Hall.

Vermesan, D., Prejbeanu, R., Laitin, R., Georgianu, V., Haragus, H., & Nitescu, S. (2014). Meniscal tears left in situ during anatomic single bundle anterior cruciate ligament reconstruction. *European Review for Medical and Pharmacological Sciences*, *18*(2), 252–256. PMID:24488916

Wang, X., Guo, F., Heller, K. A., & Dunson, D. B. (2015). *Parallelizing MCMC with Random Partition Trees*. arXiv preprint arXiv: 1506-03164

Wu, C. F. J. (1989). Bootstrap and other resampling methods in regression analysis. *Ann Stat*, *14*, 1261–1295.

Yamaguchi, K., Hazan, T., McAllester, D., & Urtasun, R. (2013). *Robustmonocular epipolar flow estimation*. CVPR.

Zeleny, M. (1987). Management Support Systems: Towards Integrated Knowledge Management. *Human Systems Management*, *7*(1), 59–70.

Zhang, A. (2017). *Data analytics: Practical guide to leveraging the power of Algorithms, data science, data mining, statistics, big data, and predictive analysis to improve business, work, and life*. Kindle Edition.

KEY TERMS AND DEFINITIONS

Analytics: Has emerged as a catch-all term for a variety of different business intelligence (BI)- and application-related initiatives. For some, it is the process of analyzing information from a particular domain, such as website analytics. For others, it is applying the breadth of BI capabilities to a specific content area (for example, sales, service, supply chain, and so on). In particular, BI vendors use the "analytics" moniker to differentiate their products from the competition. Increasingly, "analytics" is used to describe statistical and mathematical data analysis that clusters, segments, scores, and predicts what scenarios are most likely to happen. Whatever the use cases, "analytics" has moved deeper into the business vernacular. Analytics has garnered a burgeoning interest from business and IT professionals looking to exploit huge mounds of internally generated and externally available data.

Big Data: The term big data is used when the amount of data that an organization has to manage reaches a critical volume that requires new technological approaches in terms of storage, processing, and usage. Volume, velocity, and variety are usually the three criteria used to qualify a database as "big data."

Business Intelligence (BI): An umbrella term that includes the applications, infrastructure and tools, and best practices that enable access to and analysis of information to improve and optimize decisions and performance.

Data: This term comprises facts, observations, and raw information. Data itself has little meaning if it is not processed.

Data Analysis: A class of statistical methods that makes it possible to process a very large volume of data and identify the most interesting aspects of its structure. Some methods help to extract relations between different sets of data, and thus, draw statistical information that makes it possible describe the most important information contained in the data in the most succinct manner possible. Other techniques make it possible to group data in order to identify its common denominators clearly, and thereby understand them better.

Data Mining: This practice consists of extracting information from data as the objective of drawing knowledge from large quantities of data through automatic or semi-automatic methods. Data mining uses algorithms drawn from disciplines as diverse as statistics, artificial intelligence, and computer science in order to develop models from data; that is, in order to find interesting structures or recurrent themes according to criteria determined beforehand, and to extract the largest possible amount of knowledge useful to companies. It groups together all technologies capable of analyzing database information in order to find useful information and possible significant and useful relationships within the data.

Data Science: A new discipline that combines elements of mathematics, statistics, computer science, and data visualization. The objective is to extract information from data sources. In this sense, data science is devoted to database exploration and analysis. This discipline has recently received much attention due to the growing interest in big data.

Exploratory Data Analysis (EDA): In statistics, EDA is an approach to analyzing data sets to summarize their main characteristics, often with visual methods.

Garbage In, Garbage Out (GIGO): In the field of computer science or information and communications technology refers to the fact that computers, since they operate by logical processes, will unquestioningly process unintended, even nonsensical, input data ("garbage in") and produce undesired, often nonsensical, output ("garbage out"). The principle applies to other fields as well.

Hadoop: Big data software infrastructure that includes a storage system and a distributed processing tool.

Information: Consists of interpreted data, and has discernible meaning. It is lies in descriptions and answers questions like "Who?" "What?" "When?" and "How many?"

Knowledge: A type of know-how that makes it possible to transform information into instructions. Knowledge can either be obtained through transmission from those who possess it, or by extraction from experience.

Machine-to-Machine (M2M): Communications is used for automated data transmission and measurement between mechanical or electronic devices. The key components of an M2M system are field-deployed wireless devices with embedded sensors or RFID-wireless communication networks with complementary wireline access including but not limited to cellular communication, Wi-Fi, ZigBee, WiMAX, wireless LAN (WLAN), generic DSL (xDSL), and fiber to the x (FTTx).

MapReduce: A programming model or algorithm for the processing of data using a parallel programming implementation and was originally used for academic purposes associated with parallel programming techniques.

Scalability: The measure of a system's ability to increase or decrease in performance and cost in response to changes in application and system processing demands. Enterprises that are growing rapidly should pay special attention to scalability when evaluating hardware and software.

Semantic Web: (Also known as the Web 3.0) This is a network that allows machines to understand semantics, which is to say the meaning of information published online. It expands the network of web pages understandable by humans by adding metadata that is understandable by a machine and that creates links between content and different pages, which in turn allows automatic agents to access the web in a more intelligent manner and to carry out some tasks in the place of users.

Smart Data: The flood of data encountered by ordinary users and economic actors will bring about changes in behavior, as well as the development of new services and value creation. This data must be processed and developed in order to become "smart data." Smart data is the result of analysis and interpretation of raw data, which makes it possible to effectively draw value from it. It is, therefore, important to know how to work with the existing data in order to create value.

Statistical Inference: The process of deducing properties of an underlying distribution by analysis of data. Inferential statistical analysis infers properties about a population. This includes testing hypotheses and deriving estimates. The population is assumed to be larger than the observed data set; in other words, the observed data is assumed to be sampled from a larger population.

Web 2.0: The set of techniques, functions, and uses of the world wide web that have followed the original format of the web. It concerns, in particular, interfaces that allow users with little technical training to appropriate new web functions. Internet users can contribute to information exchanges and interact (share, exchange, etc.) in a simple manner.

Chapter 3
Usage of Big Data Prediction Techniques for Predictive Analysis in HIV/AIDS

Chinmayee Mohapatra
KIIT University, India

Biswaranjan Acharya
KIIT University, India

Siddhath Swarup Rautaray
KIIT University, India

Manjusha Pandey
KIIT University, India

ABSTRACT

The term big data refers to the data that exceeds the processing or analyzing capacity of existing database management systems. The inability of existing DBMS to handle big data is due to its large volume, high velocity, pertaining veracity, heterogeneous variety, and on-atomic values. Nowadays, healthcare plays a vital role in everyone's life. It becomes a very large and open platform for everyone to do all kinds of research work without affecting human life. When it comes to disease, there are so many types found all over the world. But among them, AIDS (acquired immunodeficiency syndrome) is a disease that spreads so quickly and can easily turn life to death. There are many studies going on to create drugs to cure this deadly disease, but until now, there has been no success. In cases such as this, big data is implemented for better a result, which will have a good impact on society.

DOI: 10.4018/978-1-5225-3203-3.ch003

INTRODUCTION

The rapid increase in population creates an issue in handling and analyzing the population data for the traditional data base management system. So Big data came into figure to solve the issue. Infectious disease are the disorder that happened in a normal body by organisms-such as bacteria, viruses, fungi or parasites. Some infectious diseases pass from one person to another person. Some are transmitted due to insects or animals bite. And others may happen by consuming contaminated food or water or by getting exposed to the organisms which present in the environment. AIDS (Acquired immunodeficiency syndrome) becomes a very fast spreading and turning the life to death, disease. HIV spreads from one person to another person in the population in many different ways that may be due to blood, semen and pre-seminal fluid ("pre-cum"), rectal fluids/anal mucous, vaginal fluids, breast milk. This chapter describes three types of measure those are oral meditative, Environmental Predicative and another one is a operational predicative measure. But till now there is no scope of operational measures, so it tends to null. But as if we will consider oral meditative measures then several medicines are invented for fighting with HIV/AIDS but that is only to sustain with the virus it does not eradicate the virus totally or the person cannot be cured from this disease. Environmental predicative measure includes many environmental factors, among them some factors are like poverty, cultural aspects, including religion and traditions, appear to play an essential role in the rapid and global development of AIDS epidemic. The provided measures will help the society for the better prevention of HIV/AIDS.

BIG DATA

Nowadays, data is coming in a very large and very fast manner, which becomes difficult for the traditional database to handle, so big data came to be. There are many characteristics of big data, but mostly 9v's are considered. The main characteristics of big data are volume, velocity, veracity, verity, value, validity, volatility, variability, and visualization.

- Volume indicates the amount (Hammer et al., 2008) of data that may in Gbs or Tbs or more than that.
- Velocity is considered as how fast the data are created and collected.
- Validity means till which time extend the data will be valid. And it also indicates that how much the data is valid for the computation.
- Veracity means the truthfulness of data. Value means, how much the data is valuable.

Figure 1. Characteristics of Big Data

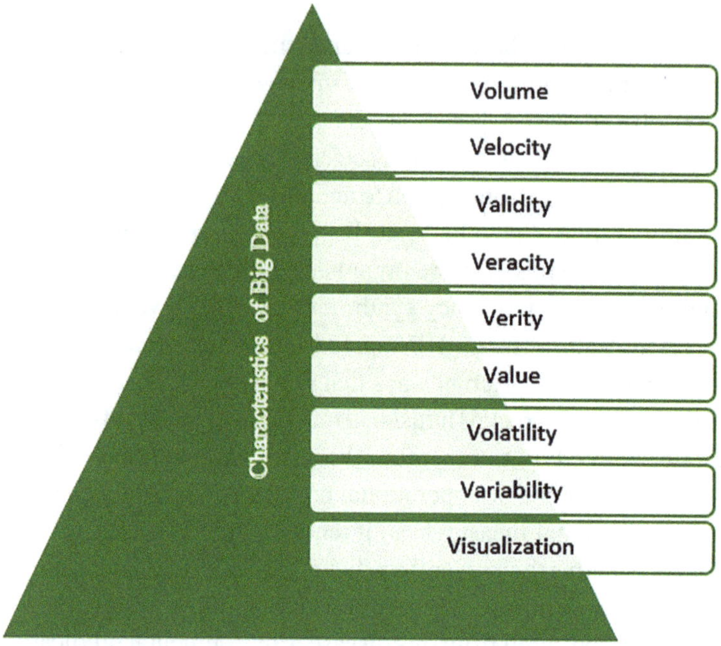

- Verity means how many types of data are present that may be structured (Oweis et al., 2015), semi-structured or unstructured. If we will consider one by one then we can say that structured data includes the data bases, the semi-structured data includes XML (Uddin et al., 2014) Files and the unstructured comes into figure in case of social media like Facebook, Twitter.
- Value deals with the valuable input. It indicates how much the data is valuable for the computation. It also includes the value that needed to be spent for storing the data. Like if we store the data in low cost storage (Toshniwal et al., 2015) then may cause some difficulties in future to access the data. Sometimes it can happen that the data will be lost forever. So, Value should be taken care of.
- Volatility means the volatile character of data i.e. the same data should be available all the time for all the users for computation and getting the result (DeRoos et al., 2014). Like there are many online shopping companies where they don't want to store some data about the customer's purchase because after one year the warranty period ends. So, after one year they delete the data from their database.

- Variability, it indicates that may be the velocity of data varies that may be at peak for some time and sometimes (Patel et al., 2012) very slow. And also, along with the velocity, the data flows may be highly inconsistent. So, it becomes a challenge to manage the data, especially when unstructured data is involved.
- Visualization is the process which helps to understand the meaning of different data values in a faster and accurate manner.

OVERVIEW OF INFECTIOUS DISEASE

Infectious diseases are disorders that occur in a normal body due to organisms-such as bacteria, viruses, fungi, or parasites. Some organisms are already present in and on our bodies; normally they are not harmful and can even be helpful, but under some circumstances, some organisms may cause disease (Barreiro-Gomez et al., 2015). Some infectious diseases pass from one person to another person, some are transmitted due to insect or animal bites, and others are caused by consuming contaminated food or water, or result from being exposed to other organisms, which are present in the environment. Signs and symptoms vary depending on the kind of organism that becomes the cause of infection, but most of the time, the disease includes fever. Mild infections may be cured by some home remedies, while some life-threatening infections may require hospitalization (Almeida et al., 2016). The ways through which infectious disease spreads are as follows:

Direct Contact

The infection can spread from one person to another person by means of exchanging the bacteria or virus through touches, kisses, coughs, or sneezes. The disease can also travel from animals to a person if the person is bitten or scratched by an infected animal. A person even can become sick due to his/her own pet. The germs can pass to an unborn baby from their mother because the unborn child resides in the womb of its mother.

Indirect Contact

Disease-causing organisms can also be passed through indirect contact. For example, someone who touches a doorknob that was handled by someone afflicted with the flu or a cold could pick up the germs that the sick person left behind. If the person who touched the doorknob proceeded to touch their eyes, mouth, or nose before cleaning hands, they can then become infected by the disease.

Spread Through Mouth

Some infections are spread through faeces that come from mouth of the infected person (Ray et al., 2016). Normally, the size of faeces are microscopic. These travel from one person's mouth to another person's mouth by air. Some examples of this kind of disease are listed below:

- Hand, foot disease
- Hepatitis-A
- Mouth disease

Spread by Skin or Mucous Membrane Contact

Infection spreads directly or indirectly when negligible particles of skin or mucous membrane come into contact with the unaffected person's skin or mucous membrane (Koçak et al., 2016).

Examples:

- Chickenpox
- Head lice
- Cold sores (herpes simplex infection)

Spread Through Blood

Blood or other fluids of body (for example: urine, saliva, breast milk, secretion from semen and vagina, etc.) plays a vital role in the transferring of infection from person to person (Chang et al., 2016). Additionally, diseases and infections can spread through the bloodstream of an infected person. This can occur in a transfer of blood or the reuse of a needle.

Examples:

- Hepatitis-B
- Human immunodeficiency virus (HIV) infection
- Hepatitis-C

Spread Through Food or Water

There are some diseases whose main cause is consumption of water or a wide variety of foods that contain disease-causing germs or related toxins (Khalid et al., 2016).

Examples:

- Typhoid and paratyphoid
- Shigella infection
- Listeria infection

Spread Through the Air by Droplets

When a person is infected with a disease or illness, they can transmit the disease by talking, coughing, or sneezing more than one small droplet containing the infectious agent goes into the air (Ray et al., 2016). And because of the droplets' size, they can travel in the air, but only for a short distance (around a meter) from the infected person. In between that time, if the droplets are inhaled by a nearby person, then the person gets the virus, which affects the normal health condition of that person. Even if a nose or mouth is touched by the hands that contain the droplet, then the infection can spread.

Examples:

- Flu
- Meningococcal disease
- Common cold

Spread Through the Air by Aerosol

The small particle that aerosols contain hold infectious agents of coughs or sneezes. But, because of their tiny size, the small particles of aerosols are sustained in air for a long time and can travel long distances. And in between the time, these particles may be inhaled by an uninfected person, which causes the person to become infected by the virus.

Examples:

- Chickenpox
- Measles
- Tuberculosis (TB)

Diseases Where Person-to-Person Spread Occurs Rarely

There are some infectious disease which very rarely spread through direct or indirect contact of person to person (Borysiak et al., 2016). Those diseases can be spread by coming into the contact with an environmental source such as animals, insects, water, or soil.

Diseases spread by contact with animals:

- Psittacosis
- Hydrated disease
- Cat-scratch Disease

Diseases spread by insects:

- Malaria
- Dengue fever
- Barmah Forest virus infection

Diseases spread by contact with water or soil:

- Tetanus.
- Amoebic meningitis

OVERVIEW OF AIDS/HIV

As everyone knows the count of people who are affected by AIDS/HIV is increasing day by day.

What Is HIV?

HIV (Human Immunodeficiency Virus) is a virus which directly targets the immune system. Once this virus goes into the body, it directly increases its cells in blood by decreasing the WBC (White Blood Cells) count; white blood cells are the fighters of immune system that help to fend off illness and disease. If a person gets infected by HIV and is not going through any type of treatment, then it's very difficult for him/her to fight off any type of infection or disease as the immune system goes down due to HIV. The spread of HIV depends on age, health, and background. But still, if HIV is left untreated for 10 to 15 years, then it damages the whole immune system. As such, HIV can be transferred through semen, blood, vaginal, anal fluids, and breast milk. It is not possible for HIV to be transmitted by sweat, saliva, or urine (Borysiak, 2016). The virus spreads from one person to another through blood transfer, sexual contact, and from infected mother to their babies during pregnancy, childbirth, and breast feeding. Some other ways in which HIV can be transmitted are through vaginal sex, oral sex, anal sex, blood transfusion, and contaminated hypodermic needles. "In the early stages of HIV infection, the most common symptoms are none," says Michael Horberg, MD, director of HIV/AIDS for Kaiser Permanent, in Oakland.

Basic Facts About HIV

- HIV stands for human immunodeficiency virus.
- There is effective antiretroviral treatment available so people with HIV can live a normal, healthy life.
- The earlier HIV is diagnosed, the sooner treatment can start – leading to better long term health.
- HIV is found in semen, blood, vaginal and anal fluids, and breast milk.
- HIV cannot be transmitted through sweat, saliva or urine.
- Using male condoms or female condoms during sex is the best way to prevent HIV and other sexually transmitted infections.
- If you inject drugs, always use a clean needle and syringe, and never share equipment.
- If you are pregnant and living with HIV, the virus in your blood could pass into your baby's body, or after giving birth through breastfeeding. Taking HIV treatment virtually eliminates this risk.

What Is AIDS?

AIDS is not a virus but a set of symptoms (or syndrome) caused by the HIV virus. A person is said to have AIDS when their immune system is too weak to fight off infection and develop certain defining symptoms and illnesses (Oweis et al., 2015). This is the last stage of HIV, when the infection is very advanced, and if left untreated, will lead to death.

Basic Facts About AIDS

- AIDS stands for acquired immune deficiency syndrome.
- AIDS is also referred to as advanced HIV infection or late-stage HIV.
- AIDS is a set of symptoms and illnesses that develop as a result of advanced HIV infection which has destroyed the immune system.
- Treatment for HIV means that more people are staying well, with fewer people developing AIDS.

Although there is currently no cure for HIV, with the right treatment and support, people with HIV can live long and healthy lives. To do this, it is especially important to undergo treatment and deal with the possible side-effects. Before going into the HIV life cycle, we should know the structure of HIV. Here Figure 2 shows a virus structure.

Figure 2. Structure of HIV

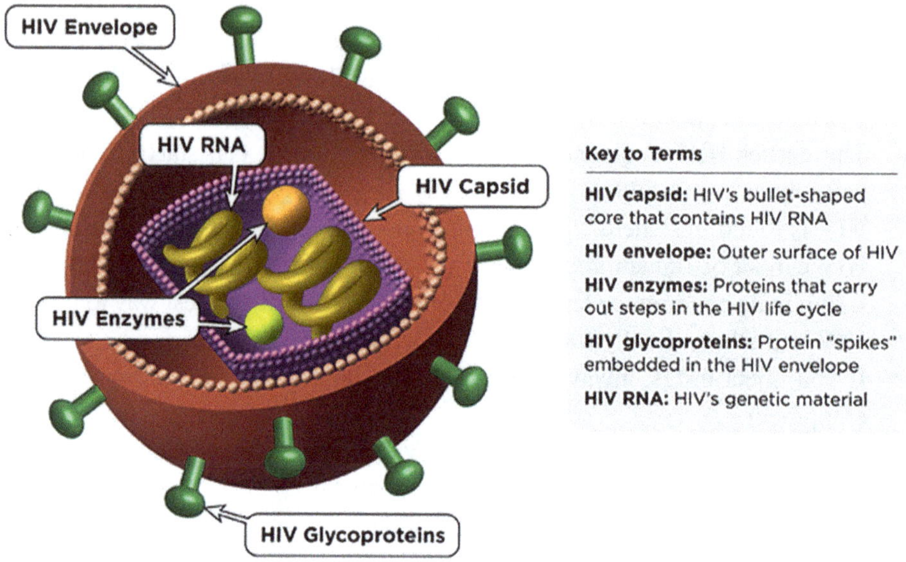

Figure 2 shows the structure of a HIV (Human Immunodeficiency Virus). The two dot marks inside the cell are HIV Enzymes which help the proteins to carry out the steps of the HIV lifecycle. Next comes HIV RNA, RNA means ribonucleic acid. It is an important molecule with long chains of nucleotides. A nucleotide contains a nitrogenous base, a ribose sugar, and a phosphate. Mostly RNA is a genetic material of HIV. HIV Capsid is the core of HIV which looks like bullet shaped and contains HIV RNA (Rutherford et al., 2016) and HIV Enzymes. HIV Envelope is the surface of HIV. HIV Glycoproteins are present at the surface of the HIV Envelope in spike shape. It plays an important role for the virus to get into the protein cell. First, it attaches itself to proteins on the surface of the cell. Then, it acts like a spring-loaded mousetrap and snaps into a new conformation that drags the virus and cell close enough that the membranes fuse. Finally, the HIV genome is released into the cell, where it quickly gets to work building new viruses.

Symptoms of AIDS

When it comes to the symptoms of AIDS, it's initially difficult to find a person affected with AIDS. But later on, there are some symptoms found in the human body which indicates that the person is affected with HIV, so below some common symptoms are given:

1. **Fever:** From a layman point of view, fever indicates the increase in body temperature due to any type of imbalance in health condition. Otherwise, fever is the initial response of a body to any type of infection. If one is infected with HIV, then he/she will experience flu-like symptoms sometime during the first four weeks, after being exposed to the virus. This is called a primary HIV infection. The range of fever can be anywhere from a mild fever to a fever of 102-degree F. Fever may also be accompanied by a sore throat, swollen lymph nodes, and nausea. When the virus moves deep into the bloodstream and starts to replicate, it disrupts the function of the immune system and cause an inflammatory reaction.
2. **Skin Rashes:** These come into figure either in the early or late stage of infection. Rashes of the eyes without any allergic reaction or drug overdose should put on an alert. They can appear in many colors: red, brown, pink, or purplish blotches on or under the skin, inside the mouth, nose, or eyelids. If the skin rash is prolonged, despite medication, then it's best to undergo an HIV test (Lu et al., 2016).
3. **Swollen Lymph Nodes:** Lymph Nodes are a part of immune system and can be affected first, in response to the inflammatory reaction of the immune system. Swollen lymph node can also indicate any other health degradation. But lingering swelling of lymph glands in the armpits, groin, or neck makes are indications that a doctor visit may be necessary.
4. **Prolonged Fatigue:** Extreme and inexplainable tiredness is a sign that indicates that there is something awry in the body. If a person gets affected by HIV, as it directly attacks the immune system of the body, then the person will feel lethargic and tired as it decreases the strength of human body.
5. **Muscle and Joint Pains:** Muscle and joint pain is another most prominent symptom for a person who get affected by HIV.
6. **Extreme Headache:** Like muscle and joint pain, headaches with fever can be a symptom for other diseases, but it cannot be neglected as it is a commonly found symptom of HIV infected people.
7. **Diarrhea:** If diarrhea continues for more than a week, then it becomes a matter of concern. Incessant diarrhea which doesn't stop, even after taking medication, could be a possible symptom of HIV infection (Sarac et al., 2016).
8. **Rapid and Unexplained Weight Loss:** Along with diarrhea, if rapid weight loss is marked, then it may be that the virus has already depleted the person's system to the maximum. If anyone is losing 10 percent of their body weight and experiences diarrhea and nausea, then it might not be good news for the person.

9. **Pneumonia:** If a person is suffering from cough, cold, weight loss, and diarrhea then it could mean that they have contracted a disease called pneumonia. If the person suffers from these symptoms for a long time, even with the medicine, then they should consult a doctor. Pneumonia is a very common occurrence for the people affected with HIV.
10. **Night Sweats:** There are some people who gets night sweats, which is not related to any temperature change or due to working out. This is also an unavoidable symptom of HIV.
11. **Fungal Infection:** A fungal infection can be identified through yellow, discolored, thickened, or brittle nails. This indicates a secondary infection after being infected with HIV. This infection can also be found as thrush in the mouth. If these symptoms are present, it could be an indication to test for HIV.
12. **Memory Loss or Depression:** This is mostly fond in the later stage of the illness, but it is an obvious sign to watch out for the infection.

Lifecycle of HIV

Lifecycle refers to the life of HIV: how it starts, spreads, and affects the human life. The HIV virus makes its target a type of white blood cell, called a T-helper cell (also called CD4 cell). These cells play an important role for having a healthy immune system as they help us to fight against diseases and infections. HIV cannot grow or reproduce on its own. Instead, it makes new copies of itself inside T-helper cells (Anelone et al., 2017). This damages the immune system and gradually weakens our natural defense. This process of infected T-helper cells multiplying is called the HIV lifecycle. Understanding the HIV lifecycle helps scientists to know how to attack the virus when it is weak and reduce its ability to multiply.

Stages of the Life Cycle

1. **Binding:** This is the initial phase of HIV/AIDS. In this phase, the virus tries to attach to the CD4(A protein present on the outside of infection- fighting white blood cells) receptor. HIV begins its lifecycle when it binds to a CD4 receptor and one of two co-receptors on the surface of a CD4+ T- lymphocyte.
2. **Fusion:** The virus then fuses with the host cell. After fusion, the virus releases RNA, its genetic material, into the host cell.
3. **Reverse Transcription:** An HIV enzyme called reverse transcript-pase converts the single strand HIV RNA to double-strand HIV DNA.

Figure 3. Life cycle of HIV

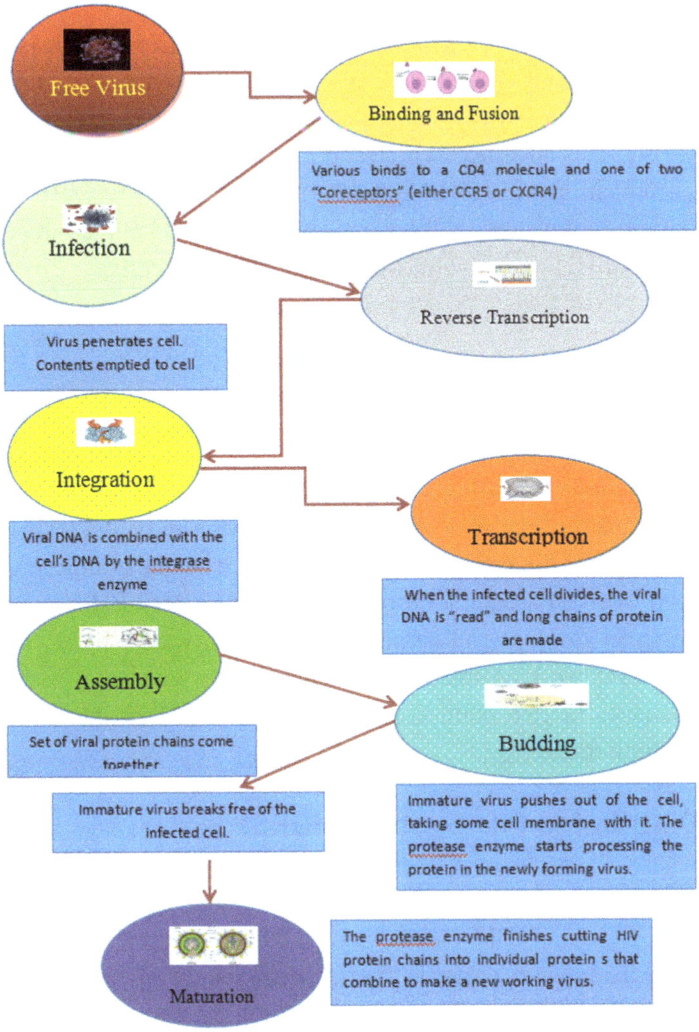

4. **Replication:** Once integrated into the CD4 cell DNA, HIV begins to use the machinery of CD4 cell to make long chains of HIV proteins. The protein chains are the building blocks for more HIV.
5. **Integration:** The newly formed HIV DNA enters the host cell's nucleus, where an HIV enzyme called integrase "hides" the HIV DNA within the host cell's own DNA. The integrated HIV DNA is called provirus. The provirus may remain inactive for several years, producing few or no new copies of HIV.

6. **Assembly:** An HIV enzyme called protease cuts the long chains of HIV proteins into smaller individual proteins. As the smaller HIV proteins come together with copies of HIV's RNA genetic material, a new virus particle is assembled.
7. **Budding:** The newly assembled virus pushes out ("buds") from the host cell. During budding, the new virus steals part of the cell's outer envelope (Young et al., 2014). This envelope, which acts as a covering, is studded with protein/ sugar combinations called HIV glycoproteins (Hotez et al., 2016). These HIV glycoproteins are necessary for the virus to bind CD4 and co- receptors. The new copies of HIV can now move on to infect other cells.

HADOOP

Hadoop is an important tool for Big Data Analytics. The origin of Hadoop came from the Google File System paper in 2003. Hadoop is a framework for storing large amount of data on clusters of commodity hardware and processing of that data (Hammer et al., 2008). A cluster is a group of interconnected computers (known as nodes) that can work on a common problem. The modules of Hadoop framework is designed with an assumption that any failure in hardware will be automatically handled by the framework (Almeida et al., 2016).

Hadoop consists of two main components: Hadoop Distributed File System (HDFS) and MapReduce.

Hadoop Distributed File System (HDFS)

Hadoop contains two main components: storage and processing. The Hadoop Distributed File System (HDFS) is the storage component. HDFS is a distributed, scalable, fault tolerant and portable file system written in Java for storing and managing huge amount of data. Hadoop creates multiple replicas of the work and distribute them among nodes (machine) in the cluster and HDFS stores the data that will be processed. It enables reliable and rapid access of the data. HDFS is a master-slave architecture in which master nodes are known as Namenode and slave nodes are known as Datanode. Namenode stores the name systems (directories and files) and manages the functioning of connected Datanodes (Uddin et al., 2014). To ensure high availability there also a secondary Namenode. The secondary Namenode is responsible for performing periodic checkpoints and keeps an up-to-date copy of the system in the memory. In the event of failure of the Namenode, checkpoints can be used to restart that Namenode. Datanode provide the actual data storage and it is where the processing is done. They are responsible for serving read and write requests of the client. Figure 4 represents the architecture of HDFS.

Figure 4. HDFS architecture

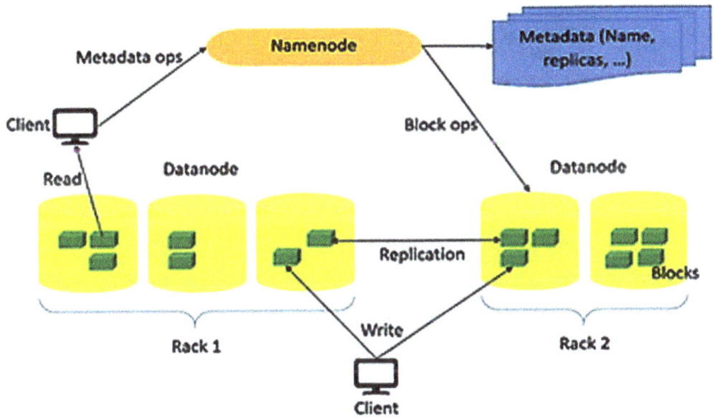

MAPREDUCE

MapReduce is a framework for performing distributed data processing using the MapReduce programming model. It is the processing component of Hadoop. The data consists of key-value pairs and computation (Oweis et al., 2015) involves two phases: the map phase and the reduce phase. The MapReduce has a single master service known as JobTracker and multiple slave services known as TaskTracker, one for each node in the cluster. JobTracker manages the job and resources and assignment of map and reduce tasks to TaskTracker. The TaskTracker is responsible for running the map and reduce tasks.

With Hadoop 2, there is an additional component known as YARN. The YARN (Yet Another Resource Manager) is a tool that enables other data processing frameworks to run on Hadoop. It provides scheduling and assignment of CPU cycles and memory to waiting applications in the Hadoop cluster. It also provides general-purpose resource management facility.

Figure 5 represents a simple example of how MapReduce works. MapReduce consists of two basic steps: a map step and a reduce step. Map step takes input tasks and splits them into smaller sub-tasks. It then performs some required operations on each sub-task and gives some intermediate outputs. Reduce step combines the intermediate outputs from the map step and gives final output. Each input and output is represented as <key, value> pair. The simple way to tell if MapReduce is working is to have it complete a word count task, which counts the number of times each word is present in a given input. As shown in the figure, the map step first splits the given input into smaller sub-tasks. Then it maps each sub-task as set of key-values in the form of <word, 1>. After that, the reduce step shuffles the <key, value> pair with same key. It then merges the pair and displays them as: <key, count>, where count is the sum of each 1 value of a key (word).

Figure 5. Example of working of MapReduce

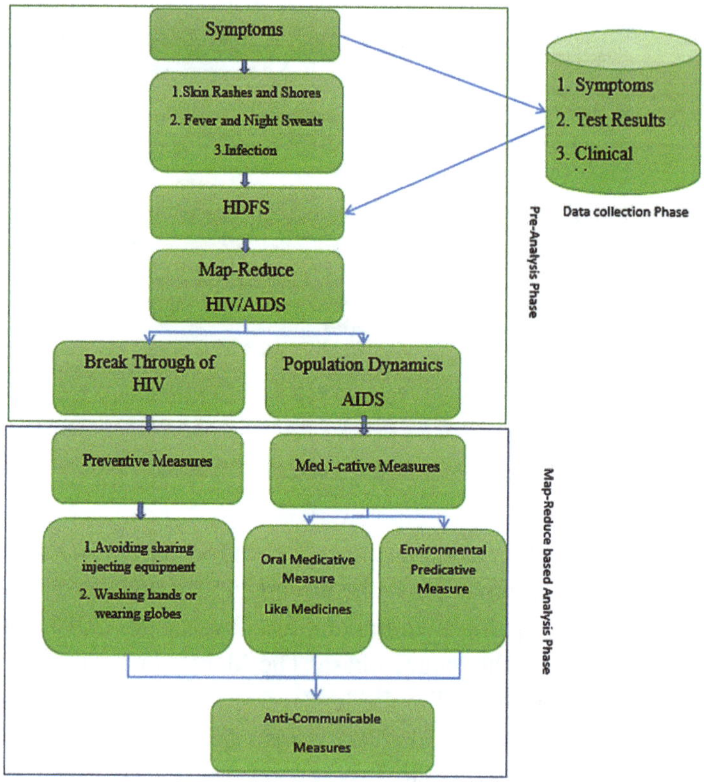

POPULATION DYNAMICS

Population dynamics is the study of any type of change in size or structure of population depending on the time. The main factors that affect population dynamics are rates of reproduction, death, and migration. As the world and technology are changing, more efficient and accurate results are needed. Big data is very useful for this because it stores and processes the data for the results that we need. Population also varies according to geographic region (e.g. there is less of a population in forests and hills in comparison to other, more urban areas). Cause of infectious disease varies with population depending on the atmosphere. Population dynamics is the study of life science, which deals with the study of changes in population with time (Radhi et al., 2016). If, in a location, a harmful disease is seen, then automatically the population of that area gets affected. For instance, Dengue fever is a very harmful disease which has a bad effect on the population. Dengue fever is mostly seen in the foresty areas where a large number of trees are present. Additionally, dengue mosquitoes are seen the most in areas where water is stored without proper care.

STATE OF THE ART

Nowadays, HIV is a serious public health problem in many communities. Till now, various research studies have been done on HIV. A supervised model has been developed to the help the literature screening of HIV. In this chapter, the author has explained that it becomes difficult for the researchers to get the accurate and most up-to-date results from the literature collected from different sources. So, for better utilization they have used the logistic tree classifier model. As a result, the system correctly labels the great majority of relevant documents, which becomes useful for the researchers to assess a greater number of documents in less time (Ray et al., 2016). This helps to improve the quality of service for HIV infection. An experiment has been conducted with Gold nano-particles and a mixture of normal salt(NaCl) and water. And according to the changes in wavelength, it is concluded that infected by HIV or not, the wavelength is measured by the change in color of the mixture. A framework has been developed for the analysis of micro-array data of three different stages of HIV-1 infection and identifies modules among co-expressed genes. The Modules are divided into three stages, then a module engine (ME) network is compiled inside the network among the modules which helps to describe the relationship between different modules (Koçak et al., 2016). Then, the relationship between gene co-expression modules is explored by comparing the ME networks between each pair of stages. This model indicates a new direction in better understanding the modular organization and preservation patterns of micro-array expression data through the different stages of HIV infection. There are various models designed for the prevention of HIV (Chang et al., 2016). Similarly, there is a model proposed, which mainly relates to the data collected from social media platforms regarding HIV. This method gives the required results in comparison to the existing machine learning methods; with this it also opens up an opportunity to validate the results obtained by using other techniques from social network analysis. A mathematical model is proposed for the analysis of eradicating viruses during the early stages of infection. With this model, they also used numerical simulation for a better result. In case of HIV infected person, drug resistance becomes a challenge for the doctor to treat the patient. It happens due to the mutation of proteins or due to the changes in gene expression level (DeRoos et al., 2014). So, this study combines both sequence and structural features for predicting HIV resistance by applying SVM and Random Forests classifiers. There are some methodologies that integrate multiple facets of biological information to identify human gene module during different stages of the HIV-1 infection. To integrate modules of different data sources into strong meta-modules, NMF based clustering is utilized. They have analyzed to show the change of co-regulation pattern of identified transcription factors (TFs) over the HIV progression stages (Rutherford et al., 2016). Nucleic acid amplification tests (NAATs) provide high diagnostic accuracy of infectious diseases, the author has described NAATs as the combination of sample preparation and amplification using isotachophoresis and recombinase polymerase amplification. And according to them this approach has the potential to reduce the cost and complexity of point-of-care (POC) NAATs (Lu et al., 2016). A strategy has been explored which helps in epidemic control through simulation. It reduces syringe sharing during injection drug use, reduced time to diagnosis, reduced time to initiation of treatment following diagnosis, and improved retention in treatment (Sarac et al., 2016). As everyone knows, nowadays drug resistance becomes a major issue in the case of many diseases, so there is some invention which combines two different drugs and result a single drug, which is more effective in comparison to the previously used drug. There are some theoretical supports of combination drug therapy for AIDS from the point of view of the dynamics theory (Anelone et al., 2017). As the disease is spreading rapidly, the number of patient is increasing, which increases the data size. Data reduction techniques are used to reduce the complexity of data and also to enhance generalization performance. An instance selection framework has been proposed, which identifies relevant and important data as a result. In this framework, the whole data-set is divided into very small chunks. Then each chunk is considered as the sample data. In this case, the most relevant and important instances of data would come up and samples would be selected before new chunk of data arrives (Young et al., 2014). So, this framework not only reduces the size of the data-set but it also helps in reducing the cost. A model of HIV infection together with an associated reach-ability analysis is used to formulate a dynamical condition for the containment of HIV infection on the manifold. Using the parameter estimates and the numerical solutions of the model, the predictions of the reachability analysis are shown to be consistent with the clinical diagnosis at the conclusion of the trial. The methodology captures the dynamical characteristics of eventual, successful, failed, and marginal outcomes. The evidence shows that the reachability analysis is an appropriate tool to monitor and develop personalized antiretroviral treatment (Patel et al., 2012).

Analytic Measure Model Based on HIV Symptoms

Here in Figure 6, a mechanism is proposed for the better prevention of HIV. In the initial stage we collect various symptoms from various resources. The information can be collected from hospitals, people's feedback, social media, or search engines, i.e. from whichever place has more searching capabilities according to experiences with HIV and the people that it affects. In the next step, the data that is collected is stored inside the HDFS (Hadoop Distributed File System). As here the data stored into small files (Young et al., 2014). Now Map-Reduce technique is used to manipulate/analyze the data. Below we have taken an example of map-reduce frame work.

Figure 6. Analytic measures

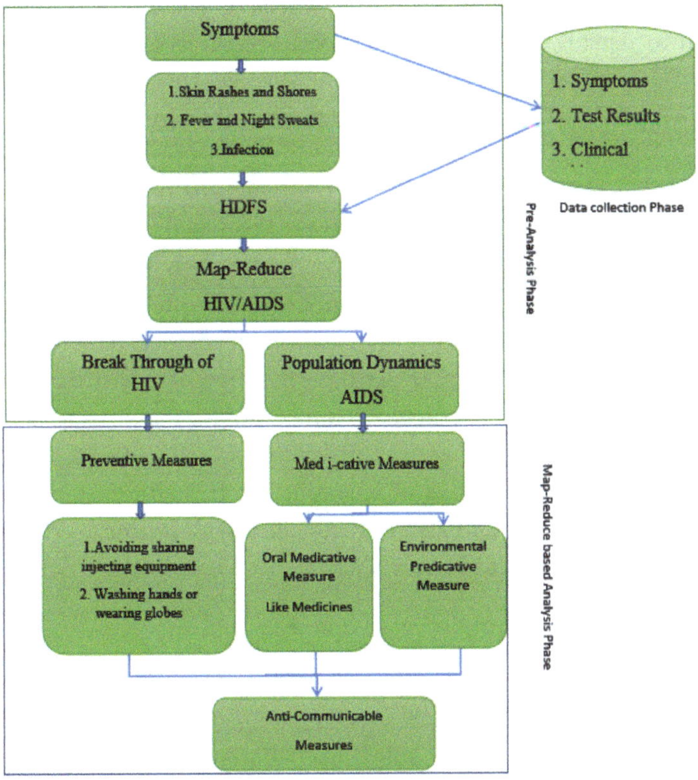

Data can be provided to the system using tools for cleansing, abstraction, and logical storage for successful mining in the further steps (Ray et al., 2016). It's become a difficult task for databases to manipulate such a large volume of data, which comes in with high velocity. So, Hadoop come into the figure, for efficient manipulation of data-set. Hadoop has two main components are HDFS and Map-Reduce. This paper use Map-Reduce methodology to save data in a globally classified manner according to the population dynamics.

In breakthrough stage of HIV, it indicates the spreading of HIV from one person to another person in the population. That may be due to

- Blood
- Semen and pre-seminal fluid ("pre-cum")
- Rectal fluids/anal mucous
- Vaginal fluids
- Breast milk.

So, it can be said that HIV spreads when the infected blood from one person transfers to the body of a person who is not infected. The blood can be transferred from person to person due to untested blood donations or untested blood for a transfusion. HIV can even spread through the syringes, needle etc. When injecting equipment is used in a sharing mode, the transfer of the virus becomes more likely. Mostly, when more than one person uses a single injecting tool, they are putting themselves in danger. If a person has sexual relations with more than one person and is also not using any type of protection, that also can lead to them getting infected by the virus. If a mother is affected by HIV, then there is a 100% chance that her child will be affected by HIV if she does not take any precautions (Khalid et al., 2016). At the time when the child is in the womb of mother, the blood droplets of the mother get attached to the child. Also, at the time of breast feeding, the milk that comes out from the mother can act as a medium for the virus to be transferred from mother to baby.

Now everyone knows the ways of spreading of HIV, the result as to how the person can suffer from HIV, and also how life ends with the Virus. So, in this case we can take some preventive measures. There are some points which can help anyone to get prevented from HIV:

- Use of condom every time vaginal, anal, or oral sex occurs.
- Sharing of needles, syringes and other injecting equipment should be avoided.
- If women is expecting a baby and is also affected from HIV, then she should undergo HIV treatment as per the doctor's advice. Because reduce the risk of passing HIV to baby during pregnancy, childbirth and breastfeeding.
- Always take the concern of a health-care professional before receiving the blood product that, the blood has been tested for HIV.
- Precautions should be taken by health-care worker, such as protection should be used like gloves and goggles, hands should be washed properly after coming into contact with blood and other bodily fluids, and the sharp equipment should be disposed safely.

Now coming to population dynamics, it indicates the change in population due to some artificial reason or due to some natural calamities. Here, it is taken into consideration, like in a particular population, how many people gets affected through the virus. Even an idea can be get that in which age the people gets more affected by the virus (Chang et al., 2016). Similarly, if it takes a particular area into consideration, then we can get a better idea as to what types of people make up that population. As it is considered, most of the patients infected by HIV are between 20 and 50 years old. Similarly, if an area is taken into consideration, then those who have less awareness about the disease may become most affected by the infection.

It can be said that initially it is HIV, but after the virus get into the human body, it starts replicating itself, which weakens the immune system. So as a result, the immune system cannot fight against small diseases.

Normally three types of measures come into figure: oral medicative, environmental predicative, and operational predicative. But till now, there aren't any operational measures that can be taken, so it tends to be left out. But, if we consider oral medicative measures then, there are several medicines. There are five major types of medicines:

- **Reverse Transcriptase (RT) Inhibitors:** Interfere with a critical step during the HIV life cycle and keep the virus from making copies of itself
- **Protease Inhibitors:** Interfere with a protein that HIV uses to make infectious viral particles
- **Fusion Inhibitors:** Block the virus from entering the body's cells
- **Integrase Inhibitors:** Block an enzyme HIV needs to make copies of itself
- **Multidrug Combinations:** Combine two or more different types of drugs into one

These medicines help people with HIV, but they are not perfect. They do not cure HIV/AIDS. People with HIV infections still have the virus in their bodies. They can still spread HIV to others through unprotected sex and needle sharing, even when they are taking their medicines. But anti-communicable measures are for all people that may or may not be affected by the virus. As with antidotes, the anti-communicable preventives should be taken by every person so that they can escape from life-threatening diseases like AIDS (Koçak et al., 2016).

As shown in the Figure 6, environmental predicative measures include many environmental factors: among them are poverty and cultural aspects (including religion and traditions), which appear to play an essential role in the rapid and global development of the AIDS epidemic. Let's consider poverty. In this case, as the people are suffering from poverty, they do not have much money or the ability spend it on treatments for disease. For example, they might use a single needle or syringe for several people. Similarly, when the cultural aspect comes into figure. In some cultures, it might be okay for a male to have more than one wife. There are so many other types of cultures that have traditions or practices that could contribute to the epidemic as well. When all these predicative measures and preventive measures are combined, they are known as anti-communicable measures.

The proposed implementation is done using some of the current existing tools and techniques of big data analysis, such as Hadoop and Map-Reduce. As the infection increases day by day, more cases of HIV are coming into figure (Ray et al., 2016). So, the data set is also increasing rapidly, so it becomes difficult for the traditional database to handle the volume of new data.

Hadoop consists of two main components that are storage and processing. The storage part deals with HDFS, Hadoop Distributed File System. HDFS leverages large blocks of data and moves the computation where data is stored. A file can be replicated several times. HDFS breaks the larger files into smaller blocks of data and stores them in a cluster. The processing part is done by the Map-Reduce framework. Map-Reduce programming helps to process massive amount of data in parallel in an efficient manner.

Now it is time to discuss the application of big data in healthcare. Here, in every step, big data is used; initially the data is collected from various resources and then all the data, regardless of its size, is stored in the storage part of Big data (i.e. HDFS). Here, the data is stored in a file format regardless of its size and structure (Structured, Semi structured or Unstructured) (Almeida et al., 2016). Then after the storage phase, it is time for the manipulation phase. For this, the data Map-Reduce framework is used. In map reduce, the data is segregated into small parts and then, by applying some conditions, we extract the information according to our need.

Map-Reduce works in two phases: mapping phase and reducing phase. By using the Map-Reduce program, a count for the number of people who are affected by dengue fever (according to population dynamics) can be completed. In Map-Reduce, the data set is divided into small chunks, then those chunks are mapped by the mapper function in a parallel manner (DeRoos et al., 2014). The output of the mappers is automatically shuffled and stored by the framework. The output is sorted based on key elements (i.e. dengue). Here, the full data set is considered. Figure 7 provides an example of Map-Reduce to better understanding its working process. In this, one file is taken into consideration, which belongs to a particular area. There are two results affected and not affected, affected means that a person is affected by HIV and not-affected means that person is not affected by HIV. According to the result it can be decided that there is the need for preventive measures, oral medicative measures, or environmental predicative measures.

Figure 7. Example of Map-Reduce

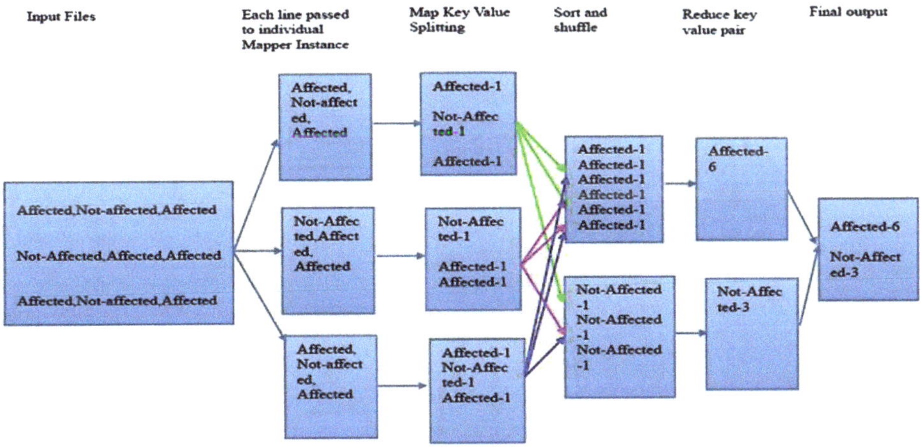

SOME MATHEMATICAL NOTATIONS FOR PREVENTION

Pre-Analysis Phase

S→ Set of symptoms of HIV
F→ Fever
D→ Diarrhea
SR→ Skin Rashes
PF→ Prolonged Fatigue
MP→ Muscle Pain
EH → Extreme headache
NS→ Night Sweats
FI→ Fungal Infection
ML→ Memory Loss
S={F, D, SR, PF, MP, EH, NS, FI, ML}
P→ Set of Population
P={P1, P2, P3…..Pn}
P← Anti-communicable Measure // The Anti-communicable measure should be provided to the total population irrespective of affected or not affected by HIV
X→ Set of instances of different populations

```
X={X1, X2,X3.......Xn}  // X1 indicates set of people of a
particular population i.e P1
X1={x1, x2,x3......xn}   // x1, x2.... xn are n Number of peoples of
X1 set.
∀X ∈ P
P ∈ S
N→ Set of nodes
N={N1, N2, N3..........Nn}          // Set of data nodes
X1, P1→ N1
X2, P2→N2
X3, P3→N3
:          :          :
:          :          :
Xn, Pn→Nn     //Here the data of each population are stored in
different nodes.
```

Map-Reduce Based Analysis Phase

By using reduce phase, the total number of people with whom the symbols found will be calculated..

Then the percentage of people affected will be calculated by considering the outcome of reduce phase and the total population.

Now for populationp1:

$$\%\ of\ people\ affected = \frac{Number\ of\ people\ with\ symptoms}{Total\ number\ of\ people\ in\ p1} \times 100$$

Similarly, % will be calculated for every population.

If 0-30% → Preventive Measure
30-60% → Oral Meditative Measure
>60% → Oral Medicative and Environmental Predicative Measures
0-100% → Anti Communicable Measures // Every person should get the anti-communicable measure.

CONCLUSION

For various kinds of research work, healthcare becomes an enormous platform for the researchers. There are many studies going on that may be for the prediction of disease, prevention of disease, providing better treatment for disease, or enhance of technology so that society can better fight the disease and model a disease free society. As described above, the analytic measure models can be used by the health welfare organization to save lives from HIV on the basis the people are educated about the common signs and symptoms. Based on the result, the preventive measures will be provided. Till now, there is no operative measure found in the case of HIV, but yes there are some medicines found as a result of medicative measure, which helps the infected person to live for a longer period of time. It can also help people who are not affected by HIV from getting the infection (Patel et al., 2012). So, as the population is increasing very rapidly, big data plays a very important role in the storing large volumes of data to get better results, which will become very useful to society. The same mechanism can be used for the diagnosis of other diseases that may be infectious or may help to protect human-life. There are so many animals that are extinct, or so endangered that they'll soon only live in books and on the internet. As such, this model can be utilized for the protection of wildlife.

REFERENCES

Almeida, H., Meurs, M. J., Kosseim, L., & Tsang, A. (2016). Data sampling and supervised learning for hiv literature screening. *IEEE Transactions on Nanobioscience*, *15*(4), 354–361. doi:10.1109/TNB.2016.2565481 PMID:28113721

Anelone, A. J., & Spurgeon, S. K. (2017). Prediction of the containment of HIV infection by antiretroviral therapy–a variable structure control approach. *IET Systems Biology*, *11*(1), 44–53. doi:10.1049/iet-syb.2016.0028 PMID:28303793

Barreiro-Gomez, J., Quijano, N., & Ocampo-Martínez, C. (2015, October). Distributed resource management by using population dynamics: Wastewater treatment application. In *Automatic Control (CCAC), 2015 IEEE 2nd Colombian Conference on* (pp. 1-6). IEEE.

Borysiak, M. D., Bender, A. T., Boyle, D. S., & Posner, J. D. (2016, November). Point-of-care HIV-1 diagnostic with integrated nucleic acid extraction and amplification from whole blood. In *Healthcare Innovation Point-Of-Care Technologies Conference (HI-POCT)*, 2016 *IEEE* (pp. 74-77). IEEE. doi:10.1109/HIC.2016.7797737

Chang, H., Moog, C., & Astolfi, A. (2016). Occurrence of HIV eradication for preexposure prophylaxis treatment with a deterministic HIV model. *IET Systems Biology*, *10*(6), 137–243. doi:10.1049/iet-syb.2016.0008 PMID:27879478

DeRoos, D., Zikopoulos, P., Brown, B., Coss, R., & Melnyk, R. B. (2014). *Hadoop for Dummies*. John Wiley & Sons, Incorporated.

Hammer, S. M., Eron, J. J., Reiss, P., Schooley, R. T., Thompson, M. A., Walmsley, S., ... Jacobsen, D. M. (2008). Antiretroviral treatment of adult HIV infection: 2008 recommendations of the International AIDS Society–USA panel. *Journal of the American Medical Association*, *300*(5), 555–570. doi:10.1001/jama.300.5.555 PMID:18677028

Hotez, P. J., Molyneux, D. H., Fenwick, A., Ottesen, E., Sachs, S. E., & Sachs, J. D. (2006). Incorporating a rapid-impact package for neglected tropical diseases with programs for HIV/AIDS, tuberculosis, and malaria. *PLoS Medicine*, *3*(5), e102. doi:10.1371/journal.pmed.0030102 PMID:16435908

Khalid, Z., & Sezerman, O. U. (2016). Prediction of HIV Drug Resistance by combining Sequence and Structural Properties. *IEEE/ACM Transactions on Computational Biology and Bioinformatics*, 1. doi:10.1109/TCBB.2016.2638821 PMID:27992346

Koçak, Y., Özyer, T., & Alhajj, R. (2016, August). Classification of HIV data by constructing a social network with frequent itemsets. In *Advances in Social Networks Analysis and Mining (ASONAM), 2016 IEEE/ACM International Conference on* (pp. 949-953). IEEE. doi:10.1109/ASONAM.2016.7752354

Lu, X., Liu, Y., Jiao, J., & Wang, R. (2016, December). Dynamic evolutions of HIV infection on treatment with combinatorial drugs. In *Bioinformatics and Biomedicine (BIBM), 2016 IEEE International Conference on* (pp. 1856-1863). IEEE.

Oweis, N. E., Owais, S. S., George, W., Suliman, M. G., & Snášel, V. (2015). A survey on big data, mining:(tools, techniques, applications and notable uses). In *Intelligent Data Analysis and Applications* (pp. 109–119). Cham: Springer. doi:10.1007/978-3-319-21206-7_10

Patel, A. B., Birla, M., & Nair, U. (2012, December). Addressing big data problem using Hadoop and Map Reduce. In *Engineering (NUiCONE), 2012 Nirma University International Conference on* (pp. 1-5). IEEE. doi:10.1109/NUICONE.2012.6493198

Radhi, M. S., Ruslinda, A. R., Fatin, M. F., Hashwan, S. S. B., Arshad, M. M., & Hashim, U. (2016, August). Colorimetric assay of HIV-1 Tat protein and peptide. In *Semiconductor Electronics (ICSE), 2016 IEEE International Conference on*(pp. 200-203). IEEE. doi:10.1109/SMELEC.2016.7573626

Ray, S., Hossain, S. M. M., & Khatun, L. (2016, September). Discovering preservation pattern from co-expression modules in progression of HIV-1 disease: An eigengene based approach. In *Advances in Computing, Communications and Informatics (ICACCI), 2016 International Conference on* (pp. 814-820). IEEE.

Ray, S., & Maulik, U. (2016). Discovering perturbation of modular structure in HIV progression by integrating multiple data sources through non-negative matrix factorization. *IEEE/ACM Transactions on Computational Biology and Bioinformatics*, 1. doi:10.1109/TCBB.2016.2642184 PMID:28029629

Rutherford, A. R., Ramadanović, B., Michelow, W., Marshall, B. D., Small, W., Deering, K., ... Vasaihexyi, K. (2016, December). Control of an HIV epidemic among injection drug users: simulation modeling on complex networks. In *Winter Simulation Conference (WSC)*, 2016 (pp. 13-37). IEEE. doi:10.1109/WSC.2016.7822077

Sarac, F., & Seker, H. (2016, October). An instance selection framework for mining data streams to predict antibody-feature function relationships on RV144 HIV vaccine recipients. In *Systems, Man, and Cybernetics (SMC), 2016 IEEE International Conference on* (pp. 003356-003361). IEEE. doi:10.1109/SMC.2016.7844752

Toshniwal, R., Dastidar, K. G., &Nath, A. (2015). Big Data Security Issues and Challenges. *International Journal of Innovative Research in Advanced Engineering*, (2).

Uddin, M. F., & Gupta, N. (2014, April). Seven V's of Big Data understanding Big Data to extract value. In American Society for Engineering Education (ASEE Zone 1), 2014 Zone 1 Conference of the (pp. 1-5). IEEE.

Young, S. D., Rivers, C., & Lewis, B. (2014). Methods of using real-time social media technologies for detection and remote monitoring of HIV outcomes. *Preventive Medicine*, *63*, 112–115. doi:10.1016/j.ypmed.2014.01.024 PMID:24513169

Chapter 4
Computational and Data Mining Perspectives on HIV/AIDS in Big Data Era:
Opportunities, Challenges, and Future Directions

Ali Al Mazari
Alfaisal University, Saudi Arabia

ABSTRACT

HIV/AIDS big data analytics evolved as a potential initiative enabling the connection between three major scientific disciplines: (1) the HIV biology emergence and evolution; (2) the clinical and medical complex problems and practices associated with the infections and diseases; and (3) the computational methods for the mining of HIV/AIDS biological, medical, and clinical big data. This chapter provides a review on the computational and data mining perspectives on HIV/AIDS in big data era. The chapter focuses on the research opportunities in this domain, identifies the challenges facing the development of big data analytics in HIV/AIDS domain, and then highlights the future research directions of big data in the healthcare sector.

DOI: 10.4018/978-1-5225-3203-3.ch004

INTRODUCTION

Recent quick raise within digital data's generation as well as the quick development concerns computational science permit us extracting recent insights from the massive sets of data, recognized as huge data, within a variety of disciplines, involving internet finance and business (Lee & Yoon, 2017; Lane et al., 2014).In the area of healthcare, discovering recent actionable insights has not been recognized widespread, even though many success achievement stories are mostly published in the academic journals and media (Edmunds et al., 2014). This postponed development of the big data technology in the sector of healthcare is unusual, taken into account a previous prediction, which is the big data technology's application that was predictable. In addition, the sector of health care could be one of the most important sectors predicted to be profited the most from the technology of big data (Murdoch & Detsky, 2013).

The growing gap among outcomes and healthcare costs is recognized as one of the most significant issues and there are many efforts under way in order to fill this gap within several developed countries (Savel & Foldy, 2012). It is demonstrated that the gap among outcomes and healthcare costs was analyzed in order to consider the poor management's result of insights from the research. The poor use of obtainable evidence, in addition to the poor imprison of care experience, each of which contributes to lead to wasted resources, missed chances in addition to possible harm to the patients (Curry, 2005). It has been proposed that the gap could be defeated through the improvement of a "continuous learning healthcare system" since an honorable cycle is shaped among the research as well as the healthcare's arms, and data could be utilized successfully (Rumsfeld, Joynt & Maddox, 2016). Consequently, an imperative demand to enhance patient outcomes and healthcare quality, developing the availability of data in addition to improving analytic capabilities are the big data era's drivers of healthcare (Rumsfeld, Joynt & Maddox, 2016; Groves et al., 2016). There are several challenges to defeat before the technology of big data has the ability to considerably enhance healthcare outcomes, quality and healthcare.

THE ERA OF BIG DATA IN THE DOMAIN OF HEALTHCARE AND MEDICINE

The Concept of Big Data

The "Big Data" term was first initiated into the computing world through Roger Magoulas from the publication of O'Reilly in 2005 to identify a huge amount of data, which the techniques of conventional data management cannot process and process because of the size and complexity of this data (Ularu et al., 2012; Chaorasiya &

Shrivastava, 2015). A conducted study on the development of Big Data as a Scientific Topic and Research indicates that the "Big Data" term was offered in the starting of research with1970s; however, has been encompassed within the publications in 2008 (Halevi & Moed, 2012; Sharma, Joshi &Manisha, 2015).

Each day, we generate 2.5 quintillion bytes of data — so much that ninety percent of the data within the world nowadays has been generated in the most recent two years only. This data arrives from each place: sensors utilized to collect climate information, place to the site of social media, videos and digital pictures, phone GPS signals in order to name a few and purchase transaction records (Mukherjee & Shaw, 2016; Jewell et al., 2014). Such massive amount of data which is being formed incessantly is what has the ability to coin as Big Data (Mukherjee & Shaw, 2016).

The decodes of Big Data formerly undamaged data in order to obtain recent insight that is incorporated into the operations of business. Nonetheless, because the amounts of data develop exponential, the recent methods are becoming outdated. Dealing with Big Data entails widespread skills of coding, statistics and domain knowledge. In spite of being Herculean within nature, the applications of Big Data are approximately ubiquitous- from the research of marketing into the scientific research to the interests of customer and so on. We have the ability to witness Big Data within action approximately every place these days (Sabia & Kalra, 2014; Kaisler et al., 2013).

In excess of a year ago, the World Bank prepared the first Innovation Challenge of WBG Big Data that promote many distinctive ideas concerning Big Data like big data in order to expect poverty as well as for climate smart agriculture and for user concentrated Identification of Road Infrastructure Condition in addition to safety and so on (Big Data Solutions, 2017). Big Data has the ability to be merely identified through the volume of 3V, variety and velocity that are considered the driving dimensions of the quantification of Big Data. Gartner analyst, Doug Laney set up the famous concept of 3 V in his 2001 Metagroup publication, Controlling the management of 3D data Controlling Velocity, Variety and Data Volume (Mukherjee & Shaw, 2016).

The following is demonstration for the 3V's of Big Data (Mukherjee & Shaw, 2016):

1. **Volume:** This fundamentally distresses huge quantities of data, which is created constantly. Originally, such data was considered problematic due to the high costs of storage. Nonetheless, with the developing costs of storage, this challenge has been reserved to some extent at bay as of now. Nevertheless, this is just a momentary solution, as well as better technology requires to be improved. Social networking websites, E-Commerce and Smartphones are recognized as examples wherever huge amounts of data are being created. This data has

Figure 1. Schematic representation of the 3V's of Big Data
Mukherjee & Shaw, 2016.

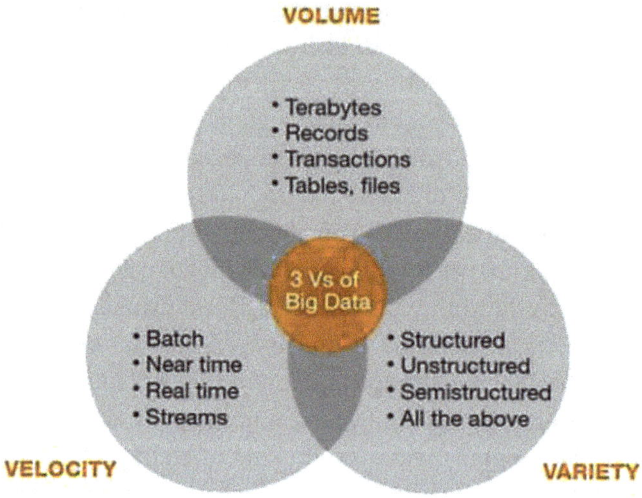

the ability to be effortlessly made differences between semi-structured data, unstructured data and structured data.

2. **Velocity:** In what recently appear like the pre-historic times, data was mostly procedure within the batches. nevertheless, this method is just possible while the rate of incoming data is slower comparing with the rate of batch processing as well as the postponed is much of an obstruction. at current days, at current days, the speed at which such massive amounts of data are being created is incredibly high. Take Facebook for instance- it creates2.7 billion like actions for every day as well as three hundreds photos among the others approximately amounting to 2.5 million pieces of content for each day at the same time as Google Now procedures over 1.2 trillion searches for every year around all over the world
3. **Variety:** Databases' Documents to excel tables to pictures and videos and audios in several formats, recently data are strongly losing structure. Structure does not have the ability to be compulsory like before data analysis. The generated data has the ability to be one of any kind- unstructured, semi-structured and structures. The traditional shape of data is known as structured data. for instance, text that is Unstructured data has the ability to be created from satellites, sensors and social networking sites.

Big Data has the ability to be depicted utilizing the model of 5Vs, which is demonstrated in the Figure 2 (Lomotey & Deters, 2014).

Figure 2. The model of 5V that presently identifies Big Data
Lomotey & Deters, 2014.

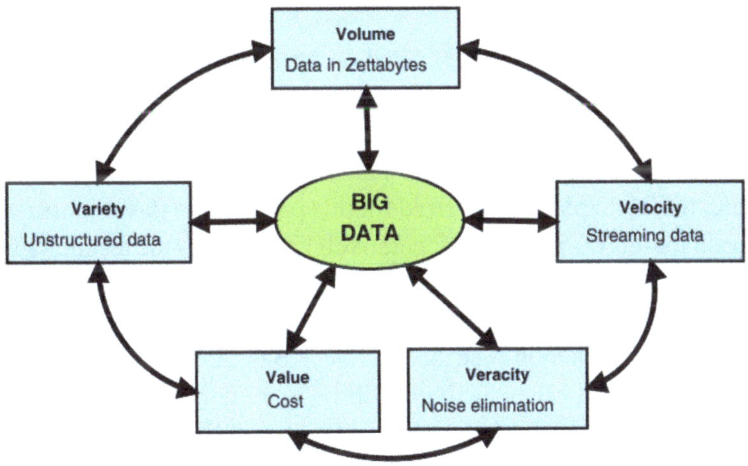

This model is an extension of the previously defined 3V model in (Laney, 2001), and involves:

1. Volume (the size's era) with the collection and generation of data masses, the scale of data becomes progressively big. The data fashioned these days is for zetta bytes order, as well as it is increasing around forty- percent for each year (Fan & Bifet, 2013).
2. Velocity (the streaming data era) indicates to the timeliness of Big Data, particularly, data analysis and collection and has to be timely and rapidly carried out, so to increase the usage of the commercial value concerns Big Data.
3. Variety (the unstructured data era) demonstrates the different kinds of data that involve unstructured and semi-structured data like text, webpage, video and audio in addition to the conventional structured data.
4. Value (the cost associated with data era) whilst the data are greatly being analyzed, collected and generated from various quarters, it is significant to demonstrate that the data of today have a number of costs. The data itself has the ability to be a "commodity" that has the ability to be sold to the third parties for proceeds. In addition, being familiar with the value or cost of the data has the ability to help in the processes of decision making concerns budget at evaluating the data storage cost.
5. Veracity (the era of data pollution, which requires cleansing) there is a great demand to ensure data's accuracy through eradicating the noise depending on the methodologies like data sanitization and pedigree. This is to make sure

about the quality of data, consequently that the decisions, which are made from the gathered data, are effective and accurate.

Implementing Big Data is recognized as an enormous task granted to large variety, velocity and volume. Big Data is known as a term surrounding the usage of method to visualize, analyze, process and process potentially huge datasets within a sensible timeframe not available to the standard technologies of IT. By expansion, the software, tools and platform utilized for this purpose are the platform, tools and software used for this purpose are cooperatively called —— the technologies of Big Data (Erdman, Keefe & Schiestl, 2013). Presently, the most normally implemented technology is Hadoop. Hadoop is defined as the conclusion of many other technologies such as the systems of Hadoop Distribution File, HBase, Pig, Hive, Etc. Nonetheless, even Hadoop as well as other methods will be extremely unable to deal with the difficulties of Big Data in the future (Lin & Ryaboy, 2013; Zicari, 2014).

Big Data Analytics' Concept

Today, the world is constructed on the base of data. The lives of these days are influenced through the ability of corporations to manage, interrogate and dispose data. The development of the infrastructure of technology for the purpose of help to create data, consequently, each of the provided service has the ability to be enhanced as they are utilized (Mitchell & Wilson, 2012). As an instance, internet these days became an enormous information-collecting platform because of online services and social media. At any time they could add data. Data explosion could not be measured in gigabytes; because data is superior; they are utilized Yottabytes (YB), Zettabytes (ZB), Exabytes (EB) and Petabytes (PB). For managing stored unstructured data's giant volume, it has been emerged the phenomena of "Big Data" (Forsyth, 2012; Stone, 2014).

It relates to the reason that the Big-Data of commercial sector had been adopted quickly in the industries of data driven such as telecommunications and financial service that could be discussed, have been experiencing a more speedy development in the volumes of data comparing to the sectors of other market, falling profitability and tighter regulatory requirements. Firstly, "Big Data" was recognized as a method to reduce and manage data management' costs. At the present, the corporations concentrate on the creation potential of value. To get benefit from further insight gained, there is a demand to evaluate execution and analytical capabilities of "Big Data" (Ventura et al., 2015; Ularu et al., 2012).

Up till the mid of 2009, the landscape of data management was simple: the systems of Online transaction processing (OLTP) (particularly databases) hold up the business processes of the company; operational data stores (ODSs) gathered the transactions of business to hold up operational reporting, as well as company data warehouses (EDWs) gathered and transformed the transactions of business in order to support both strategic and operational decision making. The Management of Big Data is mostly depended on organizing and capturing related data. Data analytics presume to be familiar that occurred, why and expect what will occur. A deeper analytics indicates recent analytical means for deeper insights (Forsyth, 2012).

The Apache Hadoop open source project and big data analytics are speedily appearing as the favored resolution to the trends of technology and business, which are unsettling the conventional processing landscape and data management. Companies have the ability to get a competitive advantage through being untimely adopters for the analytics of big data. Although big data analytics have the ability to be theoretically transforming, companies are not supposed to postpone implementation. Since mature and business intelligence (BI) tool and the Hadoop projects, the complexity of big data analytics implementation will greatly reduce; nevertheless, the untimely adopter competitive advantage will wane. The risk of Technology implementation has the ability to be lessened through adapting the existing architectural patterns and principles to the changing requirements and new technology more willingly than rejecting those (Brown et al., 2011).

Big data analytics have the ability to be distinguished from the conventional architectures of data processing through several dimensions and they are as the following (Forsyth, 2012; Russom, 2011):

- Decision making's Speed being very significant for the makers of decision
- The complexity of Processing since it makes the process of decision making very easy
- The volumes of Transactional data that are very huge
- Data structure has the ability to be unstructured and structured
- Flexibility of analysis /processing involved within the amount of analysis, which has the ability to be be performed on it
- Concurrency

The initiative of big data analytics are supposed to be combined project contains business and IT. IT is supposed to be accountable in order to deploy the right analysis tools for big data as well as implementing the management practices of sound data. Each group is supposed to that success will be evaluated through the added valuc by the improvements of business, which appears through the initiative (Nitrd, 2016).

"Big Data" is recognized as an Analytics market and Data Management opportunity driven by the requirements of recent market. Within -Database Analytics – Data Mining, there are Big Data Connectors used in order to join the data of DBMS and Hadoop. Moreover, there is a great demand to reuse the skills of SQL for applying the techniques of deeper data mining, or to re-use skills for the purpose of statistical analysis. The whole subject is about "Big Data" instead of the data of RAM-scale. This indicates to analytical learning of relationships among business events and knowledge concepts (Chen et al., 2015).

Big-Data represents an important chance for generating recent value from massive data. It is significant to specify suitable procedures for governance to manage implementations and development over the data and technology life. Not a success to believe the longer-term implications of improvement will guide to cost escalations and productivity issues (Fan, Han & Liu, 2014; Ularu et al., 2012).

The cost of actually storing great amount of data is radically lessen through the ease by which data has the ability to be loaded into the cluster of Big-Data since it is indicated that there is no longer needed a multifaceted layer of ETL seen in any more solutions of conventional Data Warehouse. Moreover, the cluster itself is characteristically constructed through the usage of commodity hardware with low cost and analysts are free for writing code in approximately any modern language through the API streaming obtainable in Hadoop (Agrawal, Joshi & Velez, 2017).

The Importance of Big Data Era in Healthcare

Health data volume mostly is predicted to raise noticeably in the future (Cottle et al., 2013). Moreover, the models of healthcare reimbursement are transforming; significant pay and usage to the performance are promising as decisive recent factors in the healthcare environment of these days. even though proceeds are not supposed to be the a main motivator, it is crucially significant for the organizations of healthcare in order to obtain available techniques, infrastructure and tools to influence big data efficiently or other risks losing many millions in profits and revenue (LaValle et al., 2011).

A report transported to the U.S. Congress in August 2012 identified big data as great volumes of high variable, complex and velocity data, which need advanced technologies and techniques in order to enable the analysis, management, distribution, storage and capture of the information (Cottle et al., 2013). Big data includes such features as velocity, variety and with respect especially to veracity, healthcare (Unit, 2012; Connolly, Wooledge & Aster, 2013; Courtney, 2012; Sagiroglu & Sinanc, 2013). Obtainable analytical methods have the ability to be applied to the enormous amount of existing (but presently unanalyzed) medical data and patient-related health in order attain outcomes' deeper understanding, which after that have the ability to be applied at the care's point. Preferably, population and individual data would notify every physician as well as her patient throughout the process of decision-making in addition to aid specifies the most suitable treatment choice for that specific patient (Raghupathi & Raghupathi, 2014).

Through using, combining and effectively digitizing big data, the organization of healthcare ranging from multi-provider groups and the offices of single-physician to great hospital networks as well as the organizations of accountable care tends to recognize important benefits (Burghard, 2012).

Possible benefits involve distinguishing diseases at earlier stages, while they have the ability to be treated more effectively and easily. Managing particular population and individual health in addition to identify health care fraud more are efficiently and quickly. Many questions have the ability to be addressed with the analytics of big data. Particular outcomes and developments may be expected or/and evaluated depended on great amounts of the historical data; for instance, length of stay (LOS); patients who will selective surgery; complications; patients who probable will not get benefit from the surgery, patients at the risk of medical complications, patients at risk for sepsis; illness/disease progression; other hospital-acquired illness; patients at risk for progression in the states of disease causal factors of disease/ illness development and probable co-morbid conditions (EMC Consulting). McKinsey evaluated that big data analytics have the ability to enable in excess of $300 billion in saving for each year in the healthcare of the United States, two thirds of this amount is through the reductions of mostly8% in the national expenditures of healthcare. R & D and Clinical operations are recognized as two of the greatest areas for possible savings with $165 billion as well as108 billion in waste correspondingly (Brown et al., 2011; Manyika et al., 2011).

Bigdata may aid decrease waste and incompetence in the subsequent three areas (Manyika et al., 2011):

1. **Clinical Processes:** Comparative research of effectiveness in order to specify more clinically cost-effective and relevant methods to treat and diagnose patients.
2. **Research & Development:** That involves:
    a. Prognostic modeling for inferior attrition as well as create a targeted, faster and leaner, R & D pipeline in the devices and drugs
    b. Statistical algorithms and tools in order to enhance clinical trial design as well as patient employment for enhanced competition treatments to patients, consequently speeding recent treatments for the market and lessening trial failures
    c. Analyzing and patient records and clinical trials in order to define the indications of follow-on as well as find out adverse influences before the products arrive at the market.

3. **Public Health:**
   a. Analyzing the patterns of disease in addition to tracking disease transmission and outbreaks in order to enhance speed response and the surveillance of public health;
   b. Earlier improvement of more precisely besieged vaccines; for instance, selecting the yearly influenza strains; and,
   c. Rotating huge amounts of data to actionable information, which has the ability to be utilized to provide services, identify needs, prevent and predict crises, particularly for the populations 'benefit

Furthermore, big data analytics in healthcare have the ability to contribute to the following (Raghupathi & Raghupathi, 2014):

1. **Evidence-Depended on Medicine:** Analyze and Combine a diversity of unstructured and structured data-EMRs, genomic data, clinical data, forecast patients at risk for readmission or disease as well as offer more well-organized care.
2. **Genomic Analytics:** Carry out gene sequencing more professionally as well as cost efficiently in addition to make genomic analysis a part of the regular processes of the medical care decision as well as the growing medical record of patient.
3. **The Analysis of Pre-Adjudication Fraud:** Quickly analyze great numbers of claim requests in order to lessen fraud, abuse and waste
4. **Remote/Device Monitoring:** Analyze and Capture in real-time great volumes of speedy-moving data from the devices of in-home and in-hospital, for safety adverse and monitoring the prediction of event.
5. **Patient Profile Analytics:** Pertain superior analytics to the profiles of patient (for example, predictive and segmentation modeling) in order to recognize persons who would get benefit from lifestyle changes or practical care, for instance, the patients at risk of improving a particular disease (e.g., diabetes) who would get benefit from defensive care

The Applications of Big Data Analytical in Medicine and Healthcare

An extensive usage of big data within the sector of health has the ability to aid help doctors make the correct choices quickly depending on the information gathered by other medical staff. Patients have the ability to benefit from more appropriate and timely treatments as well as be superior informed about the providers of health care. Moreover, a developed usage of data analysis within the sector of health sector could lead to massive cost savings throughout a more accurate recognition of needless duplication or procedures of the tests. It is demonstrated that the analysis of great clinical datasets has the ability to significantly contribute in the optimization of the cost and clinical effectiveness of recent treatments and drugs (Raghupathi & Raghupathi, 2014).

The performance analysis of many mining classification techniques of data was examined based on three major various machine learning methods and tools over the datasets of healthcare. Various data mining categorization methods have been examined depending on four diverse datasets of healthcare. The utilized standards are considered percentage of error and accuracy and rate of each applied categorization method (Gupta, Kumar & Sharma, 2011). A wide spread confusion framework, called kernelized locality sensitive hashing is used to deal with this problem in order to increase time series resemblance search by means of a series of characterized resemblance metrics. The results of Experiments indicates to the efficiency of the suggested approach (Kale et al., 2014).

Practical applications and data mining perception in healthcare was considered a way further than its stable development in the field of academic research, that raises a hypothesis, which comparatively considered a little percentage of the efforts of the academic research results in practical applications of DM in healthcare out of which they was finish that the recent interdisciplinary approach does not consider competent enough (Niakšu & Kurasova, 2012).Statistical methods for evaluating complex structure of correlation from large datasets of pharmaco-genomics. They selectively viewed many famous statistical methods and means in order to evaluate great covariance matrix for being familiar with the structure of correlation, opposite covariance matrix for the modeling of network, simultaneous tests of large-scale for choosing considerably in a different way expressed proteins and genes as well as genetic markers for multifaceted diseases in addition to elevated dimensional changeable collection for recognized significant molecules for being familiar with molecule mechanisms within pharma-cogenomics (Fan & Liu, 2013). The technique of data mining is used for diseases' prediction and develops the diagnostic accurateness. Moreover, reduced the constraint of time and cost in terms of expertise and human resources (Durairaj & Ranjani, 2013).

Medical data are frequently noisy as well as gathered in elevated dimensional format. The usage of fuzzy system aids to hold the complexity and noisiness of medical data. In addition, SAM aids to lessen the superior dimensional data (Nguyen et al., 2015). In addition, there is an intensive data incorporated framework to help with the control and prevention of silicosis (HATS), TB and HIV/AIDS in the mining industry. The purpose behind suggested big data framework is to address the requirements of prognostic epidemiology that is significant in disease control and forecasting in the mining industry (Jokonya, 2014).

Moreover, there is an approach and recent statistical model learning, which have been utilized in the statistical relationship of learning from big data in the behavioural science and medicine, which characteristically involve environmental, genomic and clinical variable. This model is very appropriate for analyzing the sets of big data that is involved with the diverse kinds of large data form environmental, genomic and clinical data (Yoo, Ramirez &Liuzzi, 2014).

This section shows instances of health-related Big Data projects, among an importance of the quantified-self movement and data from the social media (Table 1). About the big data the research related to genetic data, EMRs, omics sources and digital enterprise, readers can consult the subsequent reviews in addition to the perspectives conducted lately (Bourne, 2014; Kum et al., 2014; Shivade et al., 2013; Shoenbill et al., 2013; Tenenbaum, Sansone & Haendel, 2013).

ANALYTICAL PERSPECTIVES OF BIG DATA

Computational Perspectives

Fascinatingly, the statisticians and the computer scientists - the two researchers' communities, which are may be most frankly influenced by the phenomenon of big data-have, intended for cultural reasons, adopted separate early examples in response to it. The main interest of the computer scientists, who have to design file structures andwell-organized data is to accumulate enormous datasets as well as put into practice algorithms on them-stems from computational difficulty. It interests the needed number of the steps of computing in order to resolve an agreed problem whose difficulty is recognized in terms of input data's length as presented through a rational encoding instruments (binary string) (Pyne, Rao & Rao, 2016).

Consequently, as the volume of data develops, any technique, which needs considerably more than O (Nlog(N)) steps (that is to say greater than the time's order, which is a solitary pass in excess of the full data would demand) could be unreasonable. Whereas, some of the significant obstacles in practice with the solutions of O (Nlog(N)) are immediately concerning scalable (for example fast Fourier change), those of superior difficulty, positively involving the problems of NP-Complete class, would need help aid from the algorithmic strategies such as sampling, randomization, approximation, etc. Consequently, whereas the theory of classical complexity may think about the solutions of polynomial time the same as computational tractability's hallmark, the big data's world is required even more demanding (Fokoue, 2015).

Table 1. Some examples about the health-related Big Data projects associated to social media in addition to the quantified-self movement

Data Type	How Has It Been Used in Health?	Examples
Quantified-self data (via devices, self-reporting, or sensors)	• Permits data collection being potentially longer follow-up stages than is presently possible by standard questionnaires (Swan, 2013) • Provides richer as well as more exhaustive data on probable risk factors (behavioral, biological, environmental or physical) (Swan, 2013) • Engaged during the self-tracking of behaviors and/or signs as n=1 in groups or individual, where there is frequently a proactive position to acting on the information (Swan, 2013)	• Grin triggered electro-myogram (EMG) muscle to make unexpected joy moments in human interaction (Tasse, 2012) • Food consumption (Yau,2017) • Coffee consumption, mood and social interaction (Wolf,2017) • Information diet (McCormick, 2017) • Idea-tracking process (Chua, 2012) • Checks blood glucose levels in diabetics (e.g. Glooko) (Glooko, 2017) • Use of controller and rescue asthma medications through an inhaler sensor (e.g. Asthmapolis) (Asthmapolis, 2017) • Physical activity (e.g. FitBit; Jawbone Up, RunKeeper) (JawboneUp, 2017) • Diet (e.g. My Meal Mate) (Carter et al., 2013) • Psychological, mental and cognitive traits and states (e.g. MyCompass) (Harrison et al., 2011) • Sleep quality (e.g. Lark) (Lark, 2017) • Medication adherence (e.g. MyMedSchedule) (Dayer et al., 2013)
Location-based information	• Information based on Geographic Information Systems (GIS), Global Positioning Systems (GPS), in addition to other visualization projects and open source mapping. • Gives information on the social and environmental health determinants. • Monitors for the disease that outbreaks close to your location.	• Allergens, weather patterns, traffic patterns, pollution levels, walkability of neighborhood, water quality, in addition to access to fresh vegetables and fruit (for example supermarkets) (Cerin et al, 2013) • HealthMap(HealthMap, 2017)
Twitter (Note: a 2011 study has recommended that 8.5% of the English-language tweets are relating to illness, and 16.6% are relating to health (Paul & Dredze, 2012))	• Makes discourse easy on non-emergency healthcare (e.g. quantify medical misconception, broadcasts of public health messages) • Makes the crisis mapping easy (e.g. where eyewitness is reporting are planned on interactive maps. These data are able to assist objective areas for emergency services in addition to additional resources) • Makes the emergency services easy by permitting for the available resource wide-scale broadcast, enabling people destitute of medical help for locating help • Assesses moods and sentiments • Assesses disease extend in real-time	• Trends of resuscitation communication and cardiac arrest (Bosley et al., 2013) • Measure medical misconceptions (e.g. concussions) (Sullivanet al., 2011) • breast and Cervical cancer screening (Lyles et al.,2013) • The poor medical compliance spread (e.g., antibiotic use) (Scanfeld, Scanfeld& Larson, 2010) • 2010 Haitian cholera outbreak (Chunara, Andrews & Brownstein, 2012) • Postpartum depression (De Choudhury, Counts & Horvitz, 2013) • Boston marathon explosion Emergency situations (Chunara, Andrews & Brownstein, 2012) • Influenza A H1N1 outbreak (public concern and disease activity) (Chews & Eysenbach, 2010)
Health-related social networking sites	• Monitors the infectious diseases spread via the crowd surveillance • Makes easy of the sharing of personal health advice and data amongst consumers and patients.	• Disease surveillance locations that collect participant-reported symptoms in addition to utilize familiar online data supplies to map, disseminate and analyze, information about infectious disease outbreaks (e.g. Flu Near You, HealthMap, GermTracker, Sickweather) (HealthMap, 2017) • PatientsLikeMe (PatientsLikeMe, 2017)
Additional social networking sites (e.g. board Facebook, online discussion)	• Checks how patients are using social media for discussing their issues and concerns. • Gives awareness of what the "person in the street" says (Hill, Merchant &Ungar, 2013)	Associated medication adherence behaviors and Side effects (e.g. drug switching as well as discontinuation) (Mao et al., 2013)
Search queries plus Web logs	• "Click" stream navigational data as of web logs are establish to be educational of individual distinctiveness such as dietary preferences and mental health (West, White & Horvitz, 2013) • Search keyword choice has been critical to arrive at dependable curated health satisfied • Found to be extremely predictive for an extensive range of the population-level health behaviors	Yahoo and Google search questions have been applied for predicting epidemics of illnesses, for example: • Seasonality of depression, suicide and mental health (Ayers et al., 2013) • Influenza (Google 2013) • Lyme disease Prevalence (Seifter et al., 2010) • Prevalence of electronic cigarette use and smoking (Ayers, Ribisl& Brownstein, 2011) • Dengue fever (Chan et al., 2011)

Hill, Merchant &Ungar, 2013; Swan, 2013.

For describing big data analytics, the same as dissimilar from the common data analysis, a particular individual could propose variety of principles, particularly if the obtainable analytical strategies are not enough to solve the obstacles in hand because of particular features of data. Such features may go beyond pure volume of data (Pyne, Rao & Rao, 2016). High velocity of data has the ability to represent unparalleled problems to the statistician who could not be used to the forgoing idea (more willingly than retaining) the points of data, the same as they stream out, to convince computational challenges like single pass (the constraint of time) as well as bounded storage (the constraint of space). The variety of High data possibly will need multidisciplinary imminent in order to enable a particular individual to make rational conclusion depending on incorporation of apparently unconnected datasets. From one side, such issues are supposed to view only as cultural gaps; whereas on the other side, they have the ability to stimulate the improvement of the essential formalisms, which has the ability to bridge those gaps. Thus, a superior understanding of the cons and pros of various algorithmic choices can aid any analyst decide concerning the most appropriate of the probable resolutions objectively (Chandrasekaran & Jordan, 2013).

Data Mining Perspectives

Data mining is broadly used within fields such as medicine, science, business and engineering. With this procedure, previously concealed insights have been discovered from large quantities of data to help the business community (Che, Safran & Peng, 2013). From the time of the organizations establishment in the present era, data mining has been practical within data recording. On the other hand, Big Data is collected of not just large data amounts but as well data during different formats. Consequently, large processing speed is required (Michael & Miller, 2013). For flexible data study, there are three projected principles (Begoli & Horey, 2012):

1. Architecture must support a lot of analysis methods, for example data mining, statistical analysis, visual analysis and machine learn in.
2. Diverse storage mechanisms ought to be used since every data is notable to fit within a single form of the storage area. In addition, the data ought to be processed in a different way at different stages.
3. Data ought to be accessed proficiently.

To consider Big Data, data mining algorithms which are computer exhaustive are utilized. Like algorithms require high-performance processors. In addition, the storage as well as computing requirements of the Big Data analysis are efficiently met through cloud computing (Talia, 2013).

The aims of large data mining methods go beyond attractive the demand ed information or even finding some hidden patterns and relationships between numeral restrictions. Analyzing massive and fast stream data can lead to novel theoretical concepts and valuable insights (Berkovich & Liao, 2012). Contrasting between the results based on mining the conventional datasets, presentation the large volume of consistent heterogeneous large data has the possible for maximizing our insights and knowledge within the target domain. However, this is bringing a series of novel challenges for the research community. Defeating the challenges will redesign the data mining technology future, resulting within a spectrum of the ground-breaking data in addition to mining algorithms and techniques (Che, Safran & Peng, 2013).

One feasible advance is for improving existing algorithms and techniques by exploiting extremely parallel computing architectures. Big data mining deals with velocity, heterogeneity, privacy, extreme scale, interactiveness, accuracy and trust which existing mining algorithms and techniques are incapable of. They require of implementing and designing very-large-scale parallel mechanism learning in addition to data mining algorithms (ML-DM) has extremely increased, that accompanies the appearance of powerful parallel as well as very-large-scale data handing out platforms, e.g., HadoopMapReduce. NIMBLE is a transferable infrastructure which has been exclusively designed to enable quick execution of parallel ML-DM algorithms, running on top of Hadoop (Ghoting et al., 2011).

Apache's Mahout is a library of data mining implementations and machine learning. Also, the library is applied on top of Hadoop by the MapReduce programming form. Some significant mechanism of the library is able to run stand-alone. The most important disadvantages of Mahout are that its learning cycle is very long as well as its need of user-friendly interaction hold up. In addition, it does not apply all the required machine learning algorithms and data mining. BC-PDM (Big Cloud-Parallel Data Mining), as a cloud-based data mining stage, as well based on Hadoop, is providing access to great telecom data in addition to business solutions to the telecom operators; it is supporting parallel ETL process (load, extract and transform), text mining, data mining and social network analysis (Yu et al., 2012).

BC-PDM attempted to defeat the problem of the single function of additional approaches also to be further applicable to the Business Intelligence. PEGASUS (Peta-scale Graph Mining System) and Giraph the tow implement graph mining algorithms employing parallel computing as well as they run on top of Hadoop (Kang, Tsourakakis & Faloutsos, 2009). GraphLab is a graph-based, scalable structure, on that a number of data mining algorithms and graph-based machine learning are executed. The reported disadvantage of GraphLab is that it is requiring all data appropriate into memory (Low et al., 2012).

Machine Learning Perspectives

Machine learning methods have been found extremely effective as well as relevant to many real world requests in bioinformatics, healthcare, network security, transportations as well as finance and banking. Eventually, health related and bioinformatics data are created as well as accumulated incessantly, resultant in an unbelievable data volume. Newer appearances of big data, such as 3D imaging, biometric and genomics sensor readings, are as well fueling this exponential increase. Future requests of real-time data, for example fast application of the suitable treatments and early discovery of infections/diseases and could decrease patient mortality and morbidity. Previously, real time flowing data monitors neonates in the ICU, infectious life-threatening diseases at real time. The capability for performing real-time analytics against like large stream data crosswise all specialties would transform healthcare. There lies data with variety, volume and velocity (Kashyap et al., 2015).

Machine learning is a computer science field which studies the computational techniques which learn from data (Anzai, 2012). There are mostly a couple of types of learning techniques in machine learning, viz., supervised as well as unsupervised learning techniques (Bhattacharyya & Kalita, 2013). Within supervised learning, a technique learns from a group of things with class label, frequently called the training set. The obtained knowledge is applied to give label to unidentified objects frequently called the test objects. Alternatively, unsupervised learning techniques do not rely on the availability of training instances or prior knowledge with class labels. Every one of these machine-learning techniques needs preprocessing of datasets for effectual results. Feature collection is one of the significant preprocessing tasks, which leads to enhanced result in addition to reduced time necessity. Hybrid learning techniques, for example Deep learning, have turned into popular during the current years as well as provide significantly large accuracy. Superior data capturing technologies have guided to accumulation of an extremely high data volume, growing quickly over time. Even though the computational technologies have enhanced over time, this development is not in proportion to the increase rate in data volume. The conventional machine learning techniques are found insufficient in treatment voluminous data by the present computational resources (Floridi, 2012). Figure 3 shows the contrast among traditional data mining as well as mining of big data.

Figure 3. Traditional data mining and mining of big data
Kashyap et al., 2015.

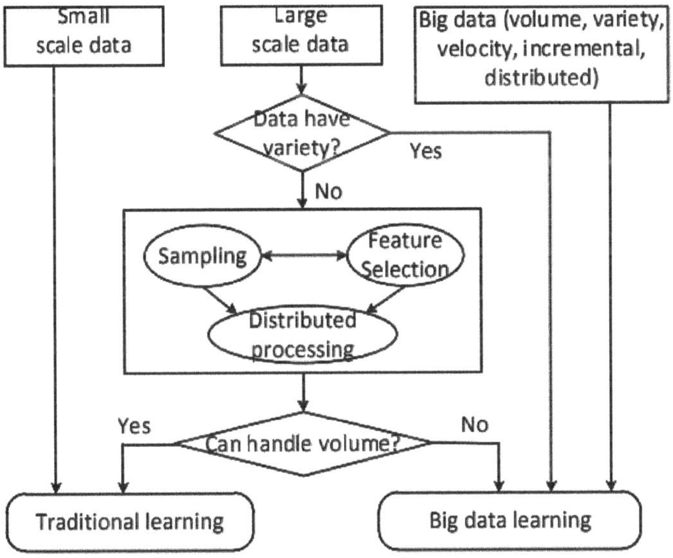

Supervised Learning

Within big data analytics, we require several advanced supervised advances for distributed and parallel learning for example divide-and-conquer SVM (Hsieh &Dhillon, 2014), Multi-hyper plane Machine (MM) classification form [49], and neural network classifiers. Amongst these SVM is one of the mainly widely and efficient used supervised learning technique and a number of modified SVM techniques have been initiated for big data analytics. Nie et al. suggest a customized SVM called New Primal SVM for big data classification (Djuric, 2013). The technique uses a new linear computational cost primitive SVM solver by two loss functions called L1-norm plus L2-norm in Augmented Lagrange Multipliers (ALM). Individual discovery of patients with Parkinson disease by SVM analysis was projected by Haller et al.,(2012).

Unsupervised Learning

Unsupervised learning does not employ the class labels of the substances for learning (Aggarwal& Reddy, 2013). Clustering is an unconfirmed technique, which is attempting to group objects for optimizing the criterion, which states that detachment among objects within the identical cluster is reduced and distance between objects in diverse clusters is exploited (Tan, Steinbach & Kumar, 2013). A most important issue within clustering is the calculation of the distance among two objects. Different proximity is measuring have been applied for this reason, such as city block distance, Euclidean and Cosine. In customary clustering, every feature is used as computing the distance among two objects. A cluster is a collection of objects, which are near to each other regarding to their common distance. That means they are alike in nature in excess of the entire set of features. However, in a number of applications, especially where number of obtainable features within a dataset is extremely large, researchers are paying attention in finding collections of objects, which are alike over division of the obtainable features (Cheng & Church, 2000). This necessity has guide to the appearance of another alternative of clustering called blustering, wherever every balusters related with a division of features (Kashyap et al., 2015).

Deep Learning

Deep learning tries to build high-level concepts in data by unsupervised or supervised learning algorithms to absorb from several abstractions levels. Deep learning utilizes data hierarchical representations for classification. Its methods are used in several applications, pattern recognition, viz., natural language processing, computer vision, besides speech recognition. Because of exponential data growth in the previous applications, this kind of learning is valuable for precise prediction from big data. Recently, academics have advanced scalable and effective parallel training deep models algorithms (Hinton et al., 2012). Several administrations use deep learning for the purpose of information retrieval, semantic indexing and decision making. The architecture of deep learning is presented in Figure 4. Input data are divided into data abstractions' multiple samples. The intermediary layers are for processing the multiple levels features for data prediction. The last prediction is done using the immediate upper layer outputs at the output layer (Kashyap et al., 2015).

Figure 4. Deep leaning architecture
Kashyap et al., 2015.

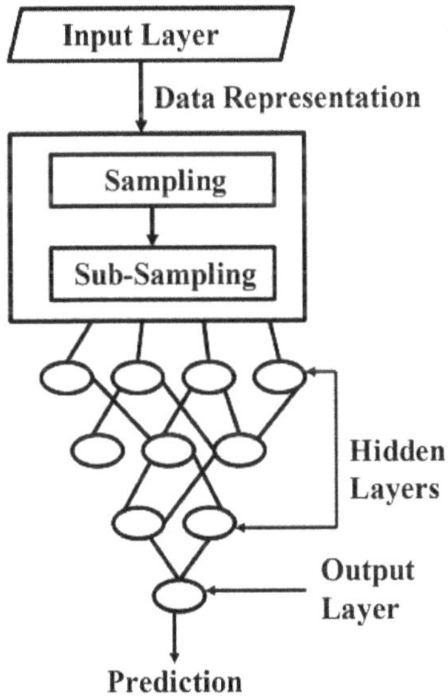

DATA TYPES OF HIV/AIDS BIG DATA ANALYTICS

Biological Data

The elements of biological data characteristically addressed involve (Geoff & Jillian, 2015):

1. The profiles of protein expression and RNA in diseased and healthy tissue at whole-organ, single cell, or regional levels
2. Inherent information concerning disease and healthy-influenced individuals, characteristically in the wide single nucleotide polymorphism (SNP)'s form, which are whole –genome sequence data (WGS) or whole exome sequence data (WES)
3. Epigenetic data on the modifications of site-specific DNA as well as his tone acetylation

This information possibly will be demanded from the models of cellular involving (iPS cells) which refers to induced pluripotent stem cells, and from vertebrate and invertebrate animal models. Moreover, it has the ability to be gained from the tissues of human, since in this case it is mostly connected to pseudononymised clinical data on cognitive function, diagnostic status, neuropath logical, neuroimaging, serological or biochemical information. Currently, this kind of compound clinical and biological data has been gathered for humble numbers of controls and cases. Instances of particular databases involve the GEO-PD, Alzheimer's Disease Genetics Consortium (ADGC), Alzheimer's Disease Neuroimaging Initiative (ADNI) in addition to different community repositories of protein expression data and cell type like Allen Brain Institute (Geoff & Jillian, 2015).

Medical and Clinical Data

Clinical data characteristically involve information concerning symptoms, diagnostic tests involving brain-imaging, CSF and blood tests; disease progression's rates, kind of treatment specified to interest's disease; the influence of that treatment, the attendance of other comorbid and illness factors; and such information concerning economic, social and physical environment. This information has the ability to be connected, within databases, to particular biological data as mentioned previously. it is predicted that, in the following one to five years, these kinds of multifaceted multimodal data will be obtained for superior numbers of controls and cases. Instances of these superior datasets involve the dementia platform of UK, Mayo clinic study of aging, DZNE Rhineland dementia project and UK 1000 Genomes projects. Several of these cohorts involve cross-sectional data and longitudinal data. Further potential resources of such detailed clinical and biological information are profitable databases taken place from trails of candidate diagnostics and new medicines (Haussleiter, Brüne & Juckel, 2009; Geoff & Jillian, 2015).

Other Types, Social, Psycho, and Demographic

Furthermore, Broad population-based information has the ability to be obtained on a great deal of persons from lasting care records, medical record as well as other population depended on epidemiological studies. even though these datasets do not typically coupled with deep biological classification, significant data has the ability to be gleaned from medical records, the recodes of lasting care institutions concerning socio-economic status, drug exposure, hospitalizations, diagnosis, exposure to different environmental risks like occupation, smoking, diet, the factors of lifestyle like exercise or cognitive engagement (Olsen & McGinnis, 2010). A number of these items (for instance, continuing cognitive engagement or early education of childhood) are already thought to the disease's progression as well as impact risk, it is predicted that, in excess of the next decade, the content of information concerning population-depended on datasets will radically develop throughout the low-cost DNA sequencing's acquisition that permits the enclosure of transcription profiling and genomics-wide sequence data on great numbers of persons (McKenzie, Neiger& Thackeray, 2016).

Other probable resources of data involve different kinds of profitable data such as social media usage, internet, mobile phone, and data on credit card. These commercial data possibly involve information about lifestyle (for instance exercise and cigarette, alcohol and diet consumption, etc) . Moreover, transformation through the time in the difficulty of such parameters like social engagement as well as shopping habits have the ability to reproduce transformations in the cognitive activities, which possibly depict the disease's early stages (Miller, Oldham & Geschwind, 2008). In addition, we are supposed to expect a more occupied public were sick individuals and healthy individuals who are sick will follow their own phenotypic data. Nowadays, there are several devices that permit sleep and exercise, blood pressure and heart rate, which present emerging instruments in order to connect the public at the same time as full partners in the diseases' developing models. Such information is probable to be produced throughout wearable devices and smart phones through three ways as the following (Zhang et al., 2013):

1. The activities of Passively-tracking like exercise utilizing the accelerometers
2. Prearranged tests wherever someone is frankly asked to perform a tests intended for properties like cognitive decline
3. Questions and surveys that the individuals have the ability to answer in real-time multiple times for every day

FUTURE WORKS AND OPPORTUNITIES

Opportunities

In the previous two decades there was an explosion within Big Data all through the health-care value chain, and the start of novel platforms, tackles, in addition to methodologies in analyzing, storing and structuring Big Data. Significant developments comprise the genomic data use within drug discovery, the clinical-trial data sharing, the electronic healthcare records use (EHRs), and the improved availability of the data from social media, mHealth applications and patient registries (Szlezák et al., 2014). The data fusion concept is gaining additional significance as on top of the set of individual data basics increases the fusing jointly of several data sets (Howell, 2014). The enormous amount of new data being produced is by now making significant contributions within epidemiology, more especially in activist public health surveillance (Salathe et al., 2012).

In the satellite sensors era, a variety of epidemiologically appropriate environmental information is able to be sourced internationally at daily periods. Big Data is allowing a closer activist matching of the disease outbreaks through covariates which can improve the mapping models accuracy. The opportunity of seasonally modified geographic baselines definitely improves conventional temporal surveillance through facilitating early caution of epidemiologically appropriate environmental changes (Hay et al., 2013).

The quantified self-concept, in that individuals deploy monitoring and sensors devices for measuring their own behavior and health, has become a truth. If aggregated and expanded at level of population, will guide to a data-driven advance of wellbeing measurement and collective health (Barrett et al., 2013). The creation of new knowledge of the treatments effectiveness as well as the outcomes prediction are of two essential applications of the big healthcare data. That means Big Data is able to be practical in retrospective and prospective research. Prospective research is product focused (for example, improvement of the disease relation to other factors for example protection factor(s) or suspected risk) and has a small recall error when it is involving longitudinal observations eventually as well as results are composed at usual time intervals. In addition, Big Data is different from tradition choice support tools when it is allowing the collection also examination real-time patient data (Murdoch & Detsky, 2013).

Novel possibilities about the discovery of the innovative pharmaceuticals, improvement of more effectual treatment protocols in addition to the improvement of personalized medicine obtain play. Statistical algorithms and tools improve clinical experiment design as well as patient recruitment for better match actions to individual patients, decreasing trial failures as well as speeding novel treatments to market. The analysis of patient records and clinical trials is allowing the classification of follow-up suggestions and the finding of adverse results before products attain the market that ultimately will develop pharmaco-vigilance in addition to patient safety (Raghupathi & Raghupathi, 2014).The assure of personalized medicine led by a considerate of every individual's genome has been advanced through increasingly powerful plus economical methods for acquiring clinically appropriate information (Pulley et al., 2012). Big Data is helping translate personalized medicine to a clinical practice through offering the chance to apply analytical capabilities which can incorporate systems biology (such as, genomics) among data of EHRs (Murdoch & Detsky, 2013). The population science integration by individual genomic measurements will allow the personalized medicine practice (Altman, 2013).

Challenges

Currently, the high variety, volume and velocity of the data collection techniques available is possible to make the society of data driven to a point in that sampling will not be essential because the whole background population is obtainable. Through working with approximately all, the information of the phenomena there is a rising capacity for expanding research questions. Additionally, Big Data includes a high messiness level in the intellect that the raise in the information amount by orders of magnitude is meaning giving up the favorite for extremely curated data for the object of having a superior sample as well as effect size (Walker, 2014). The analysis of disorganized, unstructured and voluminous data has got important discoveries (Baker, 2013; Whiteet al., 2013). However, in the lack of causality in addition to strong assumptions, is society possible to fall blindly on associations? (Lazer et al., 2014).

Still, there are a standardization problems within the healthcare sector, when data is frequently generated or fragmented within IT systems through incompatible formats. Hospital services, research, education, clinical activities as well as administrative services are siloed, furthermore, in a lot of organizations, every silo maintains its possess separate organizational (also sometimes duplicated) information and data infrastructure. The need of cross-border coordination as well as technology integration is calling for standards for facilitating interoperability amongst the Big Data value chain components (Roney, 2012).

When the quantity of health related data in addition to global digital information is growing, therefore does the number of actors' admissions in addition to using this information. Assurances have to be given in order that personal data associated with health will be employed correctly, within the context of the projected uses in addition to consistent with the related laws. Still there is skepticism in view of (where the data goes to) and (by whom it is used) moreover (for what purpose) within the EU split and excessively multifaceted legal environment. In what worries to privacy, circumstances under that data are, 10 shared to research are being conversed under the planned Data Protection Regulation (File, 2012).

Future Directions

Based on the challenges and related issues that big data scientists need to address, the following present some future research directions that can be applied to the handling of big data (Anagnostopoulos, Zeadally & Exposito, 2016):

- Big Data Curation and Cleansing
- Sharing/Storage/Transfer of Big Data
- Analysis and Collection of Big Data Results
- Ethical Considerations of Big Data

CONCLUSION

Big data is a term that defines the large amount of structured and unstructured data that have the ability to enhance the performance of the various businesses on a day-to-day basis. In the health sector, incorporating big data has a great influence in the different treatment stages and public health. However, the opportunities that big data can provide are facing some challenges including the rapid changes in the information systems and unreliable infrastructures; therefore, there must be a new direction for future research and innovations.

REFERENCES

Aggarwal, C. C., & Reddy, C. K. (Eds.). (2013). *Data clustering: algorithms and applications*. CRC press.

Agrawal, M., Joshi, A. S., & Velez, A. F. (2017). *Best Practices in Data Management for Analytics Projects*. CTO Office, Persistent Systems Ltd.

Altman, R. B. (2013). Personal genomic measurements: The opportunity for information integration. *Clinical Pharmacology and Therapeutics*, *93*(1), 21–23. doi:10.1038/clpt.2012.203 PMID:23241835

Anagnostopoulos, I., Zeadally, S., & Exposito, E. (2016). Handling big data: Research challenges and future directions. *The Journal of Supercomputing*, *72*(4), 1494–1516. doi:10.1007/s11227-016-1677-z

Anzai, Y. (2012). *Pattern recognition and machine learning*. Elsevier.

Asthmapolis. (2017). Available from: http://propellerhealth. com/

Ayers, J. W., Althouse, B. M., Allem, J. P., Rosenquist, J. N., & Ford, D. E. (2013). Seasonality in seeking mental health information on Google. *American Journal of Preventive Medicine*, *44*(5), 520–525. doi:10.1016/j.amepre.2013.01.012 PMID:23597817

Ayers, J. W., Ribisl, K. M., & Brownstein, J. S. (2011). Tracking the rise in popularity of electronic nicotine delivery systems (electronic cigarettes) using search query surveillance. *American Journal of Preventive Medicine*, *40*(4), 448–453. doi:10.1016/j.amepre.2010.12.007 PMID:21406279

Baker, E. W. (2013). Relational Model Bases: A Technical Approach to Real-time Business Intelligence and Decision Making. CAIS, 33, 23.

Barrett, M. A., Humblet, O., Hiatt, R. A., & Adler, N. E. (2013). Big data and disease prevention: From quantified self to quantified communities. *Big Data*, *1*(3), 168–175. doi:10.1089/big.2013.0027 PMID:27442198

Begoli, E., & Horey, J. (2012). Design principles for effective knowledge discovery from big data. In *Software Architecture (WICSA) and European Conference on Software Architecture (ECSA), 2012 joint working IEEE/IFIP conference on* (pp. 215-218). IEEE. doi:10.1109/WICSA-ECSA.212.32

Berkovich, S., & Liao, D. (2012). On clusterization of big data streams. In *Proceedings of the 3rd International Conference on Computing for Geospatial Research and Applications* (p. 26). ACM.

Bhattacharyya, D. K., & Kalita, J. K. (2013). *Network anomaly detection: A machine learning perspective*. CRC Press.

Big Data Solutions. (2017). *Harnessing the Power of Big Data for Trade and Competitiveness policy*. World Bank Group.

Bosley, J. C., Zhao, N. W., Hill, S., Shofer, F. S., Asch, D. A., Becker, L. B., & Merchant, R. M. (2013). Decoding twitter: Surveillance and trends for cardiac arrest and resuscitation communication. *Resuscitation*, *84*(2), 206–212. doi:10.1016/j.resuscitation.2012.10.017 PMID:23108239

Bourne, P. E. (2014). What Big Data means to me.. *Journal of the American Medical Informatics Association*, *21*(2), 194. doi:10.1136/amiajnl-2014-002651 PMID:24509599

Brown, B., Bughin, J., Byers, A. H., Chui, M., Dobbs, R., Manyika, J., & Roxburgh, C. (2011). *Big data: the next frontier for innovation, competition, and productivity*. McKinsey Global Institute.

Burghard, C. (2012). Big data and analytics key to accountable care success. *IDC Health Insights*.

Carter, M. C., Burley, V. J., Nykjaer, C., & Cade, J. E. (2013). Adherence to a smartphone application for weight loss compared to website and paper diary: Pilot randomized controlled trial. *Journal of Medical Internet Research*, *15*(4), e32. doi:10.2196/jmir.2283 PMID:23587561

Cerin, E., Lee, K. Y., Barnett, A., Sit, C. H., Cheung, M. C., & Chan, W. M. (2013). Objectively-measured neighborhood environments and leisure-time physical activity in Chinese urban elders. *Preventive Medicine*, *56*(1), 86–89. doi:10.1016/j.ypmed.2012.10.024 PMID:23137445

Chan, E. H., Sahai, V., Conrad, C., & Brownstein, J. S. (2011). Using web search query data to monitor dengue epidemics: A new model for neglected tropical disease surveillance. *PLoS Neglected Tropical Diseases*, *5*(5), e1206. doi:10.1371/journal.pntd.0001206 PMID:21647308

Chandrasekaran, V., & Jordan, M. I. (2013). Computational and statistical tradeoffs via convex relaxation. *Proceedings of the National Academy of Sciences of the United States of America*, *110*(13), E1181–E1190. doi:10.1073/pnas.1302293110 PMID:23479655

Chaorasiya, V., & Shrivastava, A. (2015). A survey on Big Data: Techniques and Technologies. *International Journal of Research and Development in Applied Science and Engineering*, *8*(1), 1–4.

Che, D., Safran, M., & Peng, Z. (2013). From big data to big data mining: challenges, issues, and opportunities. In *International Conference on Database Systems for Advanced Applications* (pp. 1-15). Springer. doi:10.1007/978-3-642-40270-8_1

Chen, X., Wang, S., Dong, Y., & Wang, X. (2015). Big Data Storage Architecture Design in Cloud Computing. In *National Conference on Big Data Technology and Applications* (pp. 7-14). Springer.

Cheng, Y., & Church, G. M. (2000). Biclustering of expression data. ISMB, 8, 93-103.

Chew, C., & Eysenbach, G. (2010). Pandemics in the age of Twitter: Content analysis of Tweets during the 2009 H1N1 outbreak. *PLoS One*, *5*(11), e14118. doi:10.1371/journal.pone.0014118 PMID:21124761

Chua, S. (2012). *Notes from the quantified self 2012 conference*. Available from: http://sachachua.com/blog/p/23723/

Chunara, R., Andrews, J. R., & Brownstein, J. S. (2012). Social and news media enable estimation of epidemiological patterns early in the 2010 Haitian cholera outbreak. *The American Journal of Tropical Medicine and Hygiene*, *86*(1), 39–45. doi:10.4269/ajtmh.2012.11-0597 PMID:22232449

Connolly, S., Wooledge, S., & Aster, T. (2013). *Harnessing the value of big data analytics*. Academic Press.

Cottle, M., Hoover, W., Kanwal, S., Kohn, M., Strome, T., & Treister, N. (2013). Transforming Health Care Through Big Data Strategies for leveraging big data in the health care industry. *Institute for Health Technology Transformation.* Retrieved from http://ihealthtran.com/big-data-in-healthcare

Courtney, M. (2012). Puzzling out big data. *Engineering & Technology*, *7*(12), 56–60. doi:10.1049/et.2012.1215

Curry, L. (2005). The Future of the Public's Health in the 21st Century. *Generations (San Francisco, Calif.)*, *29*(2), 82.

Dayer, L., Heldenbrand, S., Anderson, P., Gubbins, P. O., & Martin, B. C. (2013). Smartphone medication adherence apps: Potential benefits to patients and providers. *Journal of the American Pharmacists Association: JAPhA*, *53*(2), 172–181. doi:10.1331/JAPhA.2013.12202 PMID:23571625

De Choudhury, M., Counts, S., & Horvitz, E. (2013). Predicting postpartum changes in emotion and behavior via social media. In *Proceedings of the SIGCHI Conference on Human Factors in Computing Systems* (pp. 3267-3276). ACM. doi:10.1145/2470654.2466447

Djuric, N. (2013). *Big data algorithms for visualization and supervised learning*. Temple University.

Durairaj, M., &Ranjani, V. (2013). Data mining applications in healthcare sector: A study. *International Journal of Scientific & Technology Research, 2*(10), 29-35.

Edmunds, M., Thorpe, L., Sepulveda, M., Bezold, C., & Ross, D. A. (2014). The future of public health informatics: Alternative scenarios and recommended strategies. *EGEMS (Washington, DC), 2*(4), 3. doi:10.13063/2327-9214.1156 PMID:25848630

Erdman, A. G., Keefe, D. F., & Schiestl, R. (2013). Grand challenge: Applying regulatory science and big data to improve medical device innovation. *IEEE Transactions on Biomedical Engineering, 60*(3), 700–706. doi:10.1109/TBME.2013.2244600 PMID:23380845

Fan, J., Han, F., & Liu, H. (2014). Challenges of big data analysis. *National Science Review, 1*(2), 293–314. doi:10.1093/nsr/nwt032 PMID:25419469

Fan, J., & Liu, H. (2013). Statistical analysis of big data on pharmacogenomics. *Advanced Drug Delivery Reviews, 65*(7), 987–1000. doi:10.1016/j.addr.2013.04.008 PMID:23602905

Fan, W., &Bifet, A. (2013). Mining big data: current status, and forecast to the future. *ACM SIGKDD Explorations Newsletter, 14*(2), 1-5.

File, I. (2012). *Proposal for a Regulation of the European Parliament and of the Council on the Protection of Individuals with Regard to the Processing of Personal Data and on the Free movement of Such Data*. General Data Protection Regulation.

Floridi, L. (2012). Big data and their epistemological challenge. *Philosophy & Technology, 25*(4), 435–437. doi:10.1007/s13347-012-0093-4

Fokoue, E. (2015). *A taxonomy of Big Data for optimal predictive machine learning and data mining*. arXiv preprint arXiv:1501.00604

Forsyth, C. (2012). *For big data analytics there's no such thing as too big*. The compelling economics and technology of big data computing. White Paper.

Geoff, A. & Jillian, O. (Eds.). (2015). *Dementia Research and Care Can Big Data Help? Can Big Data Help?* OECD Publishing.

Ghoting, A., Kambadur, P., Pednault, E., & Kannan, R. (2011).NIMBLE: a toolkit for the implementation of parallel data mining and machine learning algorithms on mapreduce. In *Proceedings of the 17th ACM SIGKDD international conference on Knowledge discovery and data mining* (pp. 334-342). ACM. doi:10.1145/2020408.2020464

Glooko. (2017). Available from: http://www.glooko.com/

Groves, P., Kayyali, B., Knott, D., & Kuiken, S. V. (2016). *The'bigdata'revolution in healthcare: Accelerating value and innovation*. McKinsey& Company.

Gupta, S., Kumar, D., & Sharma, A. (2011). Performance analysis of various data mining classification techniques on healthcare data. *International Journal of Computer Science & Information Technology, 3*(4).

Halevi, G., & Moed, H. (2012). The evolution of big data as a research and scientific topic: Overview of the literature. *Research Trends*, *30*(1), 3–6.

Haller, S., Badoud, S., Nguyen, D., Garibotto, V., Lovblad, K. O., & Burkhard, P. R. (2012). Individual detection of patients with Parkinson disease using support vector machine analysis of diffusion tensor imaging data: Initial results. *American Journal of Neuroradiology*, *33*(11), 2123–2128. doi:10.3174/ajnr.A3126 PMID:22653326

Harrison, V., Proudfoot, J., Wee, P. P., Parker, G., Pavlovic, D. H., & Manicavasagar, V. (2011). Mobile mental health: Review of the emerging field and proof of concept study. *Journal of Mental Health (Abingdon, England)*, *20*(6), 509–524. doi:10.3109/09638237.2011.608746 PMID:21988230

Haussleiter, I. S., Brüne, M., & Juckel, G. (2009). Psychopathology in multiple sclerosis: Diagnosis, prevalence and treatment. *Therapeutic Advances in Neurological Disorders*, *2*(1), 13–29. doi:10.1177/1756285608100325 PMID:21180640

Hay, S. I., George, D. B., Moyes, C. L., & Brownstein, J. S. (2013). Big data opportunities for global infectious disease surveillance. *PLoS Medicine*, *10*(4), e1001413. doi:10.1371/journal.pmed.1001413 PMID:23565065

HealthMap. (2017). Available from: http://healthmap.org/

Hill, S., Merchant, R., & Ungar, L. (2013). Lessons learned about public health from online crowd surveillance. *Big Data*, *1*(3), 160–167. doi:10.1089/big.2013.0020 PMID:25045598

Hinton, G., Deng, L., Yu, D., Dahl, G. E., Mohamed, A. R., Jaitly, N., & Kingsbury, B. (2012). Deep neural networks for acoustic modeling in speech recognition: The shared views of four research groups. *IEEE Signal Processing Magazine*, *29*(6), 82–97. doi:10.1109/MSP.2012.2205597

Howell, D. R. (2014). *An examination of motor and cognitive recovery following concussion* (Doctoral dissertation). University of Oregon.

Hsieh, C. J., Si, S., & Dhillon, I. (2014). A divide-and-conquer solver for kernel support vector machines. *International Conference on Machine Learning*, 566-574.

JawboneUp. (2017). Available from: https://jawbone.com/up

Jewell, D., Barros, R. D., Diederichs, S., Duijvestijn, L. M., Hammersley, M., Hazra, A., & Portilla, I. (2014). *Performance and capacity implications for big data*. IBM Redbooks.

Jokonya, O. (2014). Towards a Big Data Framework for the prevention and control of HIV/AIDS, TB and Silicosis in the mining industry. *Procedia Technology*, *16*, 1533–1541. doi:10.1016/j.protcy.2014.10.175

Kaisler, S., Armour, F., Espinosa, J. A., & Money, W. (2013). Big data: Issues and challenges moving forward. In *System Sciences (HICSS), 2013 46th Hawaii International Conference on* (pp. 995-1004). IEEE.

Kale, D. C., Gong, D., Che, Z., Liu, Y., Medioni, G., Wetzel, R., & Ross, P. (2014). An examination of multivariate time series hashing with applications to health care. In *Data Mining (ICDM), 2014 IEEE International Conference on* (pp. 260-269). IEEE. doi:10.1109/ICDM.2014.153

Kang, U., Tsourakakis, C. E., & Faloutsos, C. (2009).Pegasus: A peta-scale graph mining system implementation and observations. In *Data Mining, 2009.ICDM'09. Ninth IEEE International Conference on* (pp. 229-238). IEEE. doi:10.1109/ICDM.2009.14

Kashyap, H., Ahmed, H. A., Hoque, N., Roy, S., & Bhattacharyya, D. K. (2015). *Big data analytics in bioinformatics: A machine learning perspective*. arXiv preprint arXiv:1506.05101

Kum, H. C., Krishnamurthy, A., Machanavajjhala, A., Reiter, M. K., & Ahalt, S. (2014). Privacy preserving interactive record linkage (PPIRL). *Journal of the American Medical Informatics Association*, *21*(2), 212–220. doi:10.1136/amiajnl-2013-002165 PMID:24201028

J. Lane, V. Stodden, S. Bender, & H. Nissenbaum (Eds.). (2014). *Privacy, big data, and the public good: Frameworks for engagement.* Cambridge University Press. doi:10.1017/CBO9781107590205

Laney, D. (2001). *3-d data management: Controlling data volume, velocity and variety.* META Group, Research Note, February 2001.

Lark. (2017). Available from: http://lark.com/

LaValle, S., Lesser, E., Shockley, R., Hopkins, M. S., & Kruschwitz, N. (2011). Big data, analytics and the path from insights to value. *MIT Sloan Management Review, 52*(2), 21.

Lazer, D., Kennedy, R., King, G., & Vespignani, A. (2014). The parable of Google Flu: Traps in big data analysis. *Science, 343*(6176), 1203–1205. doi:10.1126/science.1248506 PMID:24626916

Lee, C. H., & Yoon, H. J. (2017). Medical big data: Promise and challenges. *Kidney Research and Clinical Practice, 36*(1), 3–11. doi:10.23876/j.krcp.2017.36.1.3 PMID:28392994

Lin, J., & Ryaboy, D. (2013). Scaling big data mining infrastructure: The twitter experience. *ACM SIGKDD Explorations Newsletter, 14*(2), 6–19. doi:10.1145/2481244.2481247

Lomotey, R. K., & Deters, R. (2014). Towards knowledge discovery in big data. In *Service Oriented System Engineering (SOSE), 2014 IEEE 8th International Symposium on* (pp. 181-191). IEEE. doi:10.1109/SOSE.2014.25

Low, Y., Bickson, D., Gonzalez, J., Guestrin, C., Kyrola, A., & Hellerstein, J. M. (2012). Distributed GraphLab: A framework for machine learning and data mining in the cloud. *Proceedings of the VLDB Endowment International Conference on Very Large Data Bases, 5*(8), 716–727. doi:10.14778/2212351.2212354

Lyles, C. R., López, A., Pasick, R., & Sarkar, U. (2013). "5 mins of uncomfyness is better than dealing with cancer 4 a lifetime": An exploratory qualitative analysis of cervical and breast cancer screening dialogue on Twitter. *Journal of Cancer Education, 28*(1), 127–133. doi:10.1007/s13187-012-0432-2 PMID:23132231

Manyika, J., Chui, M., Brown, B., Buhin, J., Dobbs, R., Roxburgh, C., & Byers, A. H. (2011). *Big Data: The Next Frontier for Innovation, Competition, and Productivity.* McKinsey Global Institute.

Mao, J. J., Chung, A., Benton, A., Hill, S., Ungar, L., Leonard, C. E., & Holmes, J. H. (2013). Online discussion of drug side effects and discontinuation among breast cancer survivors. *Pharmacoepidemiology and Drug Safety*, *22*(3), 256–262. doi:10.1002/pds.3365 PMID:23322591

McCormick, T. (2012). *Video of my healthier information talk*. Available from: http://tjm.org/2012/04/17/videoof-my-healthier-information-talk/

McKenzie, J. F., Neiger, B. L., & Thackeray, R. (2016). *Planning, implementing & evaluating health promotion programs: A primer*. Pearson.

Michael, K., & Miller, K. W. (2013). Big data: New opportunities and new challenges. *Computer*, *46*(6), 22–24. doi:10.1109/MC.2013.196

Miller, J. A., Oldham, M. C., & Geschwind, D. H. (2008). A systems level analysis of transcriptional changes in Alzheimer's disease and normal aging. *The Journal of Neuroscience*, *28*(6), 1410–1420. doi:10.1523/JNEUROSCI.4098-07.2008 PMID:18256261

Mitchell, I., & Wilson, M. (2012). *Linked Data: Connecting and exploiting big data*. White paper. Fujitsu UK, 302.

Mukherjee, S., & Shaw, R. (2016). Big Data–Concepts, Applications, Challenges and Future Scope. *International Journal of Advanced Research in Computer and Communication Engineering*, *5*(2).

Murdoch, T. B., & Detsky, A. S. (2013). The inevitable application of big data to health care. *Journal of the American Medical Association*, *309*(13), 1351–1352. doi:10.1001/jama.2013.393 PMID:23549579

Nguyen, T., Khosravi, A., Creighton, D., & Nahavandi, S. (2015). Classification of healthcare data using genetic fuzzy logic system and wavelets. *Expert Systems with Applications*, *42*(4), 2184–2197. doi:10.1016/j.eswa.2014.10.027

Niakšu, O., &Kurasova, O. (2012). Data mining applications in healthcare: research vs practice. *Databases Inform Syst Baltic DB&IS, 58*.

Nitrd, N. (2016). *The Federal Big Data Research and Development Strategic Plan*. Networking and Information Technology Research and Development.

Olsen, L., & McGinnis, J. M. (2010). *Evidence Developmentfor Healthcare Decisions: Improving Timeliness*. Reliability, and Efficiency.

PatientsLikeMe. (2013). Available from: http://www.patientslikeme.com/

Patil, R. D., & Jadhav, O. S. (2016). Some Contribution of Statistical Techniques in Big Data: A Review. *International Journal on Recent and Innovation Trends in Computing and Communication, 4*(4), 293–303.

Paul, M. J., & Dredze, M. (2012). A model for mining public health topics from Twitter. *Health, 11*, 16–6.

Pulley, J. M., Denny, J. C., Peterson, J. F., Bernard, G. R., Vnencak-Jones, C. L., Ramirez, A. H., & Crawford, D. C. (2012). Operational implementation of prospective genotyping for personalized medicine: The design of the Vanderbilt PREDICT project. *Clinical Pharmacology and Therapeutics, 92*(1), 87–95. doi:10.1038/clpt.2011.371 PMID:22588608

Pyne, S., Rao, B. P., & Rao, S. B. (2016). Big Data Analytics: Views from Statistical and Computational Perspectives. In Big Data Analytics (pp. 1-10). Springer India.

Raghupathi, W., &Raghupathi, V. (2014). Big data analytics in healthcare: Promise and potential. *Health Information Science and Systems, 2*(1), 3.

Roney, K. (2012). *If Interoperability is the Future of Healthcare, What's the Delay. Becker's Hospital Review.*

Rumsfeld, J. S., Joynt, K. E., & Maddox, T. M. (2016). Big data analytics to improve cardiovascular care: Promise and challenges. *Nature Reviews. Cardiology, 13*(6), 350–359. doi:10.1038/nrcardio.2016.42 PMID:27009423

Russom, P. (2011). Big data analytics. *TDWI Best Practices Report, 19*, 40.

Sabia, S. K., & Kalra, S. (2014). Applications of big Data: Current Status and Future Scope. *SSN (Print), 3*(5), 2319–2526.

Sagiroglu, S., & Sinanc, D. (2013).Big data: A review. In *Collaboration Technologies and Systems (CTS), 2013 International Conference on* (pp. 42-47). IEEE. doi:10.1109/CTS.2013.6567202

Salathe, M., Bengtsson, L., Bodnar, T. J., Brewer, D. D., Brownstein, J. S., Buckee, C., & Vespignani, A. (2012). Digital epidemiology. *PLoS Computational Biology, 8*(7), e1002616. doi:10.1371/journal.pcbi.1002616 PMID:22844241

Savel, T. G., & Foldy, S. (2012). The role of public health informatics in enhancing public health surveillance. *MMWR. Surveillance Summaries, 61*(Suppl), 20–24. PMID:22832993

Scanfeld, D., Scanfeld, V., & Larson, E. L. (2010). Dissemination of health information through social networks: Twitter and antibiotics. *American Journal of Infection Control*, *38*(3), 182–188. doi:10.1016/j.ajic.2009.11.004 PMID:20347636

Seifter, A., Schwarzwalder, A., Geis, K., & Aucott, J. (2010). The utility of "Google Trends" for epidemiological research: Lyme disease as an example. *Geospatial Health*, *4*(2), 135–137. doi:10.4081/gh.2010.195 PMID:20503183

Sharma, V., Joshi, N. K., & Manisha. (2015). Big Data Introduction, Importance and Current Perspective of Challenges. *International Journal of Advances in Engineering Science and Technology*, *4*(3), 221–225.

Shivade, C., Raghavan, P., Fosler-Lussier, E., Embi, P. J., Elhadad, N., Johnson, S. B., & Lai, A. M. (2013). A review of approaches to identifying patient phenotype cohorts using electronic health records. *Journal of the American Medical Informatics Association*, *21*(2), 221–230. doi:10.1136/amiajnl-2013-001935 PMID:24201027

Shoenbill, K., Fost, N., Tachinardi, U., & Mendonca, E. A. (2013). Genetic data and electronic health records: A discussion of ethical, logistical and technological considerations. *Journal of the American Medical Informatics Association*, *21*(1), 171–180. doi:10.1136/amiajnl-2013-001694 PMID:23771953

Stone, M. L. (2014). *Big data for media. Reuters Institute For The Study Of Journalism*. University of Oxford.

Sullivan, S. J., Schneiders, A. G., Cheang, C. W., Kitto, E., Lee, H., & Redhead, J. (2011). What's happening? A content analysis of concussion-related traffic on twitter. *Br J Sports Med*. Available from: http://www.academia.edu/1037228/Whats_happening_A_content_analysis_of_concussion-related_traffic_on_Twitter

Swan, M. (2013). The quantified self: Fundamental disruption in big data science and biological discovery. *Big Data*, *1*(2), 85–99. doi:10.1089/big.2012.0002 PMID:27442063

Szlezák, N., Evers, M., Wang, J., & Pérez, L. (2014). The role of big data and advanced analytics in drug discovery, development, and commercialization. *Clinical Pharmacology and Therapeutics*, *95*(5), 492–495. doi:10.1038/clpt.2014.29 PMID:24642713

Talia, D. (2013). Clouds for scalable big data analytics. *Computer*, *46*(5), 98–101. doi:10.1109/MC.2013.162

Tan, P. N., Steinbach, M., & Kumar, V. (2013). Data mining cluster analysis: basic concepts and algorithms. *Introduction to Data Mining*.

Tasse, D. (2012). *Quantifiedself 2012: Some cool things. Tales 'n' ideas*. Available from: http://talesnideas.blogspot.com/2012_09_01_archive.html

Tenenbaum, J. D., Sansone, S. A., & Haendel, M. (2013). A sea of standards for omics data: Sink or swim? *Journal of the American Medical Informatics Association, 21*(2), 200–203. doi:10.1136/amiajnl-2013-002066 PMID:24076747

Ularu, E. G., Puican, F. C., Apostu, A., & Velicanu, M. (2012). Perspectives on big data and big data analytics. *Database Systems Journal, 3*(4), 3–14.

Unit, E. I. (2012). The deciding factor: Big data &decision making. *Capgemini Reports*, 1-24.

Ventura, A., Koenitzer, M., Stein, P., Tufano, P., & Drummer, D. (2015).The Future of FinTech: A Paradigm Shift in Small Business Finance. *World Economic Forum, Global Agenda Council on the Future of Financing and Capital.*

Walker, S. (2014). *Big data: A revolution that will transform how we live, work, and think*. Academic Press.

West, R., White, R. W., & Horvitz, E. (2013). From cookies to cooks: Insights on dietary patterns via analysis of web usage logs. In *Proceedings of the 22nd international conference on World Wide Web* (pp. 1399-1410). ACM.doi:10.1145/2488388.2488510

White, R. W., Tatonetti, N. P., Shah, N. H., Altman, R. B., & Horvitz, E. (2013). Web-scale pharmacovigilance: Listening to signals from the crowd. *Journal of the American Medical Informatics Association, 20*(3), 404–408. doi:10.1136/amiajnl-2012-001482 PMID:23467469

Wolf, G. (2012). The data-driven life. *The New York Times* Available from: http://www.nytimes.com/2010/05/02/magazine/02self-measurement-t.html

Yau, N. (2011). A year of food consumption visualized. *FlowingData*. Available from: http://flowingdata. com/2011/06/29/a-year-of-food-consumption-visualized/

Yoo, C., Ramirez, L., & Liuzzi, J. (2014). Big data analysis using modern statistical and machine learning methods in medicine. *International Neurourology Journal, 18*(2), 50. doi:10.5213/inj.2014.18.2.50 PMID:24987556

Yu, L., Zheng, J., Shen, W. C., Wu, B., Wang, B., Qian, L., & Zhang, B. R. (2012). BC-PDM: data mining, social network analysis and text mining system based on cloud computing. In *Proceedings of the 18th ACM SIGKDD international conference on Knowledge discovery and data mining* (pp. 1496-1499). ACM. doi:10.1145/2339530.2339764

Zhang, B., Gaiteri, C., Bodea, L. G., Wang, Z., McElwee, J., Podtelezhnikov, A. A., & Fluder, E. (2013). Integrated systems approach identifies genetic nodes and networks in late-onset Alzheimer's disease. *Cell, 153*(3), 707–720. doi:10.1016/j.cell.2013.03.030 PMID:23622250

Zicari, R. V. (2014). Big data: Challenges and opportunities. *Big Data Computing, 564*.

Chapter 5
Risks, Security, and Privacy for HIV/AIDS Data:
Big Data Perspective

Md Tarique Jamal Ansari
Babasaheb Bhimrao Ambedkar University, India

Dhirendra Pandey
Babasaheb Bhimrao Ambedkar University, India

ABSTRACT

Big data has the potential to transform healthcare systems for the prevention and treatment of HIV/AIDS by providing analytic tools that are capable of handling huge and different types of data at very fast speeds. Big data's transformative potential is also introverted by privacy and security requirements for HIV/AIDS patients' sensitive data that restrict health information exchange. Electronic health records provide the opportunity for HIV/AIDS patients to receive improved coordinated care from healthcare providers and easier access to their health information. This chapter discusses the various legal frameworks governing health information, dispels misconceptions about privacy regulations, and highlights how these legal frameworks provide privacy, confidentiality, and security to this sensitive information, and shows how EHRs can maximize the utility of big data to improve HIV/AIDS prevention and treatment.

DOI: 10.4018/978-1-5225-3203-3.ch005

INTRODUCTION

HIV is the virus that is the reason for AIDS (acquired immunodeficiency syndrome). Today's AIDS has become one of the world's most severe health and development challenges. UNAIDS/WHO estimates show that the first cases were informed in 1981 and today, there are approximately 36.7 million people currently living with HIV and tens of millions of people have passed away of AIDS-related causes since the commencement of the epidemic. However, several new cases have been reported in all regions of the world, approximately two-thirds are in sub-Saharan Africa, with 46% of new cases in Eastern and Southern Africa. According to the World Health Organization (WHO), "The human immunodeficiency virus (HIV) infects cells of the immune system, destroying or impairing their function. Infection with the virus results in progressive deterioration of the immune system, leading to "immune deficiency." The immune system is considered deficient when it can no longer fulfil its role of fighting infection and disease. Infections linked with severe immunodeficiency are known as "opportunistic infections" because they take benefit of a weakened immune system. AIDS is still a serious public health issue after three decades of prevention and treatment efforts. AIDS is the disease produced by destruction of the body's immune system from HIV. AIDS is a progressive step of HIV infection, originating when the immune system of the body no longer has the capacity to resist infections and other illnesses. Today's modern antiretroviral treatment (ART) is so effective and consistently used treatment at destroying HIV within a person's body.

Big data is revolutionizing the healthcare sector by providing effective data accessibility tools to healthcare analytics to support effective and predictive treatment. There are various big data technologies such as social networking, mobile applications any many other online tools which deliver the potential to be capable of using these data to design and develop HIV/AIDS monitoring technique.

In the United States, the Centers for Disease Control and Prevention (CDC) gather, analyzes, and distributes surveillance data on HIV infection. These huge amounts of data are one of the nation's primary sources of information on HIV. Big data tools provide reactive to proactive healthcare strategy which can result in a complete decrease in healthcare costs and eventually lead to economic growth. Big Data has the potential for significant financial and social benefits. Big data arises as a believable and cost-effective solution with the promise to transform the healthcare industry. Big data helps in prevention and control of HIV/AIDS but it also generates serious privacy, security and risk considerations. Security and privacy are always two different key concerns in information technology. In the big data era, the healthcare data volume is growing very fast. The healthcare data may contain structured EHR data, unstructured clinical data, medical imaging, genetic data and many other healthcare data. There are many severe security risks which are harmful to these healthcare data. The arrival of huge data sets from miscellaneous sources places an extra impediment to storage, processing, and communication. Security and privacy both are important to improving the public's health and maintaining the public's trust. Every stage of big data healthcare analytics in HIV/AIDS has several processes like the collection, combination, analysis, and practice has changed in current years in a way that could contemporary severe risks to individual privacy. HIV/AIDS patient faces high levels of discernment, avoidance, and disgrace around the world.

HIV/AIDS patient related all clinical and personal data are very sensitive nature of health data. Special attention should be paid to the security of data from vulnerability and dissemination of information on electronic format. Ensuring the security and privacy of HIV/AIDS personalized healthcare data are important to improving the public's health and maintaining the public's trust. Security and Privacy both are a vital concern for making the effort of prevention and treatment of HIV/AIDS successful. Sensitive health information like HIV/AIDS patient details could become more easily accessible and shareable as health records become fully automated, one can easily retrieve information over the internet. If sensitive health information is accessible by any unauthorized person, this would undoubtedly signify a breach of the HIV/AIDS patient's privacy. Healthcare providers, clinicians and other participants who are associated with such type of highly sensitive data, have a responsibility to preserve the confidentiality, privacy, and security of data and systems, and need to discourage access by unauthorized persons.

Implementation of big data analytics tools in HIV/AIDS treatment and prevention significantly increases security and patient privacy concerns. At the beginning, HIV/AIDS patient information is stored in databases with unpredictable levels of security. Furthermore, healthcare workers and clinicians need to accept by the law of privacy to guarantee patients' confidentiality, privacy, and security. Many countries have their own law and policy to protect health care data from any unauthorized access. Most HIV/AIDS data providers have HIPAA (Health Insurance Portability and Accountability) certification. HIPAA is mainly determined on authorizing security policies and procedures. In the USA, the Health Insurance Portability and Accountability Act (HIPAA) safeguards the privacy of health information, and all healthcare associations and providers are obliged to follow the privacy and security regulations of HIPAA. The Personal Information Protection and Electronic Document Act (PIPEDA) safeguard Individual's HIV/AIDS health information against use by profitable enterprises across regional and national boundaries in Canada. There are several others law and policies for the privacy and confidentiality of data like, The National HIV/AIDS Strategy and the Patient Protection and Affordable Care Act,

The Federal Data Breach Notification Law (HITECH), ISO 27799:2016, The Genetic Information Nondisclosure Act of 2008 (GINA), US freedom of information act.

INCREASING HEALTHCARE INFORMATION PRIVACY RISK

In this Big Data world while the EHRs are easily available to any authorized person over internet, huge data breaches are occurring with alarming frequency. In the following Table 1, an investigation of data breaches by industry shows that there is a need for technical and legitimate approach to make health care information more secure. The health care data breaches are now approximately 35 percent of all data breaches. Health care breaches are becoming a serious risk for the privacy for HIV/AIDS patients.

In India medical records are highly vulnerable without proper data security and privacy laws. Recently, a big healthcare breach was reported that the electronic medical records (EMR) of over 35,000 patients held by a Maharashtra based pathology lab were leaked, this shows the lack of availability of acceptable policy and procedures for security and privacy of such sensitive information. Such examples, however, are not surprising. Globally, the medical industry is extremely vulnerable to data breaches. The Office of Civil Rights under the US Department of Health and Human Services projected that in 2015 alone, over 100 million records were breached, with maximum cases being related to IT crimes and hacking (Akhil Deo, 2017). HIV/AIDS data breaches results into stigma for PLHA, is measured as a major barrier to effective responses to the HIV epidemic. However, there is little agreement among program implementers and policy-makers about how best to define, measure, and reduce the phenomenon (Mahajan et al., 2008).

Table 1. Percent of data breaches by industry sector

Industry	2005	2006	2007	2008	2009	2010	2011	2012	2013	2014	2015	2016
Business	15.9	20.9	29.1	36.1	40.6	41.4	42.0	34.4	31.8	33.6	40.1	45.2
Educational	47.8	24.9	24.9	20.0	15.7	9.8	13.5	13.4	8.8	7.3	7.4	9.0
Government/ Military	13.4	30.8	24.7	16.8	18.1	15.7	12.8	11.7	9.8	11.7	8.1	6.6
Health/Medical	10.2	13.7	14.1	15.1	14.1	24.9	24.2	35.5	44.1	42.5	35.3	34.5
Banking/Credit/ Financial	12.7	9.7	7.2	12.0	11.6	8.2	7.4	5.1	5.5	4.9	9.1	4.8

Source: Identify Theft Resource Center, Data Breach Reports, 2005–2016.

Figure 1.

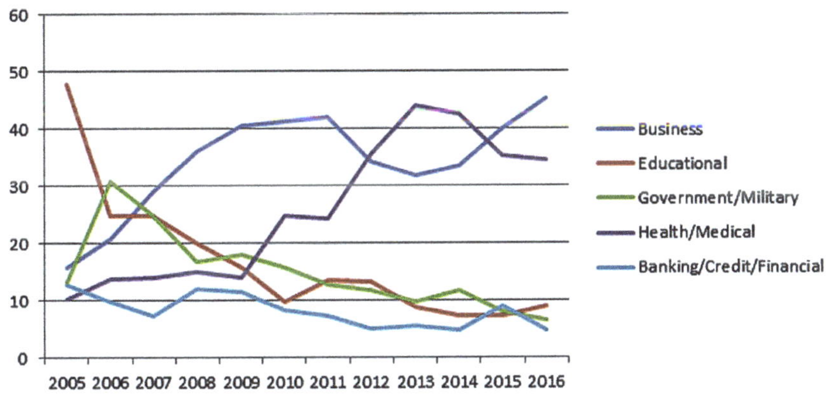

Big Data introduces security and privacy risks related to broadcasting the monitoring and sharing mechanism of HIV/AIDS sensitive data to a third-party., Risks that will need to be carefully evaluated and addressed by entities that intend to put genomic data of HIV/AIDS patients over the internet to the maintenance of the data on shared computing platforms. Safeguarding the confidentiality, integrity, availability, and privacy of data in for HIV/AIDS sensitive data is important to protecting the personal information of patients. For ensuring privacy the healthcare organization must have a systematic assessment of threats and risks that are present in a particular information system. National laws governing the privacy and security of HIV/AIDS patient sensitive health records require that government and private-sector organizations conduct a risk assessment as part of their security management processes. There is a need for the continuous monitoring system so that risks and vulnerabilities are reduced to a practical and applicable level.

BIG DATA AND HIV/AIDS

Today's patient security and privacy is a vital issue in the healthcare industry. Electronic health records (EHRs) technique is now becoming an integral part of the healthcare system and it is overbearing that EHRs are secure. It's a way to make it easier for everyone to be better informed and more involved in the patient's health care. EHRs provides several types of functionalities which consist of storage of health information and data, accessing of healthcare information, outcomes management, decision support, electronic communication and connectivity, order entry and management, patient support, administrative processes and reporting and population management (IOM, 2003). Privacy of personal health information is an important concern for many people living with HIV/AIDS. Suspicions of breaches in privacy and resultant HIV humiliation can result in patients not retrieving or adhering to care and treatment (Kempf et al., 2010). Security privacy and confidentiality are also an important concern for both individuals and society. Involvements of individuals are very rare in health research or other publically and individually valuable events, including truthful and complete disclosures of sensitive information to their physicians, if they do not have confidence in their privacy is being secure. However, it should also be noted that observations of privacy differ among individuals and groups. Information that is measured intensely private and confidential by one person may not be by others. The conception of privacy is also situation specific and acquires a different meaning depending on the stated reasons for the information being collected, the objectives of the gatherings involved, as well as the convention, politics and cultural expectations (IOM, 2009).

The mostly used way to stop the spread of HIV/AIDS is to treat those at high risk with a daily prophylactic pill but this is very expensive. It is possible to make it less expensive than the prophylactic pill with the help of big data and crackerjack software. The healthcare providers could track the outbreak in real-time and quickly help those at highest risk of infection. In June 2014, The British Columbia Centre for Excellence in HIV/AIDS (BC-CfE)'s monitoring system detected a cluster of 11 new HIV cases in a town just outside Vancouver and analyzes huge amounts of HIV genetic data to detect outbreaks (Megan Scudellari, 2016). The Solexa/ Illumina sequencing method and HiSeq instrument can produce more than 100 billion bases of sequence information in a single instrument run, and runs are collecting addressing questions in HIV research. Data from genome-wide association studies, HIV resistance testing, and epidemiological tracking all add to the flood. Given this massive volume of data, the development of digestible summaries becomes as important as generating the data itself (Frederic D. Bushman et al., 2013). In the past decade, computer-based support for therapy selection, which assesses the level of viral resistance against drugs, has become a mainstay for HIV patients (Lengauer et al., 2014).

Many healthcare organization, institutions and research laboratories have started to develop data repositories and computational tools for HIV research (Sayers et al. 2012). The Stanford HIV Drug Resistance Database hosts an easily and freely available online genotypic resistance analysis system called HIVdb to help clinicians and laboratories interpret HIV-1 genotypic resistance tests. The application's advantages are its accessibility for submitting sequences, its quality control analysis, its clearness and its widespread comments intended at educating the user. Sierra, the Stanford Algorithm web service is an extension that permits laboratories to analyze many sequences to individualize the format of their results. The ASI compiler creates and makes it conceivable for HIVdb to provide the outcome using a range of different HIV-1 genotypic resistance analysis algorithms (Tang el al., 2012).

The complexity, diversity and rich context of data being produced in healthcare are motivating the development of big data for health. Big data can help to enhancement the applicability of clinical research studies into real-world scenarios, where population heterogeneity is a problem. (Javier Andreu-Perez et al., 2015). Social networking technologies are the possible and satisfactory platform for the analysis of growing HIV and STD-related communication. Big data analytics from mobile technologies might be mainly useful in addressing HIV prevention and treatment efforts among these high-risk HIV/AIDS populations (Young et al., 2013). Today's bioinformatics, disease modeling, and digital epidemiology can be applied to address HIV prevention (Young, 2015).

Big Data in healthcare is still relatively a new tool which makes it challenging to find solid articles that provide an overview of the new technology. Big data quenches what little hope remains for the notice and choice management. Specified simply that upfront notice is not possible because new classes of goods and services reside in future and surprising uses (Cate, 2013).There are many challenges associated with big data like issues of privacy, security, compliance with rules and regulations (Jokonya, 2014). In particular, Big Data challenges the Fair Information Practices (FIPs), which is the set of standards prevailing the gathering and practice of personal data and addressing issues of privacy and accuracy (Rubinstein, 2012).

Table 2 contains the list of various HIV/AIDS data resources available over internet for researchers, clinicians, physicians and healthcare providers.

HIV/AIDS PATIENT DATA FLOW

The flow of HIV/AIDS patient data starts from the doctor's office to research laboratories, diagnostic labs, pharmacies, and other agencies working on HIV/AIDS. This data flow of HIV/AIDS patients provides many points where information security, privacy, and risk must be considered. Every point in this flow must be prepared with an information protection policy that is inclusive of Security, Privacy, and Risk Management solutions. HIV/AIDS patient electronic health care information are progressively being produced and distributed and interconnected across several points, including physician, research labs, diagnostic labs, patients, HIV/AIDS clinics, Hospitals, HIV/AIDS monitoring agencies and many other agencies working for the prevention and treatment of HIV/AIDS.

Table 2. List of HIV/AIDS data resources available over internet

Data Provider	Web Links	Description
Kaiser Family Foundation	http://kff.org/hivaids/	Provides the latest HIV AIDS data and information on the U.S. role in global health
CDC	https://www.cdc.gov/hiv/library/reports/hiv-surveillance.html	CDC provides the annual HIV Surveillance Report which is the overview on the current epidemiology of HIV disease in the United States and dependent areas.
WHO	http://apps.who.int/gho/data/node.main.617?lang=en	The world health organization provides the global health observatory data repository on HIV AIDS
UNAIDS	http://www.aidsinfoonline.org/devinfo/libraries/aspx/Home.aspx	This database contains country-reported GARPR data and Spectrum estimates
UCSF	http://hivinsite.ucsf.edu/	Developed by CHI at UCSF, This site has a broad collection of original material, including the HIV InSite Knowledge Base, a complete textbook with extensive references and related links organized by topic.
NCBI	https://www.ncbi.nlm.nih.gov/genome/viruses/retroviruses/hiv-1/interactions/	The national repository of biomedical data and literature. Provides HIV-1, human interactions database.
Los Alamos HIV Databases	http://www.hiv.lanl.gov/	Huge repository of HIV sequence and epitope information also offers access to a large number of tools that can be used to analyze and visualize these data.
Stanford University HIV Drug Resistance Database	http://hivdb.stanford.edu/index.html	Database of mutations in HIV conferring resistance to antiviral agents
NIAID	https://chemdb.niaid.nih.gov/	This database holds information mined from scientific literature on the structure and activity of compounds that have been tested against HIV, HIV enzymes or opportunistic pathogens.
BioAfrica	http://www.bioafrica.net/index.php	Provides information on HIV proteomics, subtype C distribution, and the REGA HIV-1 subtype tool
GPS-Prot	http://www.gpsprot.org/	A site for exploring interactions between, HIV and cellular proteins, with rich tools for follow-up.
HIV Replication Cycle	http://www.hivsystemsbiology.org/wiki/index.php/Introduction	A web-based account of the HIV replication cycle.
Gene Overlapper	http://www.hivsystemsbiology.org/GeneListOverlapper/	Provides output from genome-wide surveys of host-cell genes linked to HIV infection with tools for exploring overlaps

continued on following page

Table 2. Continued

Data Provider	Web Links	Description
HIV and AIDS Data Hub for Asia Pacific	http://www.aidsdatahub.org/	Provides high quality, accessible and recent data on HIV /AIDS in Asia and the Pacific.
Ryan White Services Report HRSA	https://hab.hrsa.gov/program-grants-management/ryan-white-hivaids-program-services-report-rsr	Provides HIV/AIDS program client-level data collected through the Ryan White HIV/AIDS Services Report (RSR).
Medicaid Statistical Information System	https://www.medicaid.gov/medicaid/data-and-systems/collection-systems/msis/index.html	Provides a large-scale database of all those eligible and receiving services under Medicaid and CHIP programs for every state and territory.
North American AIDS Cohort Collaboration on Research and Design (NA-ACCORD)	https://statepiaps7.jhsph.edu/naaccord/	North American regional representative of the International Epidemiologic Databases to Evaluate AIDS (IeDEA). Provides data on over 150,000 HIV-infected participants.
CFAR Network of Integrated Clinical Systems	https://www.uab.edu/cnics/	Provides electronic medical records-based network poised to integrate clinical data from the large and diverse population of HIV-infected persons.
HIV Research Network	https://cds.johnshopkins.edu/hivrn/index.cfm?do=sens.content&page=test_about_us.html	This is a network of HIV care providers from across the U.S. who provide timely demographic, clinical, and health services costs and utilization data linked to relevant clinical data on HIV-infected persons.
Clinical Case Registry: HIV	https://catalog.data.gov/dataset/clinical-case-registries-ccr	Databases designed to provide population-based data on VA patients infected with Human Immunodeficiency Virus (HIV) and/or Hepatitis C virus (HCV).
National Vital Statistics System	https://www.cdc.gov/nchs/nvss/	Provides inter-governmental data sharing in Public Health and the shared relationships, standards, and procedures.
aidsmap	http://www.aidsmap.com/	Provides a huge database of HIV prevention and treatment information, as well as a searchable global HIV/AIDS resource directory.

In general, every point must have legitimate and technical rules and regulations to provide security and privacy to HIV/AIDS patient data. This makes it challenging to break the security and privacy of patient's information across multiple points and easily recognize any attack to database when points are linked.

Figure 2. Data flow of HIV/AIDS

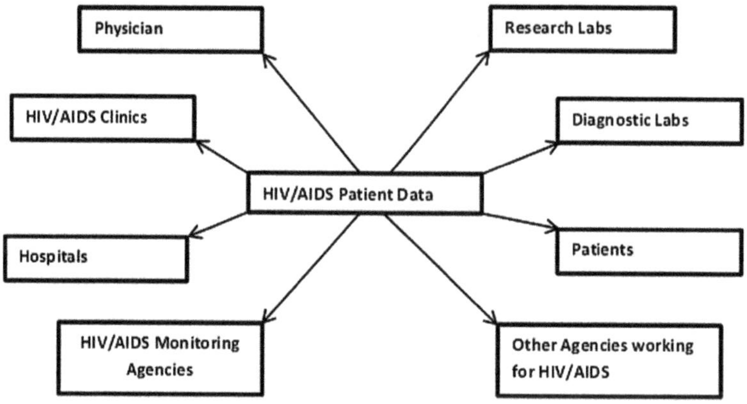

PROTECTING THE PRIVACY AND SECURITY OF HIV/AIDS PATIENT'S HEALTH RECORDS

Privacy and security are difficulties related to computer systems and applications that were not predicted until well into the second half of the present computer age. In 1976, Turn and Ware defined Privacy and Security, according to them "Privacy is an issue that concerns the computer community in connection with preserving personal information on individual citizens in computerized record keeping systems. It contracts with the civil rights of the individual regarding the collection of information in a record keeping system about his person and activities, and the processing, distribution, storage, and practice of this information in making determinations of him." They also define computer security as "Computer security includes the procedural and technical measures required to prevent illegal access, alteration, use, and dissemination of data stored or processed in a computer system. It is used to stop any thoughtful denial of service. It also includes several procedures to protect the system in its entirety from physical harm (Turn et al., 1976). There are several practices of big data presently fall into areas where there are no any proper rules and regulations. Due to the underdeveloped regulatory establishments, there is a requirement to have a secure big data policy, which must take into account the level of sensitivity of information used in predictive modeling. However, many organizations have not established best practices to ensure privacy and security of customer data. There is also the question of whose welfare, preferences and opinions are to succeed in the construction of big data related laws and policies in the future. The growing involvement of the individuals is likely to force further governing reaction to ensure that individual's information is protected (Kshetri, 2014). The increasing volume of HIV/AIDS patient's data in EHRs form, involvement of healthcare digital devices, and analytical tools that are now connected by digital networks has revolutionized the healthcare organization's ability to produce, share, transfer and access data. These electronic medical records must be protected from data breaches. The power of the international agreement over HIV/AIDS as a security issue tended to be exaggerated because of this within a few years that agreement seemed to have dissolved and important doubts had appeared over the indication for the hypothetical links between HIV and security (McInnes, 2010).

Physicians, researchers, clinicians and other health care bodies have a legitimate obligation to safeguard medical records from unauthorized and unlawful access, whether mischievous or unintended, by both insiders and hackers. To acquire this, organizations must have applicable privacy and security policies in place to protect the data, as well as risk-based management, administrative, and technical controls necessary to ensure information security. Securing personal patient information in large health care databases must be approached systematically. The majority of privacy and security risks can be addressed by conducting a risk assessment and prioritizing steps to secure an information system. As the amount of genomic information collected in electronic form continues to grow, the imperative of information security will only grow stronger.

In healthcare organization EHR systems must support the distribution of personal health care services, including care delivery, administrative processes, care management and care support processes. As individuals involve more enthusiastically in controlling of their own health, they too become important users of electronic health information. There are also important secondary uses, including education, regulation, clinical and health services research, public health and homeland security, and policy support (IOM, 2003). PLHA tend to be more worried about the social risks of treatment than about the medical outcomes of accessing counseling, testing

Figure 3. HIV/AIDS Big Data privacy and security interconnects with law, technology, and culture

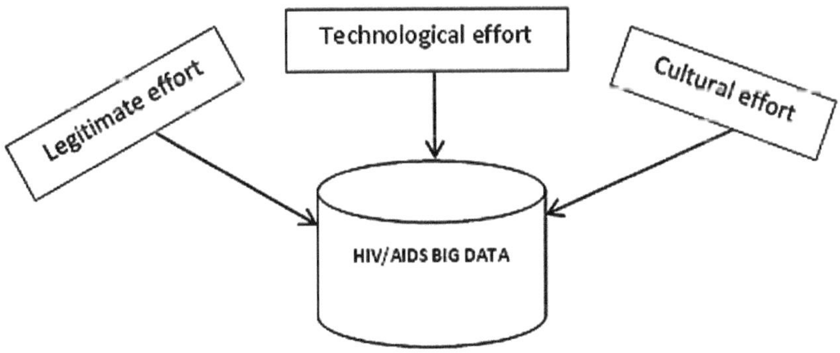

and treatment services. This type of situation is largely due to some superficial individual and organizational or structural-level gaps in the health care setting. Under ordinary situations, PLHA patients accessing health care services are involved in the required cure or treatment for their health problems, with slight attention in whether someone they know may see them in the hospital (Dapaah & Senah, 2016).

LEGITIMATE REQUIREMENTS AND CONSEQUENCES

HIV/AIDS patients strongly believe that their sensitive information should be distributed only among people involved in their treatment. They don't want to approve sharing of their health information to any third party. There are several legitimate procedures to provide Big Data security and privacy for HIV/AIDS patient's information.

Health Insurance Portability and Accountability Act

In 1996, The US Congress enacted the HIPAA (Health Insurance Portability and Accountability Act) to increase the effectiveness and efficiency of the health care system. The sharing and use of individual's health information are governed mainly by the Health Insurance Portability and Accountability Act at the national level (HIPAA, P.L. 104-191). HIPAA contains administrative simplification requirements that required HHS to adopt national standards for electronic health care transactions and code sets, unique health identifiers, and security. The US Congress recognized that advances in electronic technology could destroy the privacy of health information. Afterward, Congress merged into HIPAA requirements that instructed the adoption of National privacy protections for individually identifiable health information (Nass et. al.,2009). There are some cases in which the sturdiest safeguard of privacy, confidentiality, and security is often focused on specific areas of apprehension such as human immunodeficiency virus (HIV), AIDS, mental illness, or genetics information (Gostin, 2001). The main aim and focus of HIPAA is to assure that individuals' health information is appropriately protected while allowing the flow of health information needed to provide and promote high-quality health care and to protect the public's health and comfort. The Rule raids a balance that documents important uses of information while protecting the privacy of people who seek care and healing. HIPAA is intended to be flexible and complete to provide protection to the variety of practices and revelations that need to be addressed (Wilkes, 2014).

Health Insurance Portability and Accountability Act: Privacy Rule

The HIPAA Privacy Rule was developed under HIPAA's administrative simplification provisions by HHS, which instructed the creation of privacy standards for "protected health information" (PHI) in the absence of federal legislation. The main aim of the HIPAA Privacy Rule is to confirm that individuals' health information is accurately protected while allowing the flow of information needed to promote high-quality health care (IOM, 2009). In December 2000, HHS published a final Privacy Rule which was later amended in August 2002. This Rule is flexible and widespread to set national standards for the safeguard of independently distinguishable health information by three types of covered entities: health care providers, health plans and health care clearinghouses, and who conduct the standard health care transactions electronically. The HIPAA Privacy Rule spread over to all the entities that electronically communicate health information in connection with certain health care transactions like health plans, health care providers and health care clearinghouses (HHS, 2003). There are some data sets which differs from de-identified information in that they may comprise dates and some terrestrial information related to an individual that are absent from de-identified information. The HIPAA Privacy Rule does not apply to health information that has been de-identified in accordance with the Privacy Rule (HHS, 2003). Every health care provider should be aware that the Privacy Rule under the Health Insurance Portability and Accountability Act of 1996 (HIPAA) prescribes the use or revelation of a patient's health information, including HIV status, without the PLWHA's permission (Branson, 2006).

Health Insurance Portability and Accountability Act: Security Rule

On February 20, 2003, HIPAA Security Rule was published in which HIPAA mandate the secretary to implement security standards among other standards for certain health information (HHS, 2003). In the overview to the HIPAA Security Rule, there are many NIST publications were cited as possibly helpful resources for readers with raising vital problems and concerns related to the information security (Hash, 2005). In the case of protecting HIV/AIDS health information, HIPAA Security Rule explicitly emphases on the safeguarding of electronic protected health information (EPHI). Every healthcare organizations and HIV/AIDS patient data providers must comply with the HIPAA Security Rule, which explicitly emphases on

Figure 4. HIPAA privacy rule covered entities

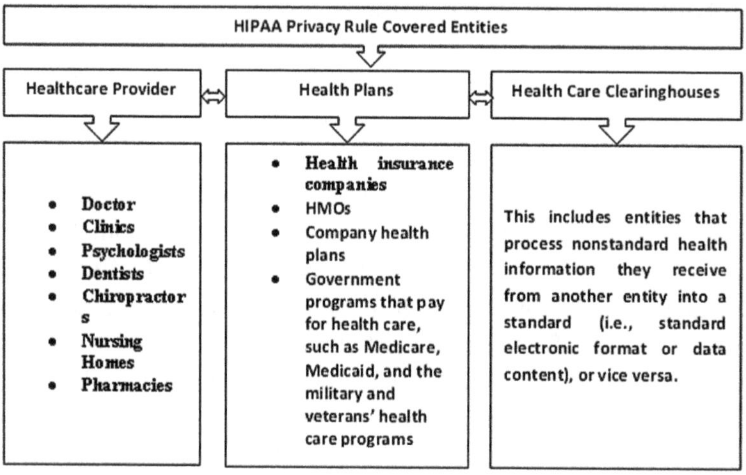

Source HHS, 2003

safeguarding the confidentiality, integrity, and availability of EPHI, as demarcated in the HIPAA Security Rule. The HIV/AIDS data providers who are responsible for creates, accepts, maintains, or communicates such sensitive information must be protected against judiciously predicted threats, vulnerabilities, and unauthorized uses and exposes. Today's the healthcare industry remains growing with the help of Big Data analytics. For the prevention and treatment of HIV/AIDS, healthcare organizations developing their strength through monitoring real time HIV/AIDS patient, scientific instrument involvement, technical approaches, following database privacy and security policy. Healthcare organizations and HIV/AIDS physicians must determine their role as factors of the confidentiality, privacy, and security of sensitive patient records.

The National HIV/AIDS Strategy and the Patient Protection and Affordable Care Act

The Patient Protection and Affordable Care Act of 2010 as revised by the Healthcare and Education Reconciliation Act of 2010, stated to collectively as the Affordable Care Act [ACA], which was signed into law in March 2010, makes an appropriate environment for implementing the National HIV/AIDS Strategy and makes its goals more achievable. Under the new law, individuals who are living with or at improved risk for HIV infection such as young marginal men will be more likely to be screened for HIV and to receive life-saving treatment and services that strengthen their ability to adhere to treatment regimens (Chen, 2012). After several challenges posed by HIV/AIDS, the White House Office of National AIDS Policy (ONAP) released a National HIV/ AIDS Strategy (NHAS) for the United States in July 2010. The primary goals of the NHAS are to reduce HIV incidence, increase access to care and optimize health outcomes for PLWHA, and reduce HIV-related health disparities (Spicer, 2012).

The NHAS is intended to build upon the Patient Protection and Affordable Care Act (ACA), which if implemented as originally planned is expected to bring millions of uninsured individuals, including many PLWHA, into the health care system. Examples of provisions of the ACA that may increase access to care for PLWHA include changes in eligibility requirements for public (e.g., Medicaid) and private health insurance, reduced out-of-pocket costs for Medicare Part D prescription drugs, expansion of coverage for preventive health services, and increased care capacity in community health centers.

The Personal Information Protection and Electronic Document Act (PIPEDA)

The Personal Information Protection and Electronics Documents Act (PIPEDA) was enacted by the Parliament of Canada, came into effect on 1 January 2001 for problems within federal jurisdiction, with the exception of the provisions on health information, which came into effect on 1 January 2002. The resolution of PIPEDA is to standardize the collection, use, and disclosure of personal information by organizations, healthcare sectors carrying on commercial activities (CMAJ, 1995). In the U.S., the Privacy Act of 1974 standardizes the collection of personal information by government agencies. There is no overarching federal law regulating private entities, but some states have their own laws, such as California's Online Privacy Protection Act of 2003. Generic privacy laws in other countries include Canada's Personal Information Protection and Electronic Documents Act (PIPEDA) and Directive 95/46/EC of the European Parliament, commonly known at the Data Protection Directive (Narayanan et. al, 2010). PIPEDA applied to personal information in the federally controlled private sector, such as broadcasting, airlines, banking sector, interregional transference, and telecommunications. PIPEDA is designed to regulate the collection, use, and disclosure of personal information in the private or commercial sector. PIPEDA is a Canadian laws and policies that support the right to privacy and the confidentiality of health record of people living with HIV/AIDS. It is anticipated for people living with HIV/AIDS and their advocates, for community-based organizations, and for legislators and policymakers. PIPEDA provides better legal privacy protections for people living with HIV/AIDS in Canada.

Health Information Technology for Economic and Clinical Health (HITECH)

On February 17, 2009, The US President Barack Obama has signed The American Recovery and Reinvestment Act (ARRA). This is commonly referred to at this juncture as the stimulus bill, includes $19.2 billion in provisions for health information technology and health information management. Title XIII of the ARRA, Health Information Technology, which is cited as the Health Information Technology for Economic and Clinical Health (HITECH) Act. This includes several amendments to HIPAA's privacy and security provisions (ARRA, 2009). HITECH Act makes stronger protections of healthcare information and also extends the privacy and security regulations of HIPAA to health care providers.

ISO 27799:2016

ISO 27799:2016 provides guidelines and best practices for healthcare information security. This also includes information security selection, implementation, and management of controls taking into consideration. The controls defined in ISO/IEC 27002 uses implementation guidelines of ISO 27799:2016 and increments them whenever there is a need to change it so that they can be effectively used for managing health information security. By implementing ISO 27799:2016, healthcare organizations and other custodians of health information will be able to ensure a minimum requisite level of security that is appropriate to their organization's circumstances and that will maintain the confidentiality, integrity, and availability of personal health information in their care. It applies to health information in all its aspects, whatever form the information takes for example words and numbers, sound recordings, drawings, video, and medical images etc. whatever means are used to store it like printing or writing on paper or storage electronically and whatever resources are used to transmit it, by hand, through fax, over computer networks, or by post, as the information is always appropriately protected (Health informatics, 2016).

The Genetic Information Non-Disclosure Act of 2008 (GINA)

GINA now will preclude insurers from doing so, the insurance industry may lack data that it believes will make insurance coverage more efficient. Some argue that since insurance companies may use other indicators, such as a manifested disease, to determine premiums and eligibility, they should be permitted to use genetic information. GINA is the first main American anti-discrimination statute in over a decade. GINA prohibits health insurers and employers from making decisions based on genetic information. While some examples do exist, both GINA's advocates and adversaries agreed that scant evidence indicated a significant history of genetic-information discrimination. (Joseph et al,2013). GINA protect the wide-ranging public from future discrimination on the basis of genetic information is sound and reasonable. Although the law still has some loopholes through which insurance providers and employers can jump, the protection provided under GINA satisfies many of the public's concerns (Donald et al., 2011). Due to GINA's inception and its demonstration genomic based healthcare data has grown tremendously and transforming approximately all areas of biomedical research especially healthcare sector.

US Freedom of Information Act

In some ways, a companion act to the FOIA, the Privacy Act of 1974, allows U.S. citizens and permanent resident aliens (but not noncitizens) certain rights with respect to information held about them by executive agencies of the federal government. These include: (1) the right to know how personal records are collected, maintained, used, and disseminated by the federal government; (2) the right to gain access to most kinds of personal information held about them; and (3) the right to amend information if it is found to be incorrect or incomplete. For the Privacy Act to apply, records have to be maintained in a system of records: In other words, records have to be grouped in a way that allows information from them to be retrieved by an identifier such as name or social security number. Information not held in this way is not subject to the Privacy Act but may be subject to the FOIA. In practice, the Privacy Act and the FOIA are often used together in making requests for information from federal agencies.

The Gramm-Leach-Bliley Act

In the US, protection of personal information privacy is a vital concern. Information privacy is a kind of commons that requires some degree of social control to construct and preserve (Janger et al., 2001) The Gramm-Leach-Bliley Act (GLBA) was enacted to make personal information more protective. The Gramm-Leach-Bliley Act (GLBA), which is also known as the Financial Services Modernization Act of 1999, provides limited privacy protections against the sale of your private financial information. Additionally, the GLBA codifies protections against pretexting, the practice of obtaining personal information by false pretenses. Gramm-Leach-Bliley Act, which generally placed restrictions on the exposé of non-public information to non-affiliated third parties, and required financial institutions, including health insurers, to provide customers or patient with notice regarding how their non-public personal information is used including an opportunity to "opt out" of certain disclosures. State departments of insurance and certain federal agencies adopted implementing regulations as required by federal law.

The Gramm-Leach-Bliley Act also gives banks and other financial institutions the ability to affiliate with insurance companies, which may lead to new competitors in the insurance and health benefits fields. It is the policy of the Congress that each financial institution has an affirmative and continuing obligation to respect the privacy of its customers and to protect the security and confidentiality of those customers' nonpublic personal information. In furtherance of the policy in subsection (a) of this section, each agency or authority described in section 6805(a) of this title shall establish appropriate standards for the financial institutions subject to their jurisdiction relating to administrative, technical, and physical safeguards (Code, 1999).

1. To ensure the security and privacy of customer and patient records especially financial and health insurance related data.
2. To safeguard against any expected threats or hazards to the security or integrity of such records
3. To safeguard against unauthorized and illegal access to such records which could result in substantial harm or inconvenience to any customer or patient.

CONCLUSION

In conclusion, this chapter has addressed the several law and policies which are available for the very sensitive big data of HIV/AIDS patients. Globally there are several organizations which are providing the data repository for HIV/AIDS data. Privacy, confidentiality, and security are dangerous issues as the health care organizations are approaching the EHRs. Protecting HIV/AIDS patient information is now becoming a global issue for the current era through continuous legislative and monitoring modifications as well as constitutional, private initiatives and technical approaches. This chapter investigates how current information security legitimate framework and policies provides adequate security, privacy, and confidentiality to HIV/AIDS EHRs. Several countries have different law and policies for implementing information security these policies should address both private and public interests to provide the maximum level of protection to highly sensitive HIV/AIDS data.

Currently, there are many legitimate frameworks provide policies for the privacy and confidentiality of PLWHA data likc privacy and security regulations of HIPAA. The Personal Information Protection and Electronic Document Act (PIPEDA) safeguard Individual's HIV/AIDS health information against use by profitable enterprises across regional and national boundaries in Canada. The National HIV/AIDS Strategy and the Patient Protection and Affordable Care Act, HITECH The Federal Data Breach Notification Law, ISO 27799:2016, The Genetic Information Nondisclosure Act of 2008 (GINA), US freedom of information act. Technologies are as yet insufficient and there is still an opportunity for improvement for the security of HIV/AIDS patient data. These types of data contain sensitive patient information which can have an impression on the patient's health and even their life. HIV/AIDS patient data involve different health information management activities for different purposes and information security is important for all these functionalities. There are ongoing discussions and progresses in the area of consent mechanisms to ensure information security of patients. As discussed earlier in this paper, requirements of consent for use of health information should not impede medical research and disease surveillance.

Consequently, there is a need for both technical and legitimate approach to address this efficiently to maintain HIV/AIDS patient privacy and fulfill the requirements of research and the epidemiology. Several risks associated with those healthcare organizations that do not follow a good security and privacy rules and regulations are primarily considerable. Several technical approaches for monitoring HIV/AIDS patient information securely incorporated into EHRs could be one of the solutions to this problem. Technically many authorization mechanisms integrating cryptographic techniques could possibly improve the information security of HIV/AIDS EHRs. Information security of these sensitive data should be considered extensively to ensure patient safety through providing secure EHRs to healthcare providers, clinicians, physicians, primary and secondary users of EHRs. Breach of information security can stem from a breach of confidentiality by authorized users and abuse of their access privileges. Therefore, ethical and legal responsibilities of users should also be considered for the information security of EHRs. This chapter focuses on the legitimate aspect of information security for HIV/AIDS sensitive EHRs and does not cover the various technical approaches for enhancing information security of HIV/AIDS EHRs.

REFERENCES

Andreu-Perez, J., Poon, C. C., Merrifield, R. D., Wong, S. T., & Yang, G. Z. (2015). Big data for health. *IEEE Journal of Biomedical and Health Informatics, 19*(4), 1193–1208. doi:10.1109/JBHI.2015.2450362 PMID:26173222

Branson, B. M., Handsfield, H. H., Lampe, M. A., Janssen, R. S., Taylor, A. W., & Lyss, S. B. (2006). Revised recommendations for HIV testing of adults, adolescents, and pregnant women in health-care settings. *MMWR. Recommendations and Reports, 55*(RR-14), 1–17. PMID:16988643

Bushman, F. D., Barton, S., Bailey, A., Greig, C., Malani, N., Bandyopadhyay, S., ... Krogan, N. (2013). Bringing it all together: Big data and HIV research. *AIDS (London, England), 27*(5), 835–838. doi:10.1097/QAD.0b013e32835cb785 PMID:23719353

Cate, F. H., & Mayer-Schönberger, V. (2013). Notice and consent in a world of Big Data. *International Data Privacy Law, 3*(2), 67–73. doi:10.1093/idpl/ipt005

Chen, M., Rhodes, P. H., Hall, I. H., Kilmarx, P. H., Branson, B. M., & Valleroy, L. A. (2012). Prevalence of undiagnosed HIV infection among persons aged≥ 13 years—National HIV Surveillance System, United States, 2005–2008. *MMWR. Morbidity and Mortality Weekly Report, 61*(02), 57–64. PMID:22695465

Code, U. S. (1999). *Gramm-Leach-Bliley Act. Gramm-Leach-Bliley Act/AHIMA*. American Health Information Management Association.

Dapaah, J. M., & Senah, K. A. (2016). HIV/AIDS clients, privacy and confidentiality; the case of two health centres in the Ashanti Region of Ghana. *BMC Medical Ethics, 17*(1), 41. doi:10.1186/s12910-016-0123-3 PMID:27422295

Deo, A. (2017). *Without Data Security and Privacy Laws, Medical Records in India Are Highly Vulnerable*. Retrieved April 20, 2017, from https://thewire.in/102349/without-data-security-and-privacy-laws-medical-records-in-india-are-highly-vulnerable/

Donald, C. G., & Sanders, A. K. (2011). The Genetic Information Nondiscrimination Act of 2008. *Journal of Diversity Management, 3*(4), 33–46. doi:10.19030/jdm.v3i4.5000

Gostin, L. O. (2001). National health information privacy: Regulations under the Health Insurance Portability and Accountability Act. *Journal of the American Medical Association, 285*(23), 3015–3021. doi:10.1001/jama.285.23.3015 PMID:11410101

Hash, J. (2005). *An introductory resource guide for implementing the health insurance portability and accountability act (HIPAA) security rule* (Doctoral dissertation). National Institute of Standards and Technology.

Health informatics – Information security management in health using ISO/IEC 27002 (2016)

HR 1, The American Recovery and Reinvestment Act of 2009 (ARRA). HITECH Provisions section 1301 et seq. Amends 42 USC section 201 et seq (Public Health Service Act (PHSA)) by adding Title XXX section 3000 et seq.

Institute of Medicine. (2003). *Committee on data standards for patient safety: board of health care services. Key capabilities of an electronic health record system: letter report*. The National Academy of Sciences.

IOM (Institute of Medicine). (2009). *Beyond the HIPAA Privacy Rule: Enhancing Privacy, Improving Health Through Research*. Washington, DC: The National Academies Press.

IOM (Institute of Medicine). (2012). *Monitoring HIV Care in the United States: Indicators and Data Systems*. Washington, DC: The National Academies Press.

Janger, E. J., & Schwartz, P. M. (2001). The Gramm-Leach-Bliley Act, Information Privacy, and the Limits of Default Rules. *Minnesota Law Review*, *86*, 1219.

Jokonya, O. (2014). Towards a Big Data Framework for the prevention and control of HIV/AIDS, TB and Silicosis in the mining industry. *Procedia Technology*, *16*, 1533–1541. doi:10.1016/j.protcy.2014.10.175

Joseph, S., Vargas, M., Johnson, J., & Timpte, C. (2013). The Genetic Information Nondiscrimination Act. BIOL, 4700, 03.

Kempf, M. C., McLeod, J., Boehme, A. K., Walcott, M. W., Wright, L., Seal, P., ... Moneyham, L. (2010). A qualitative study of the barriers and facilitators to retention-in-care among HIV-positive women in the rural southeastern United States: Implications for targeted interventions. *AIDS Patient Care and STDs*, *24*(8), 515–520. doi:10.1089/apc.2010.0065 PMID:20672971

Kshetri, N. (2014). Big data' s impact on privacy, security and consumer welfare. *Telecommunications Policy*, *38*(11), 1134–1145. doi:10.1016/j.telpol.2014.10.002

Lengauer, T., Pfeifer, N., & Kaiser, R. (2014). Personalized HIV therapy to control drug resistance. *Drug Discovery Today. Technologies*, *11*, 57–64. doi:10.1016/j.ddtec.2014.02.004 PMID:24847654

Mahajan, A. P., Sayles, J. N., Patel, V. A., Remien, R. H., Ortiz, D., Szekeres, G., & Coates, T. J. (2008). Stigma in the HIV/AIDS epidemic: A review of the literature and recommendations for the way forward. *AIDS (London, England)*, *22*(Suppl 2), S67. doi:10.1097/01.aids.0000327438.13291.62 PMID:18641472

McInnes, C., & Rushton, S. (2010). HIV, AIDS and security: Where are we now? *International Affairs*, *86*(1), 225–245. doi:10.1111/j.1468-2346.2010.00877.x

Narayanan, A., & Shmatikov, V. (2010). Myths and fallacies of personally identifiable information. *Communications of the ACM*, *53*(6), 24–26. doi:10.1145/1743546.1743558

Nass, S. J., Levit, L. A., & Gostin, L. O. (2009). *HIPAA, the Privacy Rule, and Its Application to Health Research*. Academic Press.

O'Reilly, M. (1995). Use of medical information by computer networks raises major concerns about privacy. *CMAJ: Canadian Medical Association Journal*, *153*(2), 212.

Rubinstein, I. S. (2012). Big Data: The End of Privacy or a New Beginning? *New York University Public Law and Legal Theory Working Papers*. Paper 357.D

Sayers, E. W., Barrett, T., Benson, D. A., Bolton, E., Bryant, S. H., Canese, K., ... Feolo, M. (2011). Database resources of the national center for biotechnology information. *Nucleic Acids Research*, *39*(suppl 1), D38–D51. doi:10.1093/nar/gkq1172 PMID:21097890

Scudellari, M. (2016). *Big Data Tamps Down HIV Outbreaks*. Retrieved March 30, 2017, from http://spectrum.ieee.org/the-human-os/biomedical/diagnostics/big-data-tamps-down-hiv-outbreaks

C. M. Spicer, & M. A. Ford (Eds.). (2012). *Monitoring HIV care in the United States: indicators and data systems*. National Academies Press.

Summary of the HIPAA Privacy Rule. (2017). Dep't Of Health & Human Servs. Retrieved from https://www.hhs.gov/sites/default/files/privacysummary.pdf.

Tang, M. W., Liu, T. F., & Shafer, R. W. (2012). The HIVdb system for HIV-1 genotypic resistance interpretation. *Intervirology*, *55*(2), 98–101. doi:10.1159/000331998 PMID:22286876

Turn, R., & Ware, W. H. (1976). *Privacy and security issues in information systems* (Vol. 5684). Rand Corporation. doi:10.7249/P5684

Wilkes, J. J. (2014). The Creation of HIPAA Culture: Prioritizing Privacy Paranoia over Patient Care. *BYU L. Rev.*, 1213.

Young, S. D. (2015). A "big data" approach to HIV epidemiology and prevention. *Preventive Medicine*, *70*, 17–18. doi:10.1016/j.ypmed.2014.11.002 PMID:25449693

Young, S. D., & Jaganath, D. (2013). Online social networking for HIV education and prevention: A mixed methods analysis. *Sexually Transmitted Diseases*, *40*(2), 162–167. doi:10.1097/OLQ.0b013e318278bd12 PMID:23324979

Chapter 6
Prevalence in MSM Is Enhanced by Role Versatility

Andrés J. Cortés
University of Gothenburg, Sweden & Colombian Corporation for Agricultural Research, Colombia

ABSTRACT

In the community of men who have sex with men (MSM) the prevalence of the HIV-1 infection is still high. Promiscuity and condom fatigue are making unprotected anal intercourse (UAI) more common and sexually transmitted infections (STIs) presumably harder to track. Yet, MSM communities are peculiar in the sense that men can adopt fixed (insertive or receptive) or versatile (both practices) roles. Some old theoretical work predicted that the transmission of HIV-1 would be enhanced in MSM populations engaged more in role versatility than in role segregation, in which fixed roles are predominantly adopted. These predictions were based on the assumption that the probability of acquisition from unprotected insertive anal (UIA) sex was neglectable, which is an inappropriate assumption. This chapter shows that the increase of the HIV-1 prevalence among MSM due to role versatility holds under a stronger assumption of bidirectional virus transmission.

DOI: 10.4018/978-1-5225-3203-3.ch006

BACKGROUND

The prevalence of the HIV-1 infection has decayed in the last decades in western heterosexual populations (Beyrer *et al.,* 2012). However, in the community of men who have sex with men (MSM) the prevalence is still high, despite intensive campaigns and treatment programs that keep infected men as undetectable (Beyrer *et al.,* 2012). Promiscuity and condom fatigue (Adam *et al.,* 2005), which are not unique to the MSM community, are making unprotected anal intercourse (UAI) more common and sexually transmitted infections (STIs) presumably harder to track. Yet, MSM communities are peculiar in the sense that men can adopt fixed (insertive or receptive) or versatile (both practices) roles. Some old theoretical work (Trichopoulos *et al.* 1998; Van Druten *et al.* 1992; Wiley & Herschkorn 1989) predicted that the transmission of HIV-1 would be enhanced in MSM populations engaged more in role versatility than in role segregation, in which fixed roles are predominantly adopted. These predictions were based on the assumption that the probability of acquisition from unprotected insertive anal (UIA) sex was neglectable. However, as later shown (Goodreau *et al.* 2005; Vittinghoff *et al.* 1999), this assumption is inappropriate and HIV-1 can still be acquired, although at a lower rate, via UIA sex. Here I show that the increase of the HIV-1 prevalence among MSM due to role versatility holds under a stronger assumption of bidirectional virus transmission.

I aim developing a stochastic model to demonstrate that in MSM populations that practice UAI, the prevalence of the HIV-1 infection decays when there is a transition from role versatility to role segregation without assuming that the long-term probability of acquisition from UIA sex with receptive infected partners is negligible. In other words, I will demonstrate, in a more realistic scenario that allows for bidirectional virus transmission, that the high prevalence of the HIV-1 infection in MSM populations can still theoretically be attributed to role versatility.

METHODS: A STOCHASTIC MODEL WITH DIFFERENT ROLE CLASSES

The following is assumed:

- The MSM population practices UAI.
- There is random mixing among individuals and sexual-role classes.

- A corollary of the previous assumption is that there is not role assortativity, which is when versatile MSM preferentially choose other versatile MSM as partners, or when insertive MSM preferentially choose receptive over versatile MSM as partners, or when receptive MSM preferentially choose insertive over versatile MSM as partners. Versatile individuals have the same preference of being insertive or receptive when their partners are also versatile.

By defining H as the prevalence of the HIV-1 infection at the MSM population (proportion of the population that is infected), and *B*, *V* and *T* as the proportion of males within the MSM population that have a receptive (*B*), versatile (*V*) and insertive (*I*) role (so that $B+V+T=1$), the prevalence is given by:

$$H = P(I \mid B)B + P(I \mid V)V + P(I \mid T)T \tag{1}$$

where $P(I \mid B)$, $P(I \mid V)$ and $P(I \mid T)$ are the probabilities that an individual within the population is infected given that his sexual role is receptive, versatile or insertive, respectively. These conditional probabilities are defined as follows:

$$P(I \mid B) = \rho P(I \mid V)V + \rho P(I \mid T)T \tag{2}$$

$$P(I \mid V) = \iota P(I \mid B)B + \frac{1}{2}\iota P(I \mid V)V + \frac{1}{2}\rho P(I \mid V)V + \rho P(I \mid T)T \tag{3}$$

$$P(I \mid T) = \iota P(I \mid B)B + \iota P(I \mid V)V \tag{4}$$

where ρ is the long-term probability of acquisition from URA sex with infected insertive partners and ι is the long-term probability of acquisition from UIA sex with receptive infected partners. In other words, the probability that an individual within the population is infected given his sexual role is defined by the expected prevalence of the infection at each of his potential-partners' sexual-role classes ($E(H \mid B) = P(I \mid B)B$, $E(H \mid V) = (I \mid V)V$ and $E(H \mid T) = P(I \mid T)T$) weighted by the long-term probability of acquisition from UAI with insertive ρ or receptive ι infected partners.

Notice that these very same probabilities, with some reformulation of ρ and ι, can be used to estimate the number of sexual encounters until infection (*K*) and the incidence, or the number of new infections in an interval of length *t*, *N(t)* (see section Extensions").

HIV-1 PREVALENCE AT DIFFERENT FREQUENCIES OF THE VERSATILE ROLE

For the HIV-1 infection previous models (Trichopoulos *et al.*, 1998; Van Druten *et al*, 1992; Wiley & Herschkorn, 1989) have assumed that the long-term probability of acquisition from UIA sex with receptive infected partners is negligible ($\iota \to 0$). Under this condition, $\lim_{\iota \to 0} P\left(I \mid T\right) = 0$ and equations (1-3) are simplified as follows:

$$\lim_{\iota \to 0} P\left(I \mid B\right) = \rho P\left(I \mid V\right) V \quad (5)$$

$$\lim_{\iota \to 0} P\left(I \mid V\right) = \frac{1}{2} \rho P\left(I \mid V\right) V \quad (6)$$

$$\lim_{\iota \to 0} H = \left[B + \frac{1}{2} V\right] \rho P\left(I \mid V\right) V \quad (7)$$

Observe that by assuming that the long-term probability of acquisition from UIA sex with receptive infected partners is negligible, the prevalence, as in equation (7), would tend to zero as the versatile role disappears ($V \to 0$), confirming previous predictions (Trichopoulos *et al.*, 1998; Van Druten *et al.*, 1992; Wiley & Herschkorn, 1989). However, some studies (Goodreau et al., 2005; Vittinghoff *et al.*, 1999) suggest that the assumption $\iota \to 0$ may be inappropriate. Then, in more general terms, as the versatile role disappears ($\lim_{V \to 0} \left(B + T\right) = 1$) the probabilities that an individual is infected given his sexual role (2-4), and the prevalence of the infection at the MSM population (1), would be simplified as follows:

$$\lim_{V \to 0} P\left(I \mid B\right) = \rho P\left(I \mid T\right) T \quad (8)$$

$$\lim_{V\to 0} P\left(I \mid T\right) = \iota P\left(I \mid B\right) B \tag{9}$$

$$\lim_{V\to 0} \frac{H}{\rho} = \frac{\iota}{\rho} B\left[1-B\right]\left[\rho B+1\right] P\left(I \mid B\right) \tag{10}$$

Yet, a property of the HIV-1 epidemic is that it is more likely to acquire the infection by performing URA sex with infected insertive partners than UIA sex with infected receptive partners, without the latter being negligible (Beyrer *et al.,* 2012; Goodreau *et al.,* 2005; Vittinghoff *et al.,* 1999; Bezemer *et al.,* 2015). By incorporating into the last equation this condition ($\rho \gg \iota$), which can be expressed as $\iota / \rho \to 0$, and knowing that $\rho > 0$, the prevalence *H*, as in equation (10), would then tend to zero:

$$\lim_{\substack{V\to 0 \\ \iota/\rho\to 0}} \frac{H}{\rho} = 0 \tag{11}$$

In other words, as the versatile role disappears ($V \to 0$) and is more likely to get infected by performing URA than UIA sex with infected partners ($\iota / \rho \to 0$), the prevalence of the HIV-1 infection tends to zero ($H \to 0$) (Figure 1).

DISCUSSION

Promiscuity (i.e. random mixing among individuals and sexual-role classes) is intrinsic to the present model. Therefore, I have shown that the prevalence of the infection in a promiscuous MSM population engaged in UAI would decrease as role segregation was practiced instead of role versatility without reducing the level of promiscuity and by allowing for bidirectional virus transmission. This is because in MSM populations engaged in role segregation the receptive partners, those most easily infected, are less likely to transmit the infection, while in MSM populations engaged in role versatility, the versatile individual, who is easily infected through URA sex, can rapidly transmit the infection through UIA sex. A negative feedback like this could explain why MSM populations in the Middle East, which exhibit strong role segregation because of cultural factors (i.e. anal intercourse among men is common before marriage and is a sign of manliness for the insertive partner), have a lower prevalence of the HIV-1 infection (Beyrer *et al.,* 2012).

Figure 1. Schematic representation of the prevalence of the HIV-1 infection given different proportions of the sexual roles in the MSM population. The Finetti diagram is depicting the overall prevalence (H) of the HIV-1 infection in the MSM population at different proportions of the receptive (B), versatile (V) and insertive (T) roles, so that $B+V+T=100\%$. H scores are relative because ρ and ι are undefined. High H scores are in red.

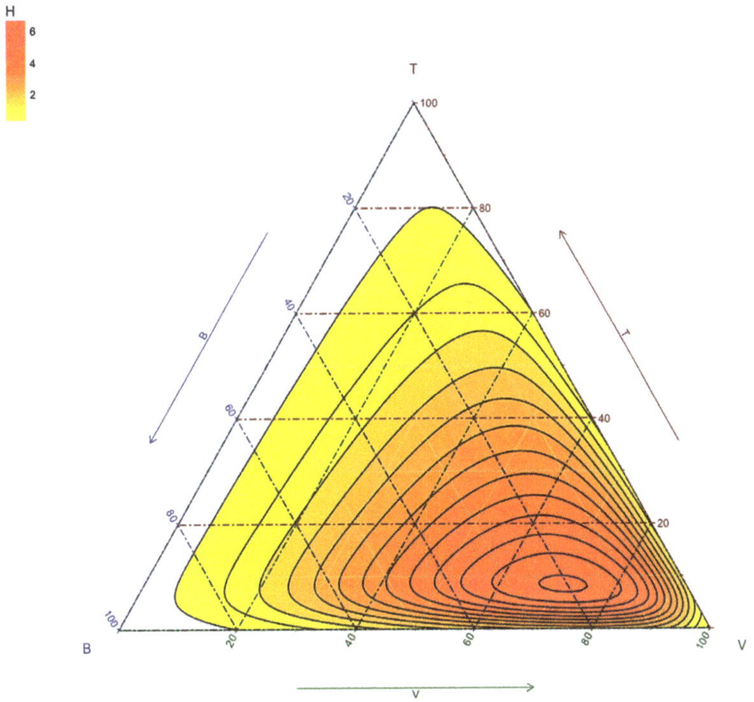

By reworking an old prediction under a more realistic scenario of role-conditioned contact risk, I demonstrated, under a strong assumption of bidirectional virus transmission, that HIV-1 prevails among MSM because of role versatility. This should raise awareness among infectiologists and the general public that besides trivial factors that may impact the prevalence of HIV-1, such as condom usage and promiscuity, sexual role segregation may drastically limit the spread of the virus in MSM populations. The suppression of role versatility, as by definition happens in heterosexual partners, is enough to drop the incidence of the HIV-1 infection.

EXTENSIONS

The original model was defined as follows:

$$\begin{bmatrix} -1 & \rho V & \rho T \\ \iota B & \frac{1}{2}(\iota+\rho)V-1 & \rho T \\ \iota B & \iota V & -1 \end{bmatrix} \begin{bmatrix} P(I \mid B) \\ P(I \mid V) \\ P(I \mid T) \end{bmatrix} = \begin{bmatrix} 0 \\ 0 \\ 0 \end{bmatrix} \tag{A}$$

By redefining ρ as the probability of acquisition from one-time URA sex with an infected insertive partner and ι as the probability of acquisition from one-time UIA sex with a receptive infected partner, it is possible to model new descriptors.

For instance, the number of sexual encounters until infection (*K*) given a specific sexual role is then described by a geometric distribution with probability $P(I \mid B)$, $P(I \mid V)$ or $P(I \mid T)$ (B), and the expected number of sexual encounters until infection $E(K)$ given a specific sexual role is $1 / P(I \mid B)$, $1 / P(I \mid V)$ or $1 / P(I \mid T)$ (C). In equations (B-E) *R* refers either to *B*, *V* or *T*.

$$P(K = k \mid R) = [1 - P(I \mid R)]^{k-1} P(I \mid R) \tag{B}$$

$$E(K \mid R) = \frac{1}{P(I \mid R)} \tag{C}$$

Similarly, the incidence, or the number of new infections in an interval of length *t*, $N(t)$, given a specific sexual role, is described by a Poisson process (D) with λ defined as $\lim_{t \to \infty} N(t) / t$, which by definition is the size of the MSM population per unitoftime(*S*)times $P(I \mid B)B$, $P(I \mid V)V$ or $P(I \mid T)T$,thatis $\lambda = P(I \mid R)RS$.

$$P_t(N = n \mid R) = \frac{[\lambda t]^n e^{-\lambda t}}{n!} \tag{D}$$

$$E(P_t \mid R) = \lambda t \tag{E}$$

and the incidence at the population level is:

$$P_t\left(N=n\right)=\frac{\left[\lambda t\right]^n e^{-\lambda t}}{n!} \tag{F}$$

$$E\left(P_t\right)=\lambda t \tag{G}$$

where $\lambda = P\left(I \mid B\right)BS + P\left(I \mid V\right)VS + P\left(I \mid T\right)TS$

ACKNOWLEDGMENT

I am grateful with Janosch Sedlacek (RIP) and Julia Wheeler for the enriching discussions that took place in the fall of 2013 in Konstanz, Germany, and that ultimately inspired the development of this model.

REFERENCES

Adam, B.D., Husbands, W., Murray, J., & Maxwell, J. (2005). AIDS optimism, condom fatigue, or self-esteem? Explaining unsafe sex among gay and bisexual men. *Journal of Sex Research*, *42*, 238-48.

Beyrer, C., Baral, S. D., van Griensven, F., Goodreau, S. M., Chariyalertsak, S., Writz, A. L., & Brookmeyer, R. (2012). Global epidemiology of HIV infection in men who have sex with men. *Lancet*, *28*(9839), 367–377. doi:10.1016/S0140-6736(12)60821-6 PMID:22819660

Bezemer, D., Cori, A., Ratmann, O., van Sighem, A., Hermanides, H. S., Dutilh, B. E., ... Fraser, C. (2015). Dispersion of the HIV-1 Epidemic in Men Who Have Sex with Men in the Netherlands: A Combined Mathematical Model and Phylogenetic Analysis. *PLoS Medicine*, *12*(11), e1001898. doi:10.1371/journal.pmed.1001898 PMID:26529093

Goodreau, S. M., Goicochea, L. P., & Sanchez, J. (2005). Sexual role and transmission of HIV Type 1 among men who have sex with men, in Peru. *The Journal of Infectious Diseases*, *191*(s1), S147–S158. doi:10.1086/425268 PMID:15627225

Trichopoulos, D., Sparos, L., & Petridou, E. (1998). Homosexual role separation and spread of AIDS. *Lancet*, *2*, 965–966. PMID:2902413

Van Druten, H., Van Griensven, F., & Hendriks, J. (1992). Homosexual role separation: Implications for analyzing and modeling the spread of HIV. *Journal of Sex Research*, *29*(4), 477–499. doi:10.1080/00224499209551663

Vittinghoff, E., Douglas, J., Judson, F., McKirnan, D., & MacQueen, K. (1999). Per-contact risk of human immunodeficiency virus transmission between male sexual partners. *American Journal of Epidemiology*, *150*(3), 306–311. doi:10.1093/oxfordjournals.aje.a010003 PMID:10430236

Chapter 7
Dissection of HIV-1 Protease Subtype B Inhibitors Resistance Through Molecular Modeling Approaches:
Resistance to Protease Inhibitors

Ameeruddin Nusrath Unissa
National Institute for Research in Tuberculosis (NIRT), India

Luke Elizabeth Hanna
National Institute for Research in Tuberculosis (NIRT), India

ABSTRACT

Protease (PR) is an important enzyme required for the posttranslational processing of the viral gene products of type-1 human immunodeficiency virus (HIV-1). Protease inhibitors (PI) act as competitive inhibitors that bind to the active site of PR. The I84V mutation contributes resistance to multiple PIs, and structurally, this mutation affects both sides of the enzyme active site. In order to get insights about this major resistance site to PR inhibitors using in silico approaches, in this chapter, the wild-type (WT) and mutant (MT) I84V of PR were modeled and docked with all PR inhibitors: Atazanavir, Darunavir, Indinavir, Lopinavir, Nelfinavir, Saquinavir, and Tipranavir. Docking results revealed that in comparison to the WT, the binding score was higher for the MT-I84V. Thus, it can be suggested that the high affinity towards inhibitors in the MT could be due to the presence of energetically favorable interactions, which may lead to tight binding of inhibitors with the MT protein, leading to the development of PR resistance against PIs in HIV-1 eventually.

DOI: 10.4018/978-1-5225-3203-3.ch007

INTRODUCTION

Protease (PR) is an essential enzyme that is required for the posttranslational processing of the viral gag and gag-pol polyprotein gene products, which yields the structural proteins and enzymes of the type-1 human immunodeficiency virus (HIV-1) particle. HIV-PR is a dimeric aspartic protease that consists of two identical, non-covalently associated subunits of 99-amino acid residues (Wlodawer & Erickson, 1993). The active site is covered over by two P-hairpin structures, or "flaps," that are highly flexible and undergo large localized conformational changes during the binding and release of inhibitors and substrates (Collins, Burt, & Erickson, 1995). To date several crystal structures of HIV-PR inhibitor complexes have been solved to aid the process of inhibitor design, these complexes enables to understand the mechanisms of resistance at an atomic level (Appelt, 1993; Fitzgerald & Springer, 1991). Mutations of specificity-determining residues that would directly interfere with inhibitor binding constitute an obvious mechanism for resistance to PR inhibitors which are otherwise known as PI. On the other hand, mutations at the non-active site of the enzyme that indirectly interfere with inhibitor binding via long-range structural perturbations represent other resistance pathways. Such mutations that eventually result in an enzyme with enhanced catalysis and cleavage site mutations that lead to enhanced processing by mutant enzymes, and "regulatory'' mutations elsewhere in the genome that lead to improved viral growth in the presence of PR inhibitors (Erickson, Gulnik, & Markowitz, 1999).

Clinically resistance to PIs such as Atazanavir ATV, Darunavir (DRV), Indinavir (IDV), Lopinavir (LPV), Nelfinavir (NFV), Saquinavir (SQV) and Tipranavir (TPV) has been well documented. More mutations are selected by the PI than by any other class of anti-retro virals. The effect of PI resistance mutations on individual PI may be difficult to quantify when many mutations are present in the same virus isolate or when mutations occur in unusual patterns. The effect of PI resistance mutations on drug susceptibility can also be modulated by gag cleavage site mutations and possibly other parts of gag that influence Gag-Pol processing (Guha & Haldar, 2012).

Twenty-three mutations in 16 codons of the PR gene related to major drug-resistance to PIs were identified by phenotypic resistance assays according to the estimates of International AIDS Society (Rhee et al., 2003). Differences in polymorphisms in the protease gene have been reported among different subtypes. For examples, the D30N mutation is associated with subtype B viruses and the L90M mutation is favored in the subtypes G, CRF02_AG, and CRF02_AE isolates with treatment failure (Santos & Soares, 2011).

Major mutations site of PR are 30, 46, 50, 83, 84, 90, while minor mutations sites are 10, 20, 24, 32, 35, 54, 71, 73, 77, etc., (Guha & Haldar, 2012; Rhee et al., 2003; Wainberg, Zaharatos, & Brenner, 2011). Amongst the major drug-resistance to PIs, the signature D30N mutation causes high-level resistance to NFV (Santos & Soares, 2011) and R8Q/K confers high-level resistance to some of the earliest PIs. L90M mutation is associated with resistance to many PIs (Shafer et al., 2001). V32I is associated to reduce susceptibility to all PIs, except SQV (Shafer et al., 2001). Further, the drugs such as LPV and DRV shows high genetic barrier for resistance (Guha & Haldar, 2012). V82A/T/F/S cause resistance to IDV, RTV, and LPV, when present with other mutations, these mutations contribute resistance to NFV, ATV, and SQV. V82I is a polymorphism that does not appear to be associated with drug resistance (Shafer et al., 2001).

Of significance, when compared to others the I84V mutation contributes resistance to each of the PIs (Shafer et al., 2001). In addition, on the basis of the structural parameters of PR also, the most intriguing mutation is the I84V that affects both sides of the enzyme's active site because of the symmetry of the enzyme. Since the inhibitor is asymmetric, the two mutations were predicted to have different effects, but the net result was a loss of interaction in going from the bulky isobutyl side chain of Ile to the smaller isopropyl side chain of Val (Erickson & Burt, 1996; Antunes et al., 2014). In line with this discussion, in our study, to understand the differences in the binding affinity between this clinically essential mutant (MT- I84V) and wild-type (WT) of HIV-1 protease protein which eventually lead to PR resistance. The MT- I84V of PR was allowed to interact with seven drugs such as ATV, DRV, IDV, LPV, SQV, NFV and TPV using *in silico* approaches in comparison to WT.

MATERIALS AND METHODS

Template Selection and Homology Modeling of Mutant PR

In the present study, the target PR protein sequence (P03369) was obtained from the Uniprot database (http://www.uniprot.org/) and submitted to protein alignment program (BLASTp) (Altschul et al., 1997) wherein the program searched the sequence against protein database (PDB) (http://www.rcsb.org/pdb/home/home.do). From the search, the crystal structure of PR enzyme of HIV-1 known as 4HVP was found as template and wild-type (WT) (Miller et al.,1989).

Model Building

The residue Ile at position 84 of PR of HIV-1 in template was substituted to Val to create the MT (I84V) protein. Further, in the synthetic template protein 4HVP, A chain was retained and the heteroatoms such as water and others were removed, and command line options were provided for sequence alignment between WT and template, followed by a series of commands for model building using software MODELLER9v14 were provided (Sali, 1995).

Model Evaluation

Validation of the models was done by Ramachandran plot (Lovell et al., 2003). Further the deviation between the WT and the models upon structural superimposition was calculated using PDBeFOLD (Krissinel & Henrick, 2003).

Ligands

The ligands ATV, DRV, IDV, LPV, NFV, SQV and TPV used in this study were obtained from Chemspider database [http://www.chemspider.com]. Chemsketch software (ACD/Chemsketch version 10.0) was used to obtain the structure of the ligand in Mol format and the ligand was saved as Mol2 file using software Discovery Studio (Jones, Willett, & Glen, 1995).

Discovery Studio (DS)

The software v-2.0 was used for visualization purpose of modeled proteins, and docking data Jones, Willett, & Glen, 1995).

Docking Protocol

Docking was carried out with the help of software-GOLD (Discovery Studio, version 2) The GOLD protocol is based on the concept of genetic algorithm wherein the receptor is held rigid while the ligands are allowed to flex during the refinement process. *The input files for both the protein (WT and MT) and the ligands were generated.* Followed by energy minimization, Hydrogen atoms were added to the model and ligands using auto edit option in GOLD before docking. The cavity atom file containing the atom number of binding residues was prepared for ligands such as ATV, DRV, IDV, LPV, NFV, SQV and TPV (Arg 8, Asp 25, Ala 28, Gly 27, Asp 29, Gly 48, Gly 49, Ile 50, Pro 81, and Ile 84. The binding residues were selected based on comparison between the binding regions of 4HVP (Miller et al., 1989).

Dockings were performed under 'Standard default settings' mode- number of islands was 5, population size was 100, number of operations was 100,000, niche size was 2, and selection pressure was 1.1. Ten docking poses were obtained for each ligand. Poses with highest GOLD score were used for further analysis. The docked poses of the ligands were visualized using DS. The scoring function of GOLD provides a way to rank the ligands relative to one another. Ideally, the score should correspond directly to the binding affinity of the ligand for the protein, so that the best scoring ligand poses are the best binders.

RESULTS

Template Selection and Homology Modeling of MT of PR

4HVP was identified as the template as it displayed maximum identity with the PR protein (Figure 1) using BLASTp search against PDB. Mutant model of PR was built based on substitution at codon 84 in the WT- protein sequence (P03369) of PR of HIV-1, using MODELLER 9v14 (Figure 2) respectively.

Evaluation of Residues

- Number of residues in favoured region (~98.0% expected): 89 (93.7%)
- Number of residues in allowed region (~2.0% expected): 5 (5.3%)
- Number of residues in outlier region: 1 (1.1%)

Figure 1. BLASTp result showing 92% identity between template (4HVP) A chain and the target WT-PR sequence (P03369) of HIV-1

NCBI Blast:Protein Sequence (99 letters)

Chain A, Structure Of Complex Of Synthetic Hiv-1 Protease With A Substrate- Based Inhibitor At 2.3 Angstroms Resolution

Sequence ID: 4HVP_A **Length:** 99 **Number of Matches:** 1

e 1 more title(s)

Range 1: 1 to 99 GenPept Graphics Next Match Previous Match

Related Information

Structure - 3D structure displays

PubChem BioAssay - bioactivity screening

Identical Proteins - Identical proteins to 4HVP_A

Score	Expect	Method	Identities	Positives	Gaps
184 bits(467)	2e-67	Compositional matrix adjust.	91/99(92%)	96/99(96%)	0/99(0%)

```
Query  1   PQVTLWQRPLVTIKIGGQLKEALLDTGADDTVLEEMSLPGRWKPKMIGGIGGFIKVRQYD  60
           PQ+TLWQRPLVTI+IGGQLKEALLDTGADDTVLEEM+LPG+WKPKMIGGIGGFIKVRQYD
Sbjct  1   PQITLWQRPLVTIRIGGQLKEALLDTGADDTVLEEMNLPGKWKPKMIGGIGGFIKVRQYD  60

Query  61  QILIEICGHKAIGTVLVGPTPVNIIGRNLLTQIGCTLNF  99
           QI +EI GHKAIGTVLVGPTPVNIIGRNLLTQIG TLNF
Sbjct  61  QIPVEIXGHKAIGTVLVGPTPVNIIGRNLLTQIGXTLNF  99
```

Figure 2. Ramachandran Plot of MT of PR

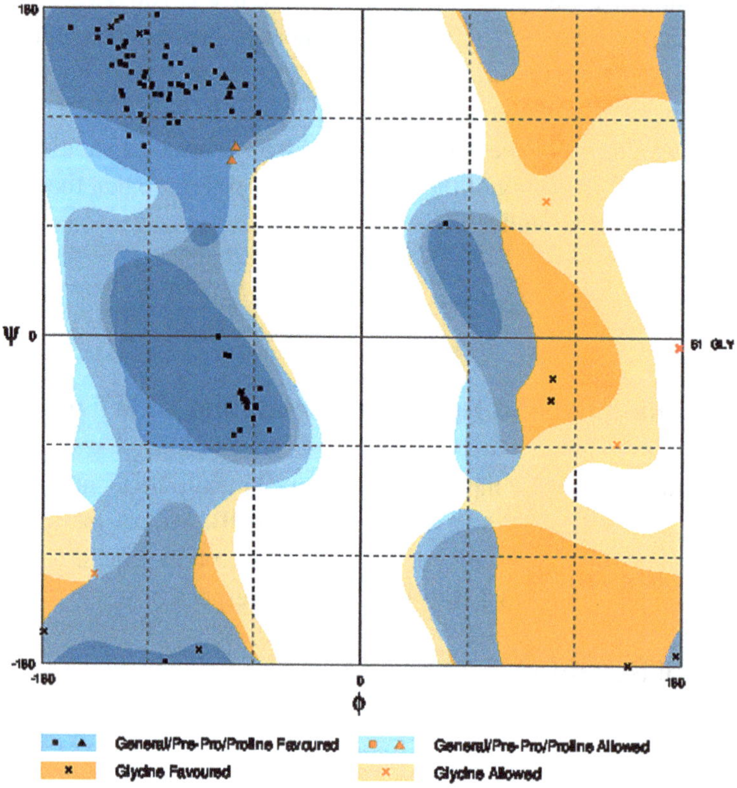

The created model was validated by structural superimposition that showed the root mean square deviation (RMSD) between the WT and MT as 0.6 Å, which suggests minimal deviation of WT compared to the MT model (Figure 3). Further, Ramachandran plot analysis (Figure 4) showed 93% of residues of the MT protein were in the most favored region indicating the good quality of the model.

Docking Between PR and Inhibitors

The three-dimensional model and WT proteins were used for docking with seven inhibitors such as ATV, DRV, IDV, LPV, NFV, SQV and TPV and the docked complexes were seen using DS (Figure 5-11). Docking of inhibitors with PRs resulted in ten poses. Of the ten poses, the best ligand pose was selected based on top GOLD score. In case of MT-I84V PR, the score was high for all the inhibitors and the score was low in case of WT (Figure 12).

Figure 3. Superimposition of template-4HVP (green) and MT of PR (pink) showing an RMSD of 0.6 Å

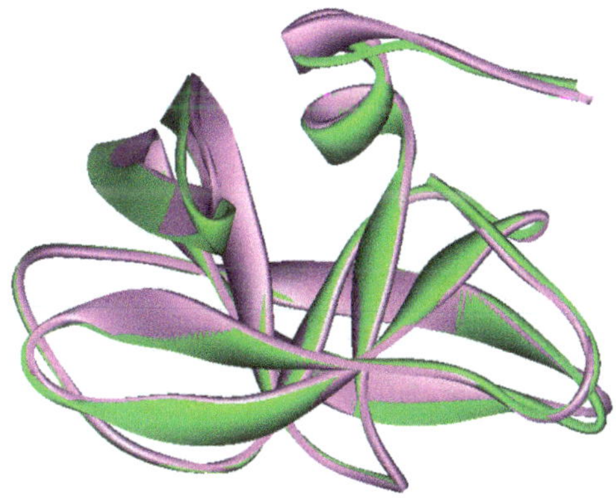

Figure 4. Structure of PR -WT (green) and 3-D model of MT (pink), the residues at position 84 is displayed in stick model (dark blue)

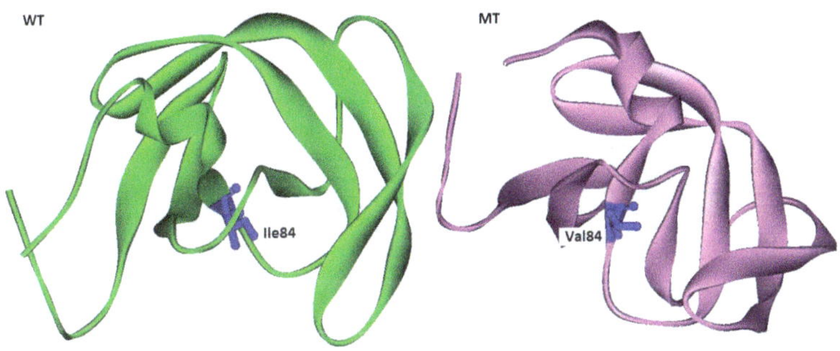

Figure 5. Docking complex WT and MT of PR with ATV (green)

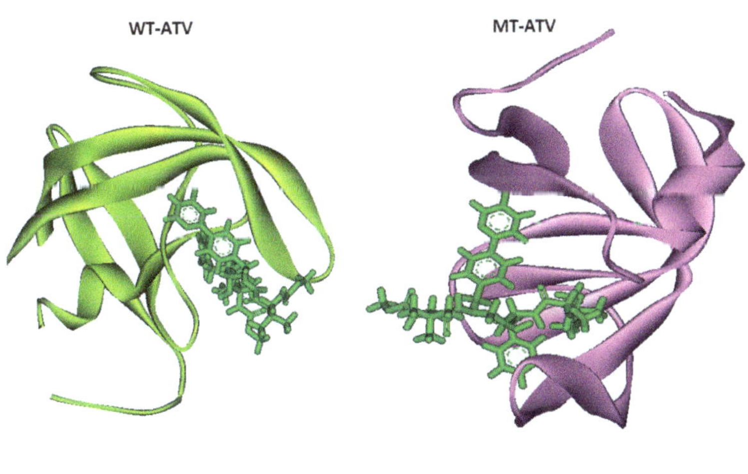

Figure 6. Docking complex of WT and MT of PR with DRV (red)

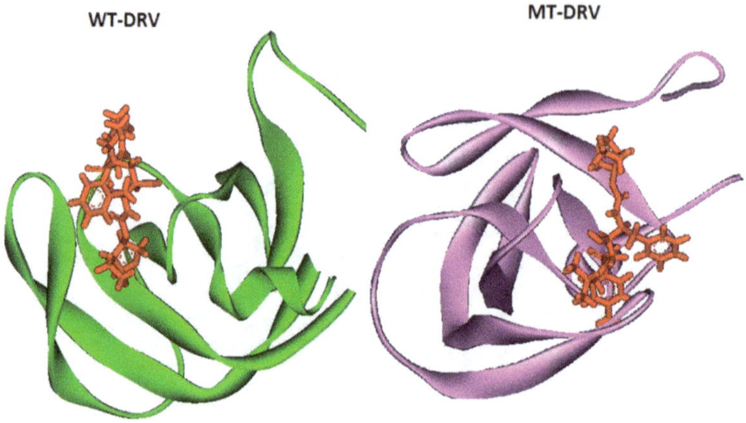

Figure 7. Docking complex of WT and MT of PR with IDV (cyan)

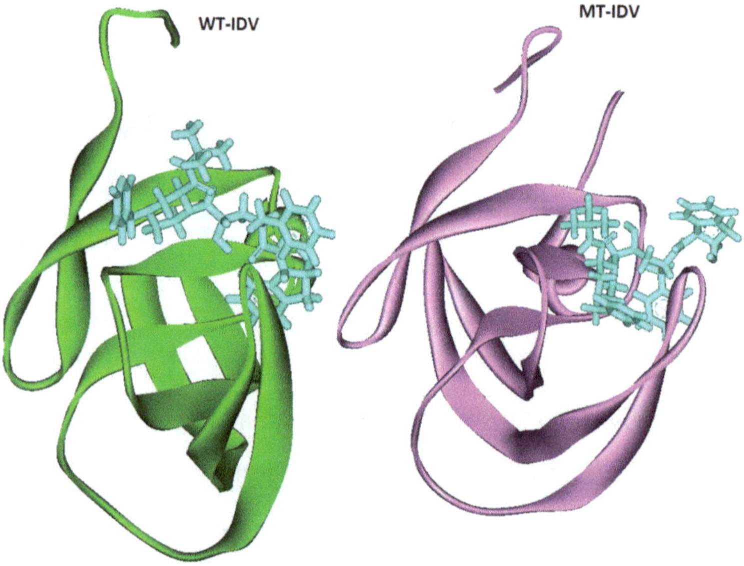

Figure 8. Docking complex of WT and MT of PR with LPV (magenta)

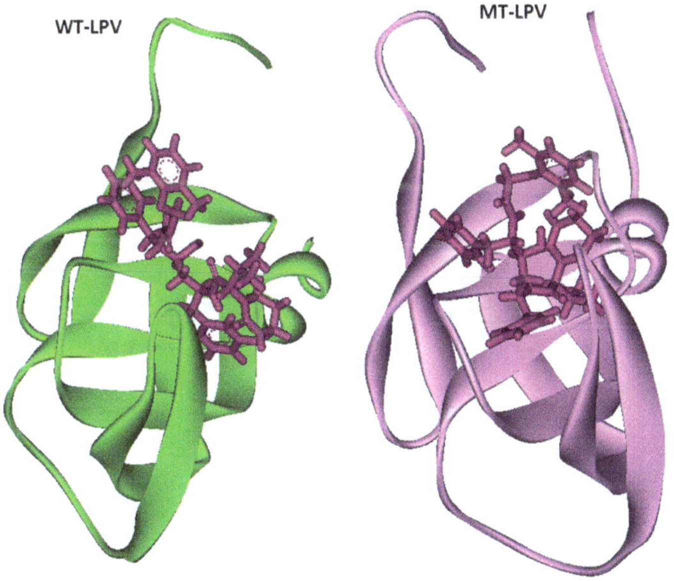

Figure 9. Docking complex of WT and MT of PR with NFV (mustard)

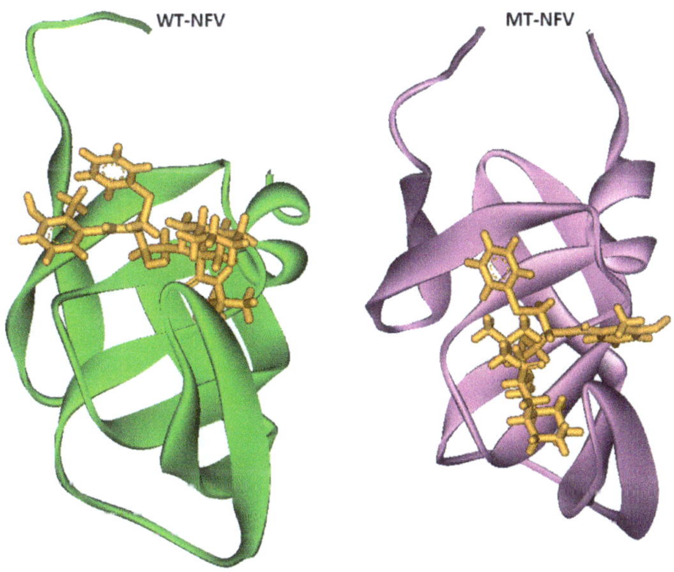

Figure 10. Docking complex of WT and MT of PR with SQV (dark blue)

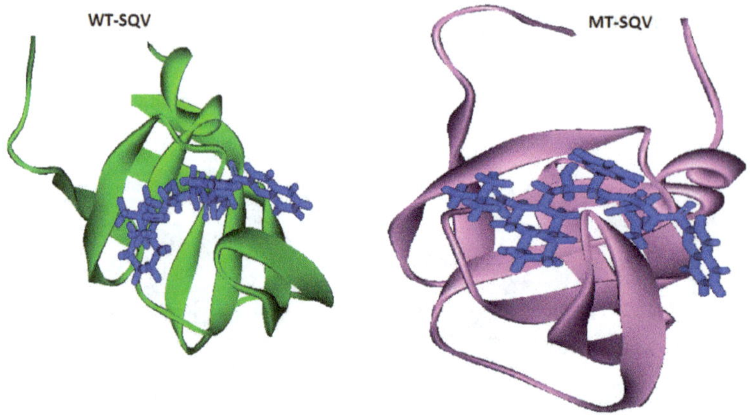

Figure 11. Docking complex of WT and MT of PR with TPV (light blue)

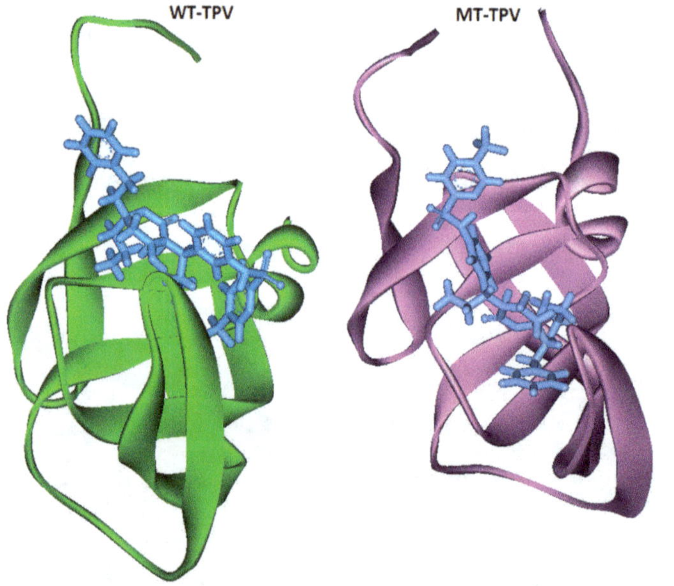

Figure 12. Docking score of WT and MT of PR with all PIs

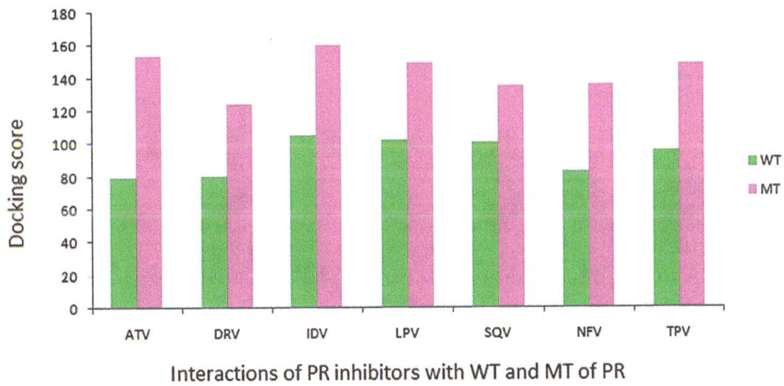

Interactions Between PRs and Ligands at Their Ligand Binding Site

The interactions profile of WT and MT-PRs with seven PIs at their binding site is illustrated in Figures 13-19 and Table 1. In general, the inhibitor and enzyme make a pattern of complementary hydrogen (H) bonds between their respective backbone atoms. In case of WT-PR complexed with ATV, the number of H bonds was less (10) compared to the MT (18). Notably, the clinically essential residue Ile84 is catalytically significant as it was present in the active site. Residues: Arg8, Asp29, Gly27, Gly48 were directly involved in interactions with the drug-ATV in WT. While in case of MT-ATV complex, Arg8 and 105, Ile50 and 147, Gly48 and 145 were involved in interactions, other types of residual interactions are shown in Table 1.

Surprisingly, same numbers of H bonds (8) were found in WT and MT docked with DRV. In WT-DRV complex, Arg8 and 105, Asp30 and 127 were involved in direct interaction with DRV. In MT-DRV complex, Asp25, Gly27 and Ile50 were directly involved.

In WT-PR docked with IDV the number of H interactions was half (8) in number in comparison to MT (16). In WT-IDV complex, residues such as Asp29 and Gly27 were directly involved in interactions, while in case of MT-IDV complex Asp25 and 122, Gly49 and146 were involved in interactions with IDV.

In WT complcxcd with LPV, the numbers of H bonds were 8 in comparison to MT containing 14 bonds. In WT-LPV complex, Asp25 and Gly27 were directly involved in interactions. In MT complex, Asp25 and Asp122 were involved in interactions with the LPV. Of importance, the structurally relevant residue Val84 was found to occur in this complex at the ligand binding site.

Figure 13. Interactions of WT and MT of PR with ATV (green) at its binding site

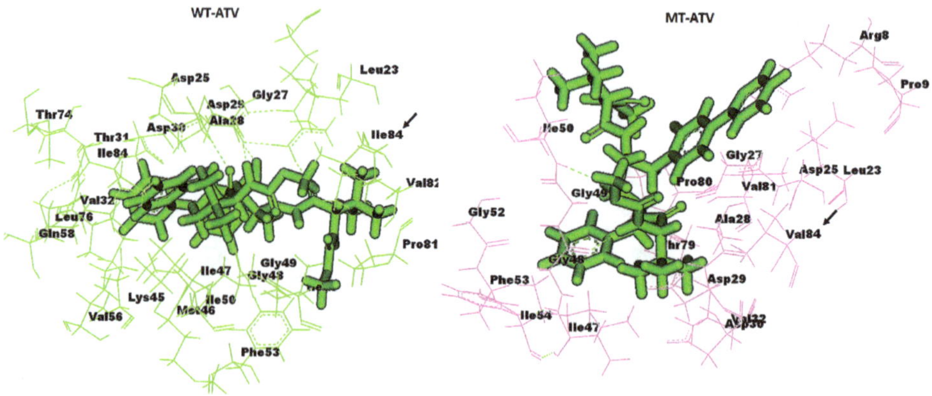

Figure 14. Interactions of WT and MT with DRV (red) at its binding site

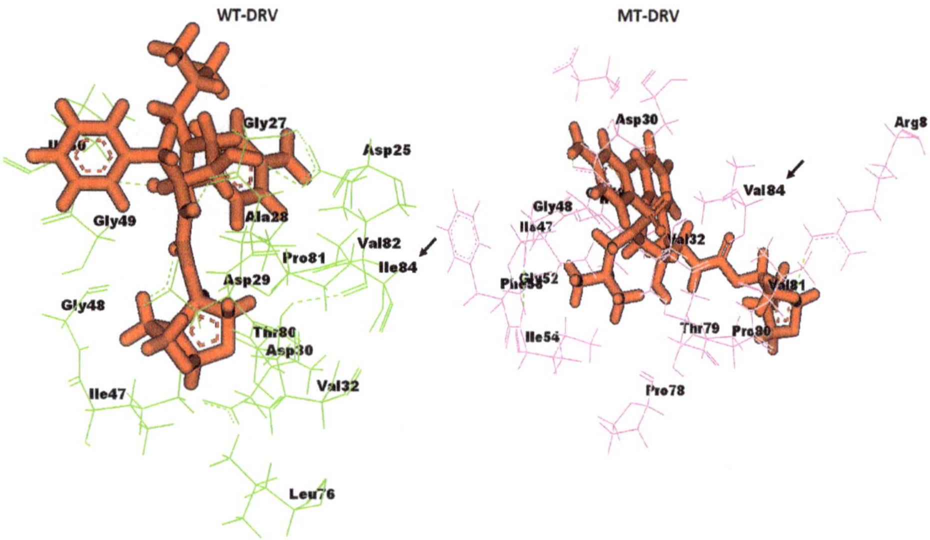

In case of WT complexed with NFV, the bonding pattern was very different with only 2 H bonds in WT in comparison to 12 H bonds in MT. The residue Ile50 was directly interacting with the drug in WT and in MT complex, in addition to residue Ile50 as like in WT, residues Asp29, Asp126 and Ile147 were involved in direct interactions.

In contrast to other PIs, in case of WT-PR complexed with SQV, the occurrence of more number of H bonds (12) compared to MT (6). Residues Asp25, 29 and 30, Gly27 and 48 were directly involved in the interactions. In case of MT-SQV complex,

Figure 15. Interactions of WT and MT of PR with IDV (cyan) at its binding site

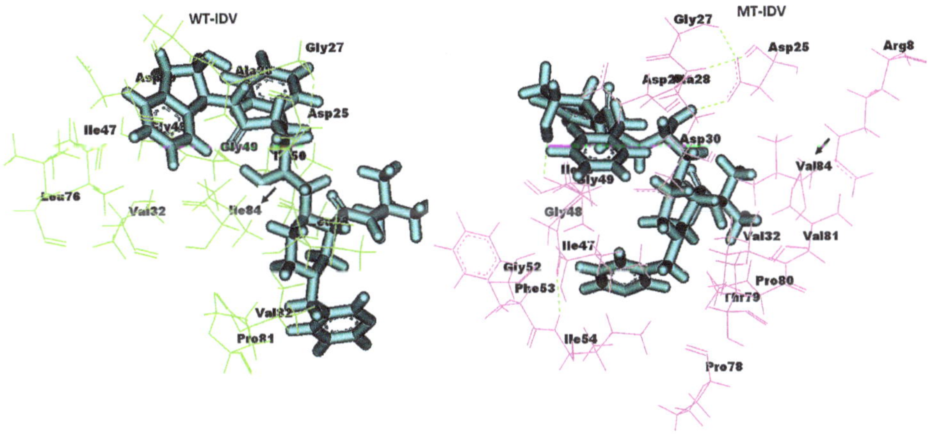

Figure 16. Interactions of WT and MT of PR with LPV (magenta) at its binding site

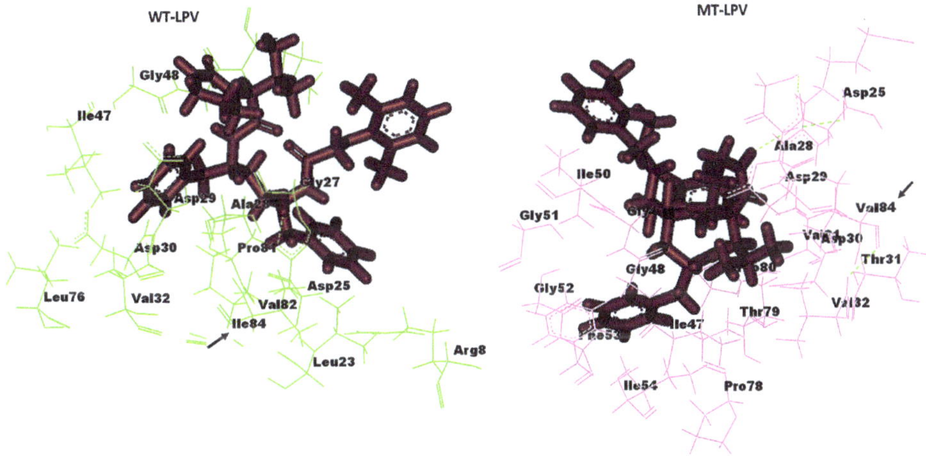

more number of residues in addition to residues Asp29 and 30, other residues such as Asp126, 127 and Gly145, 146 were directly involved in the interactions.

Similar to the number difference WT complexed with LPV, in WT complexed with TPV the number of H bonds were less (7) compared to the numbers (12). In WT-TPV complex, the commonly seen residues like Asp30 and Ile50 were found in direct interactions, while in case of MT-TPV complex, also the frequently seen residues such as Arg8 and 105 were involved in interactions (Table 1).

Figure 17. Interactions of WT and MT of PR with NFV (mustard) at its binding site

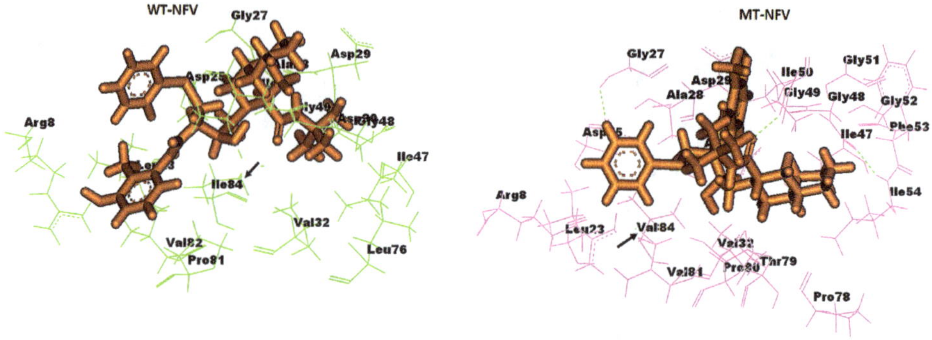

Figure 18. Interactions of WT and MT of PR with SQV (dark blue) at its binding site

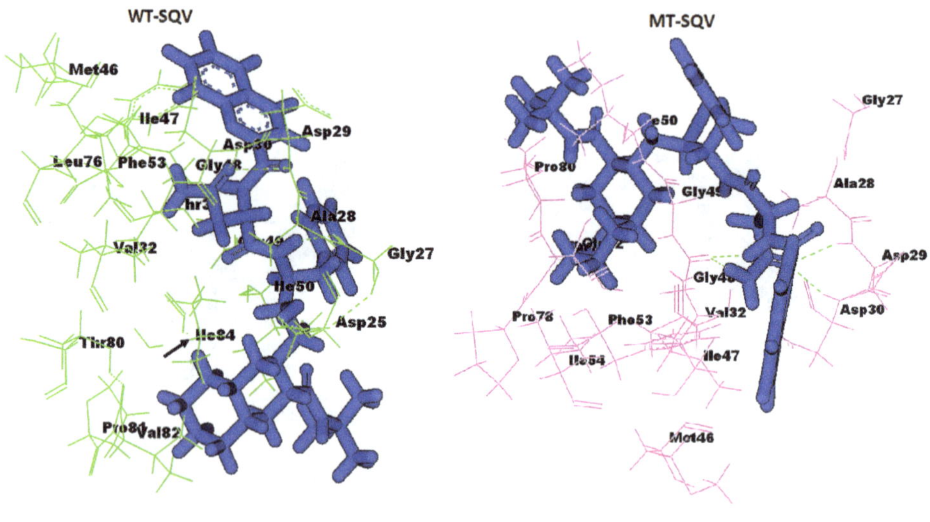

DISCUSSION

PR of HIV-1 is a crucial enzyme which is required for the replication of the HIV-1 and responsible for chronic infection of the virus. The enzyme contains a conserved triad, Asp-Thr-Gly, at positions 25-26-27, respectively (Erickson, Gulnik, & Markowitz, 1999; Shafer et al., 2001). The hydrophobic substrate cleft of the PR recognizes and cleaves 9 different sequences to produce the matrix, capsid, nucleocapsid, and p6 proteins from the Gag polyprotein and the protease, RT, and integrase proteins from the Gag-Pol polyprotein (Erickson, Gulnik, & Markowitz, 1999). Therefore, this most important enzyme of HIV-1 is targeted by several inhibitors (ATV, DRV,

Figure 19. Interactions of WT and MT of PR with TPV (light blue) at its binding site

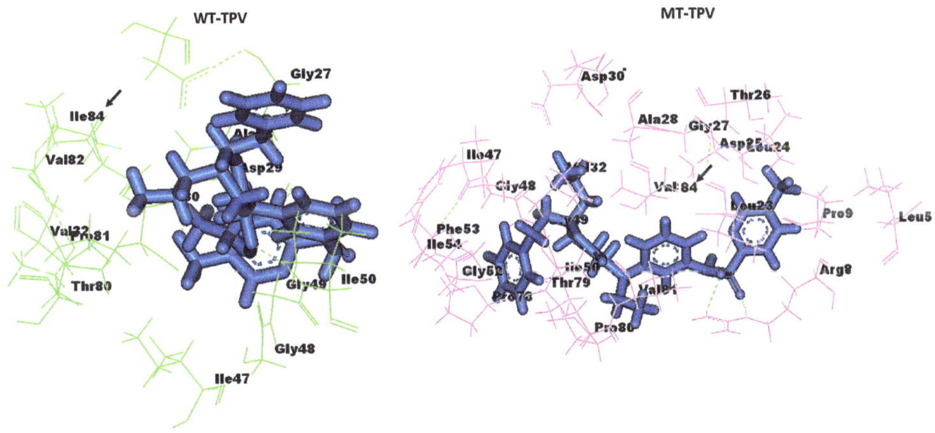

IDV, LPV, SQV, NFV and TPV); however, resistance has also been observed to all these PIs.

Mutations sites of PR gene are classified as major and minor mutations sites, the major drug-resistance sites were associated with high-level resistance, while minor sites with low-level. It was found that around 23 mutations in 16 codons of the PR gene were the major drug-resistance sites (Rhee et al, 2003). In addition, differences in polymorphisms in the PR gene have been reported among different subtypes (Santos & Soares, 2011). Of all other mutations, the I84V mutation contributes resistance to multiple PIs (Shafer et al., 2001) and structurally, this mutation affects both sides of the enzyme active site. Thus, it is of interest to know

Table 1. H bond formation at PIs binding site

PR With Inhibitors	No. of HB	HB Donor	HB Acceptor	Bond Distance (A°)
WT-ATV	10	A:ASP29:HN	ATV:O	2.10
		A:VAL32:HN	A:ILE84:O	2.04
		A:LEU76:HN	A:THR31:O	1.97
		A:ARG87:HH11	A:ASP29:OD1	1.86
		B:ARG8:HE	A:ASP29:OD1	1.93
		B:ARG8:HH12	ATV:OAL	1.90
		ATV:H4	A:GLY27:O	1.72
		ATV:H15	A:GLY48:O	1.45
		ATV:H25	A:ASP29:OD2	1.94
		B:ARG8:HH11	A:ASP29:OD2	1.78

continued on following page

Table 1. Continued

PR With Inhibitors	No. of HB	HB Donor	HB Acceptor	Bond Distance (A°)
MT-I84V-ATV	18	ARG8:HH21	ATV:NBD	2.04
		GLY27:H	ASP25:OD1	2.09
		GLY27:H	ASP122:OD1	2.09
		ILE47:H	ILE54:O	2.23
		ILE47:H	ILE47:H	2.23
		ILE50:H	ATV:OAM	2.25
		ILE54:H	ILE47:O	2.10
		ILE54:H	ILE144:O	2.10
		ARG105:HH21	ATV:NBD	2.04
		GLY124:H	ASP25:OD1	2.09
		GLY124:H	ASP122:OD1	2.09
		ILE144:H	ILE54:O	2.23
		ILE144:H	ILE151:O	2.23
		ILE147:H	ATV:OAM	2.25
		ILE151:H	ILE47:O	2.10
		ILE151:H	ILE144:O	2.10
		ATV:H4	GLY48:O	2.02
		ATV:H4	GLY145:O	2.02
WT-DRV	8	ARG8:HH22	DRV:O26	2.33
		ILE54:H	ILE47:O	2.10
		ILE54:H	ILE144:O	2.10
		ARG105:HH22	DRV:O26	2.33
		ILE151:H	ILE47:O	2.10
		ILE151:H	ILE144:O	2.10
		DRV:H1	ASP30:OD2	2.07
		DRV:H1	ASP127:OD2	2.07
MT-I84V-DRV	8	A:GLY27:HN	A:ASP25:OD1	2.37
		A:ILE50:HN	DRV:O9	2.18
		A:THR80:HG1	A:VAL82:O	2.24
		B:ARG8:HH11	A:ASP29:OD2	1.78
		B:GLY27:HN	B:ASP25:OD2	2.03
		B:ILE50:HN	DRV:O9	1.72
		DRV:H19	A:ASP25:OD2	2.10
		DRV:H21	A:GLY27:O	1.99

continued on following page

Table 1. Continued

PR With Inhibitors	No. of HB	HB Donor	HB Acceptor	Bond Distance (A°)
WT-IDV	8	A:GLY27:HN	A:ASP25:OD1	2.37
		A:ASP29:HN	IDV:O4	2.05
		A:ARG87:HH11	A:ASP29:OD1	1.86
		B:ARG8:HE	A:ASP29:OD1	1.93
		B:ARG8:HH11	A:ASP29:OD2	1.78
		B:GLY27:HN	B:ASP25:OD2	2.03
		IDV:H32	A:GLY27:O	1.90
		IDV:H35	A:GLY27:O	1.99
MT-I84V-IDV	16	GLY27:H	ASP25:OD1	2.09
		GLY27:H	ASP122:OD1	2.09
		ALA28:H	ASP25:O	2.40
		ALA28:H	ASP122:O	2.40
		ILE54:H	ILE47:O	2.10
		ILE54:H	ILE144:O	2.10
		GLY124:H	ASP25:OD1	2.09
		GLY124:H	ASP122:OD1	2.09
		ALA125:H	ASP25:O	2.40
		ALA125:H	ASP122:O	2.40
		ILE151:H	ILE47:O	2.10
		ILE151:H	ILE144:O	2.10
		IDV:H21	ASP25:OD2	2.04
		IDV:H21	ASP122:OD2	2.04
		IDV:H35	GLY49:O	2.08
		IDV:H35	GLY146:O	2.08
WT-LPV	8	A:GLY27:HN	A:ASP25:OD1	2.37
		A:ARG87:HH11	A:ASP29:OD1	1.86
		B:ARG8:HE	A:ASP29:OD1	1.83
		B:ARG8:HH11	A:ASP29:OD2	1.78
		B:ARG8:HH11	A:ASP29:OD2	1.78
		B:ARG8:HH11	A:ASP29:OD2	1.78
		B:GLY27:HN	B:ASP25:OD2	2.03
		B:ARG87:HH21	B:ASP29:OD1	2.28
		LPV:H32	B:GLY27:O	2.09
		LPV:H35	A:ASP25:OD2	1.94

continued on following page

Table 1. Continued

PR With Inhibitors	No. of HB	HB Donor	HB Acceptor	Bond Distance (A^{O})
MT-I84V-LPV	14	GLY27:H	ASP25:OD1	2.09
		GLY27:H	ASP122:OD1	2.09
		ALA28:H	ASP25:O	2.40
		ALA28:H	ASP122:O	2.40
		VAL32:H	VAL83:O	2.17
		VAL32:H	VAL180:O	2.17
		GLY124:H	ASP25:OD1	2.09
		GLY124:H	ASP122:OD1	2.09
		ALA125:H	ASP25:O	2.40
		ALA125:H	ASP122:O	2.40
		VAL129:H	VAL84:O	2.17
		VAL129:H	VAL180:O	2.17
		LPV:H5	ASP25:OD2	1.85
		LPV:H5	ASP122:OD2	1.85
WT-NFV	2	B:GLY27:HN	B:ASP25:OD2	2.03
		B:ILE50:HN	NFV:O21	1.95
MT-I84V -NFV	12	GLY27:H	ASP25:OD1	2.09
		GLY27:H	ASP122:OD1	2.09
		ILE50:H	NFV:O17	2.11
		ILE54:H	ILE47:O	2.10
		ILE54:H	ILE144:O	2.10
		GLY124:H	ASP25:OD1	2.09
		GLY124:H	ASP122:OD1	2.09
		ILE147:H	NFV:O17	2.11
		ILE151:H	ILE47:O	2.10
		ILE151:H	ILE144:O	2.10
		NFV:H37	ASP29:OD2	1.84
		NFV:H37	ASP126:OD2	1.84

continued on following page

Table 1. Continued

PR With Inhibitors	No. of HB	HB Donor	HB Acceptor	Bond Distance (A°)
WT-SQV	12	GLY27:HN	ASP25:OD1	2.37
		ASP29:HN	SQV:O	1.87
		ASP29:HN	SQV:OD1	2.46
		ASP30:HN	SQV:OD1	1.82
		A:THR80:HG1	A:VAL82:O	2.24
		A:ARG87:HH11	A:ASP29:OD1	1.86
		B:ARG8:HE	A:ASP29:OD1	1.83
		B:ARG8:HH11	A:ASP29:OD2	1.78
		B:GLY27:HN	B:ASP25:OD2	2.03
		SQV:H7	A:GLY48:O	2.09
		SQV:H14	A:ASP25:OD2	1.86
		SQV:H16	A:GLY27:O	2.10
MT-SQV	6	ASP29:H	SQV:OD1	2.24
		ASP30:H	SQV:OD1	2.23
		ASP126:H	SQV:OD1	2.24
		ASP127:H	SQV:OD1	2.23
		SQV:H7	GLY48:O	1.75
		SQV:H7	GLY145:O	1.75
WT-TPV	7	A:GLY27:HN	A:ASP25:OD1	2.37
		A:ASP30:HN	TPV:F40	2.45
		A:ILE50:HN	TPV:O	1.96
		A:THR80:HG1	A:VAL82:O	2.24
		B:ARG8:HH11	A:ASP29:OD2	1.78
		B:GLY27:HN	B:ASP25:OD2	2.03
		B:ILE50:HN	TPV:O8	2.01
MT-I84V -TPV	12	ARG8:HE	TPV:O31	1.96
		ARG8:HH21	TPV:O32	2.23
		GLY27:H	ASP25:OD1	2.09
		GLY27:H	ASP122:OD1	2.09
		ILE54:H	ILE47:O	2.10
		ILE54:H	ILE144:O	2.10
		ARG105:HE	TPV:O31	1.96
		ARG105:HH21	TPV:O32	2.23
		GLY124:H	ASP25:OD1	2.09
		GLY124:H	ASP122:OD1	2.09
		ILE151:H	ILE47:O	2.10
		ILE151:H	ILE144:O	2.10

HB = Hydrogen bond; Å = Angstrom

the interactions of one such clinically and structurally relevant variant of PR such as V84I in comparison to WT with all PIs.

In the light of which, the MT-V84I was modeled and docked with 7 PIs in this study. The docking score suggest that in comparison to the WT, the binding score was higher for the MT-I84V with respect to all inhibitors. In general, an enzyme contains number of well-defined pockets, or subsites, in its active site region into which inhibitor side chains protrude, resulting in tight binding interactions between enzyme and inhibitor. In the present context, the high affinity of MT-PR towards inhibitors could be due to the presence of energetically favorable interactions between the MT protein and the ligands, which may lead to tight binding of inhibitors with the MT-I84V protein, this in turn may lead to slow release or no release of inhibitors which may lead to the development of PR resistance in mutant variants of HIV-1 eventually.

Amongst all other types of protein-ligand interactions, hydrogen (H) bond interactions are of prime importance, as it contributes to the stability and integrity of ligand and protein complex. Similarly, in the present study, the presence of more number of H bonds in the MT in comparison to WT would be a probable reason for the high affinity as evident in all cases of PIs except in SQV, whose interaction profile was more in WT in comparison to MT. In case of NFV, many H bonds (12) in comparison to only 2 in WT, suggest that it could contribute more resistance compared to other PIs for this particular mutation- V84I. Besides H bonding, high score in MT could be attributed to less number of torsions in the MT's side chain atoms and increased van der Waals, desolvation and electrostatic energy contributions.

The residues Arg8, Arg105, Asp29, Gly27, Gly48, and Ile50 were commonly involved in direct interactions with the respective PIs in WT and residues Asp25, Asp122, Gly27 and Ile50 were frequently observed in case of MT-PI (Table1). Further, in almost all interactions of PIs with WT and MT of PR, the presence of V84 and I84 is highly acknowledged (Figures 13-19).

Molecular dynamics (MD) is a most powerful method to determine the protein or enzyme's binding activity during dynamic state of the protein in the current scenario. Although, in this study MD simulations was not performed due to lack of facility, yet, an effort to determine the binding affinity of WT and the structurally relevant MT-I84V protein of PR with almost seven PIs was undertaken for the first time to our knowledge. In short, presence of more number of H bonds somehow influences the high docking score leading to high affinity which will be reflected by the tight binding and slow or no release of inhibitors leading to resists the effect of inhibitors, as in case of MT-PR with inhibitors in comparison to WT may eventually lead to the development of PR resistance to PIs in HIV-1.

REFERENCES

Altschul, S. F., Madden, T. L., Schäffer, A. A., Zhang, J., Zhang, Z., Miller, W., & Lipman, D. J. (1997). Gapped BLAST and PSI-BLAST: A new generation of protein database search programs. *Nucleic Acids Research*, *25*(17), 3389–3402. doi:10.1093/nar/25.17.3389 PMID:9254694

Antunes, D. A., Rigo, M. M., Sinigaglia, M., de Medeiros, R. M., Junqueira, D. M., Almeida, S. E., & Vieira, G. F. (2014). New insights into the in silico prediction of HIV protease resistance to nelfinavir. *PLoS One*, *9*(1), e87520. doi:10.1371/journal.pone.0087520 PMID:24498124

Appelt, K. (1993). Crystal structures of HIV-1 protease-inhibitor complexes. *Perspectives in Drug Discovery and Design*, *1*(1), 23–48. doi:10.1007/BF02171654

Collins, J. R., Burt, S. K., & Erickson, J. W. (1995). Flap opening in HIV-1 protease simulated by 'activated' molecular dynamics. *Nature Structural & Molecular Biology*, *2*(4), 334–338. doi:10.1038/nsb0495-334 PMID:7796268

Erickson, J. W., & Burt, S. K. (1996). Structural mechanisms of HIV drug resistance. *Annual Review of Pharmacology and Toxicology*, *36*(1), 545–571. doi:10.1146/annurev.pa.36.040196.002553 PMID:8725401

Erickson, J. W., Gulnik, S. V., & Markowitz, M. (1999). Protease inhibitors: Resistance, cross resistance, fitness and the choice of initial and salvage therapies. *AIDS (London, England)*, *13*(Suppl A), S189–S204. PMID:10885776

Fitzgerald, P. M. D., & Springer, J. P. (1991). Structure and function of retroviral proteases. *Annual Review of Biophysics and Biophysical Chemistry*, *20*(1), 299–320. doi:10.1146/annurev.bb.20.060191.001503 PMID:1651087

Guha, S. K., & Haldar, S. N. (2012). Drug Resistance in HIV. Medicine Update, 84–88.

Jones, G., Willett, P., & Glen, R. C. (1995). Molecular recognition of receptor sites using a genetic algorithm with a description of desolvation. *Journal of Molecular Biology*, *245*(1), 43–53. doi:10.1016/S0022-2836(95)80037-9 PMID:7823319

Krissinel, E., & Henrick, K. (2003). Protein structure comparison in 3D based on secondary structure matching (PDBeFold) followed by Cα alignment, scored by a new structural similarity function. *Proceedings of the 5th International Conference on Molecular Structural Biology*, 88.

Lovell, S. C., Davis, I. W., Arendall, W. B. III, de Bakker, P. I., Word, J. M., Prisant, M. G., ... Richardson, D. C. (2003). Structure validation by Cα geometry: Φ, ψ and Cβ deviation. *Proteins, 50*(3), 437–450. doi:10.1002/prot.10286 PMID:12557186

Miller, M., Schneider, J., Sathyanarayana, B. K., Toth, M. V., Marshall, G. R., Clawson, L., ... Wlodawer, A. (1989). Structure of complex of synthetic HIV-1 protease with a substrate-based inhibitor at 2.3 A resolution. *Science, 246*(4934), 1149–1152. doi:10.1126/science.2686029 PMID:2686029

Rhee, S. Y., Gonzales, M. J., Kantor, R., Betts, B. J., Ravela, J., & Shafer, R. W. (2003). Human immunodeficiency virus reverse transcriptase and protease sequence database. *Nucleic Acids Research, 31*(1), 298–303. doi:10.1093/nar/gkg100 PMID:12520007

Sali. (1995). *MODELLER: Implementing 3D Protein Modeling, mc2, vol. 2:5.* Burlington, MA: Molecular Simulations Inc.

Santos, A. F., & Soares, M. A. (2011). The impact of the nelfinavir resistance-conferring mutation D30N on the susceptibility of HIV-1 subtype B to other protease inhibitors. *Memorias do Instituto Oswaldo Cruz, 106*(2), 177–181. doi:10.1590/S0074-02762011000200010 PMID:21537677

Shafer, R. W., Dupnik, K., Winters, M. A., & Eshleman, S. H. (2001). A guide to HIV-1 reverse transcriptase and protease sequencing for drug resistance studies. *HIV Sequence Compendium, 2001*, 1. PMID:22324021

Wainberg, M. A., Zaharatos, G. J., & Brenner, B. G. (2011). Development of antiretroviral drug resistance. *The New England Journal of Medicine, 365*(7), 637–646. doi:10.1056/NEJMra1004180 PMID:21848464

Wlodawer, A., & Erickson, J. W. (1993). Structure-based inhibitors of HIV-1 protease. *Annual Review of Biochemistry, 62*(1), 543–585. doi:10.1146/annurev.bi.62.070193.002551 PMID:8352596

Chapter 8
HIV-Associated Neurocognitive Disorder:
The Interaction Between HIV-1 and Dopamine Transporter Structure

Ahmed Abd Elkader Elrashedy
National Research Center, Egypt

ABSTRACT

In the last two decades, several advancement studies have increased the care of HIV-infected individuals. Specifically, the development for preparation of combination antiretroviral therapy has resulted in a dramatic decline in the rate of deaths from AIDS. The term "HIV-associated neurocognitive disorder" (HAND) has been used to distinguish the spectrum of neurocognitive dysfunction associated with HIV infection. HIV can pass to the CNS during the early stages of infection and last in the CNS. CNS inflammation and infection lead to the development of HAND. The brain can serve as a sanctuary for ongoing HIV replication, even when the systemic viral suppression has been achieved. HAND can remain in patients treated with combination antiretroviral therapy, and its effect on survival, quality of life, and everyday functioning make it a significant unresolved problem. This chapter discusses details of the computational modeling studies on mechanisms and structures of human dopamine transporter (hDAT) and its interaction with HIV-1 trans activator of transcription (Tat).

DOI: 10.4018/978-1-5225-3203-3.ch008

INTRODUCTION

About 36.7 million people in the world suffer from the acquired immune deficiency syndrome (AIDS) disease caused by human immunodeficiency virus (HIV) and about 1.1 million people have died from this disease, according to the 2016 report of United Nations Programme on HIV/AIDS (UNAIDS) (Who, UNICEF, 2016). (See Figure 1 and Figure 2.) 70% of HIV-infected individuals suffer from HIV-associated neurocognitive disorders (HAND) (Ernst et al., 2009; Zhu et al., 2009; Midde, Gomez, & Zhu, 2012; Robertson et al., 2007).

Even though our knowledge is improving and we're learning more about HAND, there is no specific treatment for curing HAND. HAND affects survival, quality of life, and everyday activities, so the development of a HAND treatment remains important for HIV patients (Heaton et al., 1994).

All over the world, HAND is the major cause of cognitive impairment and persists, even in individuals who've received combination antiretroviral therapy (Heaton et al., 2010a; Tozzi et al., 2007). The spectrum of neurological complications in HAND are generally segregated into three main groups: asymptomatic neurocognitive impairment (ANI; 33%), mild neurocognitive disorders (MND, 20–30%), and severe, albeit rare, HIV-associated dementia (HAD; 2–8%) (Heaton et al., 2010b; McArthur et al., 2010).

The clinical impairments in HAND include attention, memory, learning, motor function, and behavioral changes. As combination antiretroviral therapy becomes more widely distributed in resource-limited settings, survival will improve and the long-term global impact of HAND will become even more important.

Adding to that, early HIV infection of the CNS is believed to contribute to the development of HAND. Evidence shows that the CNS can subsequently serve as a storage tank for ongoing HIV replication, so that limits the opportunity for a complete cure or eradication of the infection (Fois & Brew, 2015). Additionally, the incidence and progression of HAND are usually combined with the intake of recreational drugs like cocaine and methamphetamine (Buch et al., 2011). If HAND can be prevented at early infection stage, the quality of life for the patient will be improved and the economic burden will be lessened on the healthcare system.

Joining together lines of clinical observation, supported by imaging, (Wang et al., 2004; Chang et al., 2008) neuropsychological performance testing (Meade et al., 2011; Kumar et al., 2011) and postmortem examinations (Gelman et al., 2012), have implicated dopamine (DA) dysregulation with the abnormal neurocognitive function observed in HAND (Berger & Arendt, 2000). DA-rich brain regions (basal ganglia and related structures) are highly sensitive to the effects of both HIV infection and substance use.

During the course of HAND, at the early stage, HIV-1 infects the monocyte, then it is passes to the brain through the blood-brain barrier (BBB) and becomes present in cerebrospinal fluid after approximately 2-3 weeks (asymptomatic infection) (Scheller et al., 2010) of being exposed to the primary infection (Davis et al., 1992; Nath & Clements, 2011; Williams et al., 2013). After that, the virus spreads perivascular macrophages and microglia and establishes a reservoir within the brain. These infected cells eliminate a large number of viral particles daily, which ultimately extend the viral load in the CNS. Furthermore, these cells secrete neurotoxic HIV-1 viral proteins that include structural protein gp120 and nonstructural protein Tat (trans-activator of transcription) as well as pro inflammatory cytokines and chemokines (Mattson, Haughey, Nath, 2005). Many studies observed that HIV-1 cannot immediately infect dopaminergic neurons but extracellularly discharged viral proteins through direct binding which lead to progressively destruct the neurons and cause subsequent neurodegeneration (Nath et al., 2000b; Ferris, Mactutus, & Booze, 2008). Among these proteins, Tat has been highly linked to progressive neuronal dysregulation, which leads to the development of HAND.

Tat can be present in DA-rich brain areas (Hudson et al., 2000; Del Valle et al., 2000; Lamers et al., 2010) and in the sera (Xiao et al., 2000; Westendorp et al., 1995) of HIV-1 infected patients. Long-term viral exposure can improve damage in the mesocorticolimbic DA system (Nath, Jankovic, & Pettigrew, 1987; Koutsilieri, 2002) and to the brain pathways controlling motivation (Wise & Bozarth, 1987; Everitt & Robbins, 2005; Berridge, 2007). Lastly, Dopamine (DA) dysregulation has been combined with cognitive deficits in HIV-1 positive people (Purohit, Rapaka, & Shurtleff, 2011; Jacobs et al., 2013).

RISK FACTORS FOR HAND

Cardiovascular Risk Factors

These factors were attached to the declining in the cognitive performance in the Multicenter AIDS Cohort Study (MACS), adding to that the obesity, and diabetes are important factor for HAND in the CNS HIV Antiretroviral Therapy Effects Research (CHARTER) cohort (McCutchan et al., 2012; Becker et al., 2009). There were a study carried on 245 HIV individual in Italy suffered from diabetes, carotid intima-media thickness and cardiovascular risk factors including hyperlipidemia and tobacco use and they found that this factors were greatly compared with the lower cognitive performance (Fabbiani et al., 2013).

Figure 1. People living with HIV

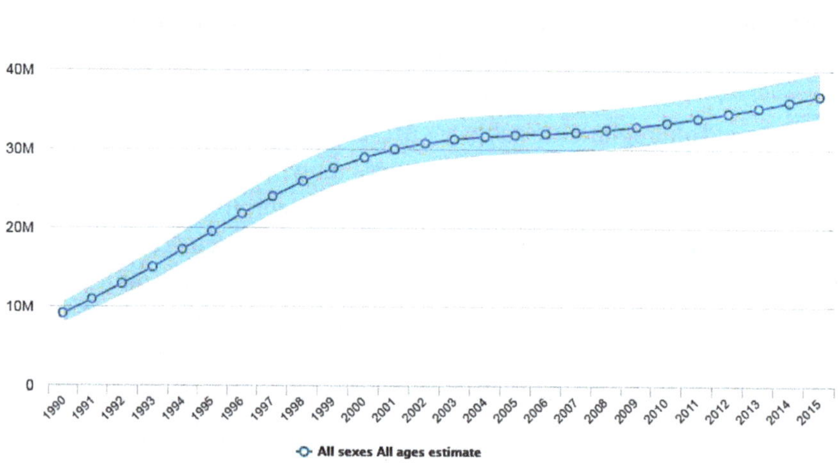

Figure 2. AIDS related deaths: 1,100, 000
Source: UNAIDS Estimates July 2016.

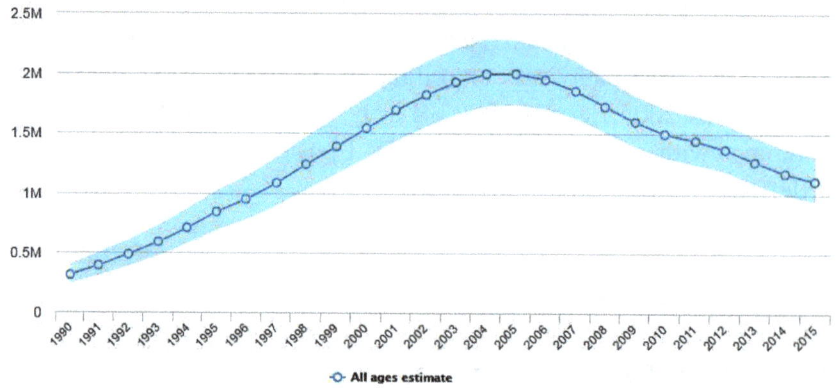

Figure 3. Timeline of advances in neuro-AIDS research [HIV-associated neurocognitive disorder (HAND)]
Note: AZT, azidothymidine; HNRC, HIV Neurobehavioral Research Center; MACS, Multicenter AIDS Cohort Study; UCSD, University of California San Diego

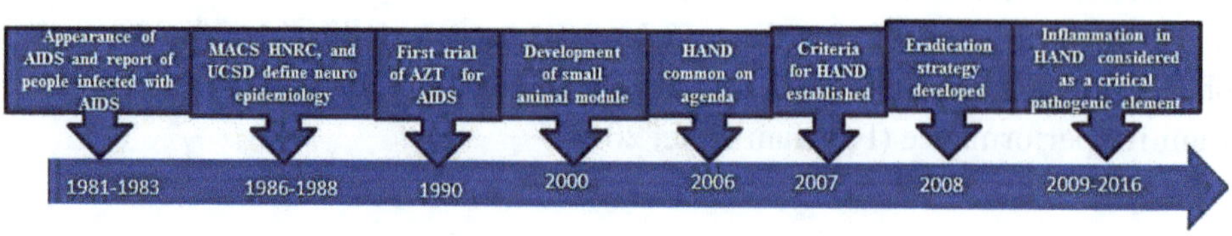

Age

Elderly people (>50 years) are strongly associated with HAND (Fazeli et al., 2015; Valcour et al., 2004; Joska et al., 2011; Joska et al., 2012) this resulted from the fact that HAND risk is likely confounded by elevated the prevalence of cerebrovascular risk factors at older ages (Marquine et al., 2014) in the CNS HIV Antiretroviral Therapy Effects Research (CHARTER) cohort, Older HIV+ adults, increased systolic blood pressure, high Body mass index (BMI), high serum cholesterol, and a diagnosis of AIDS, all this factor were contributed with worse global neuropsychological performance, suggesting that small or large vessel atherosclerotic disease could be associated to cognitive impairment in older HIV+ individuals (Heaton et al., 2012).

Hepatitis C Virus Infection

Hepatitis C co-infection with HIV was found to double the risk of cognitive impairment in HIV+ individuals comparing with those without hepatitis C (Vivithanaporn et al., 2012).

HUMAN DOPAMINE TRANSPORTER

DA transporter (DAT)-mediated DA reuptake is important for normal DA homeostasis. Human dopamine transporter (hDAT) is particular clinical importance because its convoluted in many dieses such as Parkinson's disease, schizophrenia and drug dependence . Dopamine (DA) is the native substrate for this receptor and it's a critical neurotransmitter for both reward systems and locomotor control. Torres *et al.* (2003), found that hDAT plays an important role in controlling the spatial and temporal extra neuronal DA concentration. Its familiar that Cocaine is one of the most abuse drug all over the world and hDAT is the main target for cocaine in the neuronal system (Sulzer, 2011), its act through binding of cocaine to hDAT, cocaine blocks the reuptake of dopamine from CNS synapses and thus increased the duration of dopaminergic neurotransmission in brain areas associated with reward (Figure 4). Many people all over the world are addict with cocaine and up to now no US FDA approved medication for cocaine abuse (Uhl, 2003; Chen et al., 2006). Adding to that, hDAT is also associated with transactivator of transcription (Tat) of HIV-1 this because HIV-1 Tat protein has been detected in the brain and the sera of HIV-1 patients (Del Valle et al., 2000; Hudson et al., 2000; Lamers et al., 2010). HIV-1 Tat plays a vital role in HIV-associated neurocognitive disorders (HAND) (Aksenova et al., 2006; Zhu & Reith, 2008; Zhu et al., 2009; Ferris et al., 2010; Purohit, Rapaka, Shurtleff, 2011; Midde, Gomes, & Zhu, 2012; Bagashev &

Sawaya, 2013; Ferris et al., 2009) by disrupting intracellular communication (Kim, Yoon, & Kim, 2013).Through interaction with some important protein in the CNS receptors such as monoamine (dopamine, norepinephrine, and serotonin) transporters and N-methyl-D-aspartate NMDA) that are targets of some abused drugs including cocaine and methamphetamine (Ferris, Mactutus, & Booze, 2008; Ferris et al., 2010; Purohit, Rapaka, & Shurtleff, 2011; Bagashev & Sawaya, 2013; Heaton et al., 2010c; Gaskill et al., 2009; Buckner et al., 2006; Nath et al., 2001; Meade et al., 2011a; Meade et al., 2011b; Chang et al., 2008; Kumar et al., 2011; Berger & Arendt, 2000; Sardar, Czudek, Reynolds, 1996; Kumar et al., 2009; Scheller et al., 2010; Beuming et al., 2008; Koutsilieri et al., 2000; Koutsilieri, Meulen, & Reiderer, 2001; Ernst et al., 2010; Ferrarese et al., 2001; Aksenov et al., 2012; Silverstein et al., 2012). By binding to hDAT, the HIV-1 Tat can block the DA uptake by hDAT.

So that, it is worthy to design and synthesis a drug which capable to block HIV-1 Tat binding with hDAT without affecting the normal function of hDAT. Knowledge of the detailed 3D structure of hDAT is important for understanding the molecular mechanisms concerning how hDAT interact with with HIV-1 Tat and DA-transporting

Figure 4. Schematic representation of dopamine synaptic terminals. HIV-1 penetrates the brain at the early infection stage and infects macrophages and microglial cells. These cells exude viral proteins that including Tat and other neurotoxic factors. Cocaine, a major psycho stimulant blocks DAT to inhibit DA translocation. Both Tat and cocaine elevate synaptic DA levels byinhibiting DA reuptake into presynaptic terminal. This increased DA induces further replication of virus in infected cells. Persistent exposure to the viral proteins, oxidative stress induced by increased DA levels and other chemokines aggravate the severity of the neurocognitive deficits in HIV-1 positive population.

Note: dopamine is synthesized in the presynaptic neuron starting from tyrosine to L-DOPA, and then the aromatic amino acid decarboxylase (AADC) catalyzes the formation of dopamine.

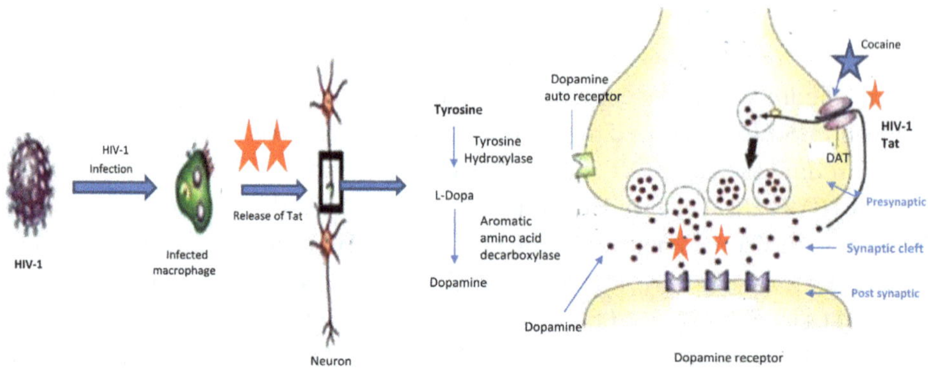

process in hDAT, etc. This study may lead to rational drug design for new treatment used for drug addiction and HIV-associated neurocognitive disorders (HAND). Although there is no x-ray crystal structure reported for hDAT, but there is a large computational modeling and simulations on the hDAT mechanisms and structures have been reported in literature. These studies will be a good starting point for further studies on the structures and mechanisms of hDAT and rational drug design.

The hDAT Structure Modeling

Similar to other members of neurotransmitters like sodium symporters (NSS) family (Ragin et al., 2015), hDAT binds with dopamine released from the synaptic cleft and transports DA into presynaptic neurons (Vo et al., 2013; Janssen et al., 1992; Heaton et al., 2011).

This process can be divided into three conformational states of hDAT

1. Outward – open state (the extracellular side of binding site is opened while the intracellular is closed).
2. Outward occluded state (both extracellular and intracellular side are closed)
3. Inward—open state (the extracellular side of binding site is closed while the intracellular is opened). See Figure 5.

Early X-ray structures of Na/H antiporter or lactose permease (LacY, e.g., PDB entry of 1PV7 with a resolution of 3.6 A^0) were used as a template for homology modeling studies for the 3D structure of hDAT, but later Huang *et.al* (2007) found that this model was not suitable for homology modeling of any member of the NSS family. Instead of this, Huang X *et.al* (2007) used an x-ray crystal structure of leucine transporters from Aquifex aeolicus ($LeuT_{Aa}$) as a template for homology Modeling (Huang & Xhan, 2007). The x-ray crystal structure of leucine transporter from Aquifex aeolicus ($LeuT_{Aa}$) was considered a much more reasonable template because of the bacterial homolog of NSS, $LeuT_{Aa,}$ which has a structural folding and physiological features that are similar to other NSS family members (Singh et al., 2008; Krishnamurthy & Gouaux, 2012; Yamashita et al., 2005). Based on the $LeuT_{Aa}$ structures, many computational and experimental studies have been done on the structures of hDAT and its related transporters (Huang & Zhan, 2007; Stockner et al., 2013; Guptaroy et al., 2009; Gelman et al., 2012; Huang, Gu, & Zhan, 2009; Sucic, 2010; Gedeion et al., 2010; Koldsø et al., 2011; Henry et al., 2011; Shan et al., 2011; Midde et al., 2013). The LeuTAa-based 3D structures of hDAT have been established to be used in predicting the hDAT-Tat interaction (Purohit, Rapak, & Shurtleff, 2011). On the other hand, these structures are not executive; this is because the sequence identity is less than 25% between LeuTAa and hD_{AT}.

Figure 5. Schematic representation of the mechanisms regarding dopamine-transporting cycle of human dopamine transporter. For the purpose of clear, conversion of hDAT conformation is reduced to the turning of an L-shape switch. Extracellular and intracellular lipid interfaces are represented by red and blue lines, respectively.(i) (A) Holo hDAT in outward-open state. Extracellular dopamine molecules are available to the hDAT-interaction site. (i) Holo hDAT in outward-occluded state. The binding site is closed and no longer accessible for dopamine. (iii) Holo inward-open state with DA. The intracellular side of binding site is opened. (iv) Apo inward-open state without DA. Dopamine is released to the intracellular cytoplasm. (v) Apooutward-occluded state without DA. (vi) Apo outward-open state without DA.

DA: Dopamine; hDAT: Human dopamine transporter.

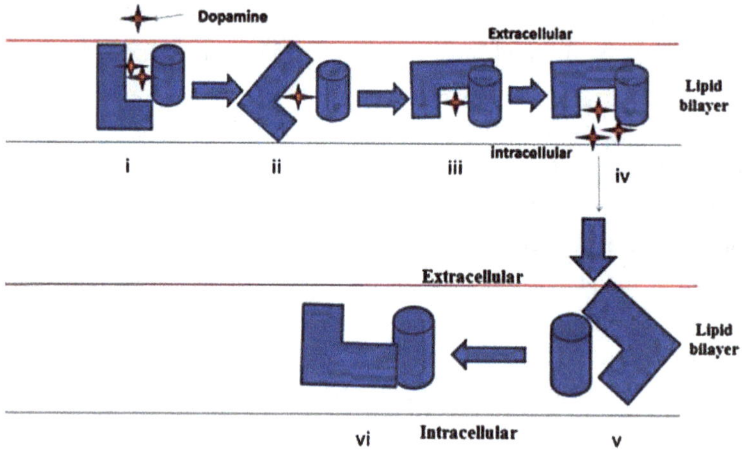

Recently, there are many x-ray crystal structures of drosophila DAT (dDAT) in its outward-open state (PDB entry: 4XNX, 4XPT, 4XPH, 4XP4, 4XP5, 4XP9,4XPA, 4XPB, 4XPG, 4XP1, 4XP6, 4XPF, 4XNU and 4M48) (Jacobs et al., 2013; McCutchan et al., 2012; Becker et al., 2009). These structures have provided an extraordinary chance to refine and remodel the hDAT structure in the outward-open state.

Recently, Yuan Y *et al.* (2015) have reported the first homology model of hDAT settled on the dDAT structure. The resulted dDAT-based hDAT model in the outward-open state is similar to LeuTAa-based model in the outward-open state, but with some more accurate details in the remodeled structure. Its considered as a refined model to the LeuTAa-based model in the outward-open state. Adding to that, it is important to understand the detailed mechanism of the DA-transporting cycle in hDAT to model the 3D structures of hDAT in the outward-occluded and inward-open states. However, all the recent x-ray crystal structures of the dDAT study only provide 3D structure of dDAT in the outward-open state, so there is no x-ray crystal structure of dDAT in the inward-open or outward-occluded state.

Nevertheless, there are x-ray crystal structures of $LeuT_{Aa}$ in all of the 3D conformational states (the outward-occluded, outward open and inward-open), and it is notable that the majority of differences in structures between the dDAT and $LeuT_{Aa}$ in the outward-open state exist in the regions that are not engaged in the conformational motion from the outward-open state

to the outward-occluded and inward-open states. They were able to build up a reasonable model of hDAT in the outward-occluded and inward-open states through combination using all these available x-ray crystal structures of dDAT and $LeuT_{Aa}$ (Yuan et al., 2015).

Outward-Open State Modeling

The dDAT structure was used as a template to module the outward-open state based on aforementioned x-ray crystal structures. Yuan *et al.* (2015) used the Modeler module (version 9v7) of Discovery Studio 2.5.5 to build the structure of the outward-open state of hDAT. The PROMALS3D server was used to make a complete multiple-sequence alignment (Pei, Tang, & Grishin, 2008) on the amino-acid sequences of the human serotonin transporter and the human norepinephrine transporter, $LeuT_{Aa}$, hDAT, dDAT. The result from the sequence alignment indicates that that hDAT is highly homologous to dDAT with identity 46% (a sequence similarity of 59%). In addition, the amino acid sequence alignment between hDAT and dDAT showed that 12 regions with high homology can be assigned to 12 transmembrane (TM) because the helices are 60% similar. Because of that 40% sequence identity between the target protein and template so that the similarity is sufficient for building up a satisfactory homology model (Šali et al., 1995; Nayeem, Sitkoff, & Krystek, 2006). Recently, Yuan *et al (2015)* created the initial structure model of hDAT and for missing residue they made conformational sampling and homology modeling (including 19 residues located at extracellular loop 2 of hDAT, the first 57 residues on the N-terminal and the last 20 residues on the C-terminal) and they added the Zn^{+2} to build up the Zn^{+2} binding site of this hDAT model (Yuan et al., 2015; Midde et al., 2015), which would contribute to the understanding for mechanism of Zn^{+2} regulation on hDAT transporting DA (Loland, Norgaard-Nielson, & Gether, 2003; Norregaard et al., 1998).

Outward -Occluded and Inward-Open States Modeling

Because all the accessible x-ray structures of dDAT represent the outward-open state of the DAT so that this crystal structure are not enough for routine homology modeling of the inward –open state and the outward occluded of hDAT. In principle, there are many computational methods that are used for constructing different conformation based on the starting conformation for example random-expulsion MD, enhanced sampling MD, normal mode analysis, and coarse-grained simulation (Lüdemann, Lounnas, & Wade, 2000). Because of the bias in the conformational conversion mode, some atomic details of stating conformation could be lost during the use of this method.

Luckily, according to available x-ray crystal structures, there is a pseudo twofold symmetry axis between TM1-TM5 and TM6-TM10 of the NSS members, and TMs 2–5 and TMs 7–10 form a tube-like supporting frame for TM1 and TM6. Likely, the folding pattern of the 5 (TM1-TM5) + 5 (TM6- TM10) repeat is maintained between the $LeuT_{Aa}$ and the NSS members, and also has been conjoined by other non-NSS members (Loland, 2014). See Figure 6.

Based on the recent finding, the x-ray crystal structures of other NSS members, including those for different conformational states (i.e., the outward- open, outward-occluded and inward-open states) of $LeuT_{Aa}$ (Singh et al., 2008; Krishnamurthy & Gouaux, 2012), and the mechanistic studies on monoamine transporters (Krishnamurthy, Piscitelli, & Gouaux, 2009; Wang & Lewis, 2010), they suggest that these NSS members should share the synonymous structural architecture and features for uptake of substrate and binding of ions, and they share the typical conformational states combined with the substrate transporting process.

Although it is acceptable to module both the inward-open states and outward-occluded states of hDAT, starting from $LeuT_{Aa}$ x-ray crystal structures wouldn't be reasonable due to the quality of this module (because of the lower sequence similarity between $LeuT_{Aa}$ and hDAT compared with the high sequence similarity between hDAT and dDAT). Therefore, by combining all x-ray structures for both dDAT and Leu T_{Aa} a more reasonable model for hDAT in the outward-occluded and inward-open states were constructed. As the structure differentiates between the dDAT and $LeuT_{Aa,}$ the structures in the outward-open state exist only in the regions that are not involved in the conformational motion from the outward-open state, outward-occluded, and inward-open states. This lead to a total homology model of hDAT: homology models 1-4 (HM1-4), HM1 (dDAT-based outward-open state model of hDAT) and HM2 ($LeuT_{Aa}$-based outward-open state model of hDAT), of HM3 ($LeuT_{Aa}$-based outward-occluded state model of hDAT) and HM4 ($LeuT_{Aa}$-based inward-open state model of hDAT and this strategy was validated by testing

Figure 6. Structural representation of the LeuT in the outward occluded conformation. The 5 + 5 structural repeat is emphasized by TMs 1 to 5 shown in blue and TMs 6 to 10 in green. TMs 11 and 12 are gray. The bound leucine is located in themiddle (brown spheres).

Reprinted with permission of Elsevier from Loland CJ (2014). The use of LeuT as a model in elucidating binding sites for substrates and inhibitors in neurotransmitter transporters. Biochim. Biophys. Acta 1850(3), 500–510 (2014).

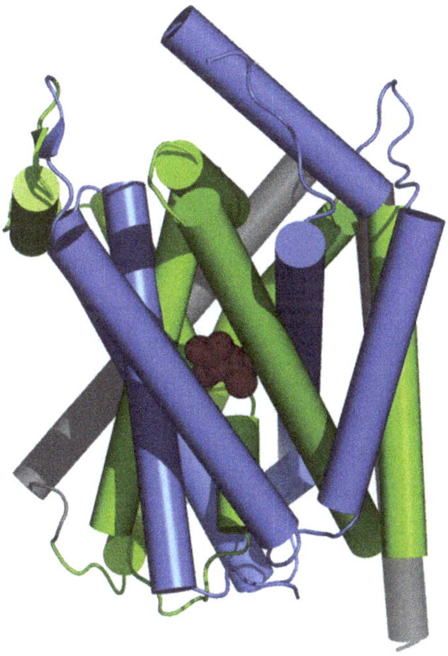

conformational conversion induced by targeted molecular dynamics simulations (Yuan et al., 2015).

Although the dDAT and $LeuT_{Aa}$ are similar in their x-ray structures, the dDAT is better template than $LeuT_{Aa}$ for homology modeling (PDB entries as 3F3A [Singh et al., 2008], 2A65 [Yamashita et al., 2005] and 3TT3 [Krishnamurthy & Gouaux, 2012]) this because there are some significant differences between the dDAT-based hDAT models (Yuan et al., 2015; Yuan et al., 2016) and the $LeuT_{Aa}$-based ones (Hudson et al., 2000; Westendorp et al., 1995; Purohit, Rapaka, & Shurtleff, 2011; Heaton et al., 2012). The Zn $^{+2}$ coordinate residue, H375, is present on the extracellular end of TM7 in the dDAT based hDAT models into the loop region in the LeuTAa-based hDAT model, which is significant for fair modeling of the Zn^{2+} binding site (Yuan et al., 2015). Besides, a short U-turn loop in EL6, there was the hydrophobic residues, tyrosine 551,548,470 (Y551, Y548, Y470) and F553 in the dDAT based hDAT models, whereas this structural feature was missing in EL6 of the $LeuT_{Aa}$-based hDAT model (Yuan et al., 2015). Reasonable modeling of this U-turn loop is significant for better understanding the role of many key residues, such as Y470 and H547 (Yuan et al., 2016). Moreover, TM12 in the dDAT based hDAT model is bound significantly by residue P573 at the middle-point of the helix (Yuan et al., 2015), making TM12 twisted away from the helical bundle and moved much more toward the lipid bilayer (Penmatsa, Wang, & Gouaux, 2015), whereas TM12 in the $LeuT_{Aa}$-based models was geometrically straight (Krishnamurthy & Gouaux, 2005).

Lysine 92 [K92] and Tyrosine 470 [Y470] in Dopamine Transporting

In the dopamine transporting process, TM1 and TM6 prove a significant motion during conformational conversion according to computationally modeled hDAT structures as TM1a and TM6b being significantly different in the outward-open and outward occluded states (Yuan et al., 2015; Midde et al., 2015). In addition, R85-D476 salt bridge was reported to be a key indication for the conformational conversion from the outward open to the outward-occluded state of hDAT (Schmitt & Reith, 2011; Manepalli et al., 2012). This because that TM1b (containing R85) also contacts directly with TM10 (containing D476) in the outward occluded state so that any structure change will affecting the interaction of TM1b with EL4, TM10, and TM10 and this will influence the motion of TM1b and effect the Dopamine uptake by hDAT (Yuan et al., 2015).

From MD simulation study, There are a slat bridge between D313(TM6a) and K92 (TM1b) and side chains in all of three typical conformational states of hDAT (Yuan et al., 2011; Midde et al., 2015), in addition, the motion of both TM1b and TM6a are required for the elimination, conformational conversion, of K92-D313 salt bridge by K92M mutation is expected to isolate TM1b with TM6a, which may damage the DA uptake process (Midde et al., 2015), adding to that, TM1b also plays an important role in inducing the conformational conversion of hDAT . For the conformational conversion of hDAT from the outward-open state to the other states during the dopamine-transporting process its required a stable D476-R85 salt bridge (Schmitt & Reith, 2011; Manepalli et al., 2012). The positively charged side chain R85(TM1b) forms direct intramolecular interaction with the negatively charged D476(TM10) side chain in the outward-occluded and inward-open state indeed the outward-open state hDAT so that by disturbing the D476-R85 salt bridge this would damage the TM1b and TM10 motion- related conformational conversion of hDAT (Yuan et al., 2016).

To confirm the computational insight, Midde *et al* (2015) made *in vitro* pharmacological activity assays, and they found that K92M mutation will decrease the maximal velocity (V_{max}) for DA uptake by approximately threefold (Midde et al., 2015), which is consistent with the computational insight. Adding to that, Chen *et al.* (2006) made a D313N mutation and they found that fourfold decrease in the V_{max} for DA $_{uptake}$, which further supports the interaction between K92 and D313. Adding to that, the, K92 is not involved in DA binding based on the computation model (Yuan et al., 2015), which is consistent with the watching that the K92M mutation did not significantly change the K_m (Midde et al., 2015). Adding to that, according to the mentioned computational models, residues Y470of TM10 was formed by the hydrophobic and aromatic residues including L224, I230, I469, Y548, Y551 and F553 and stayed at the center of the local hydrophobic regions (Yuan et al., 2015; Yuan et al., 2016). In this region, residues Y548 (on EL6) and Y551 (on EL6) compact the aromatic side chain of Y470, so that, the tight interaction between Y548, Y470 and Y551 are anticipated to hold the position of Y470, and then stabilize TM10, which is significant for the hDAT activity (Yuan et al., 2016). In particular, the stable Y548-Y470-Y551 interaction (YYY motif) are present in all three typical conformational states of hDAT so that the stability of this motif is significant for the dopamine-transporting process (see Figure 7) (Yuan et al., 2016; Quizon et al., 2016), so that the hDAT mutation can occur. For example, Y470A or Y470H is expected to attenuate the hydrophobic interaction among the three residues in the YYY motif, which would decline the effectiveness of dopamine transporting (Yuan et al., 2016). Midde et al. (2015) confirmed by pharmacological testing that Y470H or Y470A mutation only significantly declined the V_{max} without a significant change on the K_m, which is in agreement with the computational model. Based on the overall data collected from the computations and experiments (Yuan et al., 2015; Midde et al., 2015; Schmitt & Reith, 2011) on the effects of mutations Y470 and K92, the computational model on the dDAT template has helped to better our understanding of the DA transporting mechanism and the regulation of hDAT activity.

Modeling of hDAT–Tat-Binding Mode

It would be a great challenge to determine the hDAT–Tat-binding complex, especially when there are no available x-ray crystal structures of hDAT–Tat-binding complex in the physiological membrane environment. On the other hand, the molecular modeling techniques provide useful tools to module the possible hDAT–Tat interaction, this module (Huang & Zhan, 2007; Huang, Gu, Zhan, 2009; Yuan et al., 2015) has helped to determine how hDAT interacts with Tat. In 2013, Midde *et.al* published the first computational modeling study on the possible hDAT–Tat interaction, the LeuTAa-based hDAT model (Huang & Xhan, 2007; Huang, Gu,

Figure 7. Structural details of the residues Y470, Y551, H547, D476, and R85 on hDAT. hDAT is represented as a cyan ribbon, while the first part of trans membrane helix 10 (TM10a) and extracellular loop 6 (EL6) are colored in green and orange. Reprinted with permission from Quizon PM, Sun WL, Yuan Y, Midde NM, Zhan CG, Zhu J, Molecular mechanism: the human dopamine transporter histidine 547 regulates basal and HIV-1 Tat protein-inhibited dopamine transport, Scientific Reports 6, 39048, 1-14. Copyright 2016 American Chemical Society (Quizon et al., 2016).

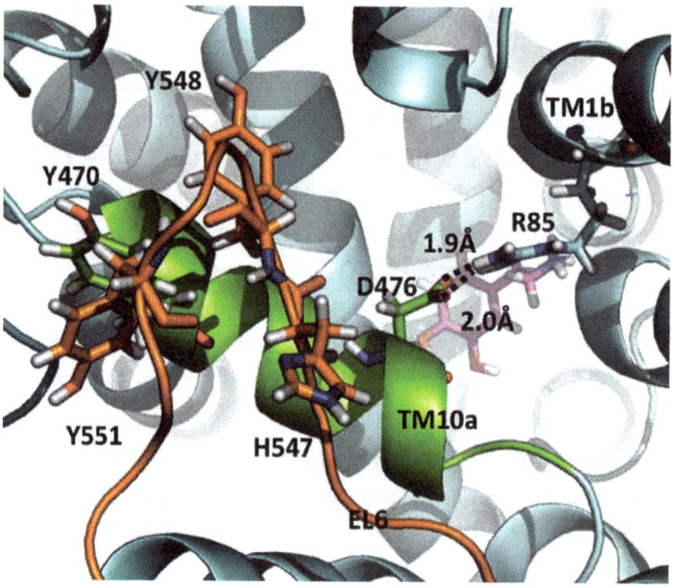

Zhan, 2009) was used. This modeling provided a mechanistic insight concerning how HIV-1 Tat interacts with hDAT and inhibits dopamine uptake by hDAT. This study also proved that the hDAT–Tat binding does not interfere with hDAT–DA binding, but stopped the conformational changing from the outward-open state to the other states (outward-occluded and inward-open states), so that they block the DA uptake by hDAT. Adding to that, this study confirmed that the Y470 of hDAT contains key residue that is involved in the interaction between hDAT and Tat, and the Y470H mutation would reduce the hDAT–Tat binding (Midde et al., 2013).

The MD-simulated hDAT–Tat-binding structure has showed that K92, Y88, and Y470 of hDAT are involved in the binding between hDAT and Tat (see Figure 8). The role of the K92, Y88, and Y470 of hDAT has been validated by DA uptake assays and site-directed mutagenesis. This agreement between both the computational and experimental data suggests that the computation predicted for hDAT–Tat-binding mode and mechanistic insights are acceptable and provide a new starting point to design pharmacological studies on the molecular mechanism of HIV-associated neurocognitive disorders (HAND).

Figure 8. The key residues involved in the binding between HIV-1 trans activator of transcription and human dopamine transporter in the outward-open state. Atomic interactions on the binding interface of the typical hDAT–Tat-binding structure. HIV-1 Tat protein is shown as ribbon and colored in gold, and hDAT is shown as cyan ribbon. Residues T-M1, T-P18 and T-K19 of HIV-1 Tat are shown in ball-stick style and colored in yellow. Residues D-Y470, D-Y88 and D-K92 are shown in ball-stick style and colored in green. Dashed lines represent intermolecular hydrogen bonds with labeled distances. For D-Y470, the red point indicates the center of its aromatic ring, and the dashed line pointing to the red ball represents the cation–π interaction with labeled distance.

Reprinted with permission from Yuan Y, Huang X, Midde NM et al. Molecular mechanism of HIV-1 Tat interacting with human dopamine transporter. ACS Chem. Neurosci. 6(4), 658–665 (2015). Copyright 2015 American Chemical Society (Yuan et al., 2015).

hDAT: Human dopamine transporter; Tat: Transactivator of transcription

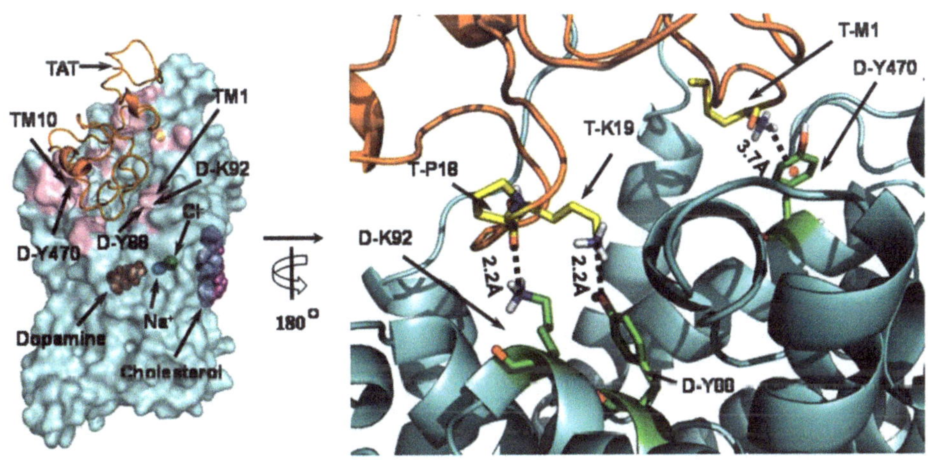

GENE THERAPY FOR HAND

Many mutations on hDAT residues not only interfere with hDAT–Tat binding, but also decline the dopamine uptake activity of hDAT, for example K92M, Y470H and Y88F (Yuan et al., 2016), a combined experimental and computational study has demonstrated that residue H547 of hDAT plays an important role in the dopamine uptake by hDAT and the hDAT–Tat interaction as H547 forms a hydrogen bond with residue R49 of HIV-Tat (see Figure 9). The hydrogen bond with the H547 side chain is expected to be broken with the H547A mutation and the mutation of this residue H547A not only attenuate Tat-induced inhibition of dopamine uptake, but also increase the V_{max} of hDAT for dopamine uptake (196% increase in DA uptake). H547A displays a differential sensitivity to protein kinase C (PKC) (activator (PMA) or inhibitor (BIM)), which leads to either activation or inhibition of DAT function relative to hDAT, which indicates a change in basal PKC activity in H547A.

These findings demonstrate that histidine 547 on hDAT plays an important role in stabilizing basal DA transport and Tat-DAT interaction (Yuan et al., 2016; Quizon et al., 2016). This study may help to develop novel concepts for therapeutic treatment of HAND. For example, gene therapy as the HAND-related abnormal neurocognitive function is associated with dysfunctions in dopamine neurotransmission (Purohit, Rapaka, Shurtleff, 2011; Bagashev & Sawaya, 2013), so that by improving dopamine uptake through effective delivery of a gene for an engineered hDAT mutant (such as one including the H547A mutation) will improve dopamine update activity without binding with HIV-1 Tat. For development of effective gene therapy, it's essential to have an hDAT mutant which doesn't bind with Tat. Therefore, Tat will not affect the dopamine uptake activity of the hDAT mutant. Adding to that, the higher the dopamine uptake activity of the hDAT mutant, the more effective the gene therapy would be. On the other hand, one may develop a small molecule drug which can bind with hDAT to affect the hDAT functions in a way similar to the effects of the H547A mutation, so that interferes with the hDAT binding with Tat and improves the normal dopamine uptake activity of native hDAT (Yuan et al., 2016).

Figure 9. A local view of DAT residue H547 and its direct interaction with Tat residue R49, the hydrogen bond with the H547 side chain is expected to be broken with the H547A mutation, which is consistent with decreased inhibitory activity of Tat on hDAT-H547A.

Reprinted with permission from Pamela M. Quizon, Wei-Lun Sun, Yaxia Yuan, Narasimha M. Midde, Chang-Guo Zhan, Jun Zhu, Molecular mechanism: the human dopamine transporter histidine 547 regulates basal and HIV-1 Tat protein-inhibited dopamine transport, Scientific Reports 6, 39048, 1-14. Copyright 2016 American Chemical Society (Quizon et al., 2016).

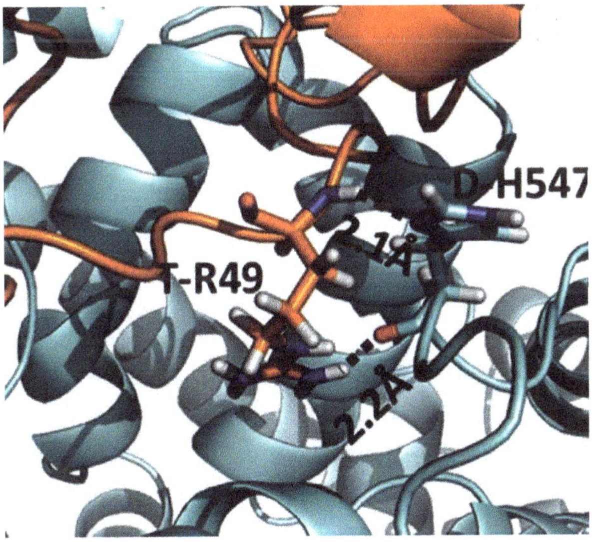

DRUG ABUSE THERAPY

A typical target of a psycho stimulant, such as cocaine, is the dopamine transporter, which becomes the preclinical target in the early stages of drug abuse therapy. So that, by selective inhibition to dopamine reuptake that interacts with hDAT lead to effective therapy for cocaine abuse (Carroll et al., 2008; Carroll et al., 2009; Kimmel et al., 2007; Froimowitz et al., 2007; Yohn et al., 2016). The mechanism of this medication is based on the fact that dopamine can partially substitute for cocaine, thus declining cocaine self-administration and decreasing the desire for cocaine (Liu & Molino, 2007; Runyon & Carroll, 2006; Papakostas, 2006). It is also possible to make potent allosteric hDAT modulators that can partially interfere with DA uptake by hDAT without affecting the hDAT–DA interaction (Richard et al., 2015). X-ray crystal structures of dDAT and LeuT-based hDAT models have been used to learn how the inhibitors interact with the transporter (Koldsø, Grouleff, & Schiøtt, 2015; Forrest et al., 2008; Severinsen et al., 2012; Seddik et al., 2013; Claxton et al., 2010; Beuming et al., 2008; Dahal et al., 2014; Grouleff et al., 2015; Kristensen et al., 2011; Koldsø et al., 2012). Recently developed hDAT models may be used to rationally design more active dopamine reuptake inhibitors so that the more active inhibitor binds with hDAT in any of the three conformational states.

CONCLUSION

Although there is no x-ray crystal structure available for human dopamine transporter (hDAT) but the, docking, molecular modeling, and dynamics simulations have provided a good 3D structural models of hDAT in its three typical conformational states, its binding with HIV-1 Tat, and its DA uptake mechanism. Particularly, the computational studies have greatly predicted the first-ever hDAT–Tat binding model, and this module has been supported by all of the experimental validation tests so that the 3D structures of hDAT in different conformation states and the complex between both HIV-1 Tat and DA have given a more detailed structural and mechanistic insights related to how hDAT uptakes DA and how HIV-1 Tat increase the normal function of hDAT. The general of the 3D modeled structures of hDAT and its binding with DA and Tat are reproducible with available experimental data in literature, and have been supported by the experimental validation tests. The detailed structure and mechanistic insight resulted from the computational studies on hDAT and hDAT–Tat interactions since HIV-1Tat and DA do not compete in their binding with hDAT, this will be great for future rational drug design of novel strategies for the cure of HIV associated neurocognitive disorders (HAND) which can prevent Tat from interaction with hDAT without blocking the DA uptake by hDAT.

REFERENCES

Aksenov, M. Y., Aksenova, M., Mactutus, C., & Booze, R. M. (2012). D1/NMDA receptors and concurrent methamphetamine+ HIV-1 Tat neurotoxicity. *Journal of Neuroimmune Pharmacology*, *7*(3), 599–608. doi:10.1007/s11481-012-9362-3 PMID:22552781

Aksenova, M. V., Silvers, J. M., Aksenov, M. Y., Nath, A., Ray, P. D., Mactutus, C. F., & Booze, R. M. (2006). HIV-1 Tat neurotoxicity in primary cultures of rat midbrain fetal neurons: Changes in dopamine transporter binding and immunoreactivity. *Neuroscience Letters*, *395*(3), 235–239. doi:10.1016/j.neulet.2005.10.095 PMID:16356633

Bagashev, A., & Sawaya, B. E. (2013). Roles and functions of HIV-1 Tat protein in the CNS: An overview. *Virology Journal*, *10*(1), 358. doi:10.1186/1743-422X-10-358 PMID:24359561

Bagashev, A., & Sawaya, B. E. (2013). Roles and functions of HIV-1 Tat protein in the CNS: An overview. *Virology Journal*, *10*(1), 358. doi:10.1186/1743-422X-10-358 PMID:24359561

Becker, J. T., Kingsley, L., Mullen, J., Cohen, B., Martin, E., Miller, E. N., ... Visscher, B. R. (2009). Multicenter AIDS Cohort Study.Vascular risk factors, HIV serostatus, and cognitive dysfunction in gay and bisexual men. *Neurology*, *73*(16), 1292–1299. doi:10.1212/WNL.0b013e3181bd10e7 PMID:19841381

Berger, J. R., & Arendt, G. (2000). HIV dementia: The role of the basal ganglia and dopaminergic systems. *Journal of Psychopharmacology (Oxford, England)*, *14*(3), 214–221. doi:10.1177/026988110001400304 PMID:11106299

Berger, J. R., & Arendt, G. (2000). HIV dementia: The role of the basal ganglia and dopaminergic systems. *Journal of Psychopharmacology (Oxford, England)*, *14*(3), 214–221. doi:10.1177/026988110001400304 PMID:11106299

Berridge, K. C. (2007). The debate over dopamine's role in reward: The case for incentive salience. *Psychopharmacology*, *191*(3), 391–431. doi:10.1007/s00213-006-0578-x PMID:17072591

Beuming, T., Kniazeff, J., Bergmann, M. L., Shi, L., Gracia, L., Raniszewska, K., ... Loland, C. J. (2008). The binding sites for cocaine and dopamine in the dopamine transporter overlap. *Nature Neuroscience*, *11*(7), 780–789. doi:10.1038/nn.2146 PMID:18568020

Beuming, T., Kniazeff, J., Bergmann, M. L., Shi, L., Gracia, L., Raniszewska, K., ... Loland, C. J. (2008). The binding sites for cocaine and dopamine in the dopamine transporter overlap. *Nature Neuroscience, 11*(7), 780–789. doi:10.1038/nn.2146 PMID:18568020

Buch, S., Yao, H., Guo, M, Mori, T., Su, T.P., & Wang, J (2011). Cocaine and HIV-1 interplay: molecular mechanisms of action and addiction. *Journal of Neuroimmune Pharmacology, 6*, 503-515.

Buckner, C.M., Luers, A.J., Calderon, T.M., Eugenin, E.A., & Berman, J.W. (2006). Neuroimmunity and the blood-brain barrier: molecular regulation of leukocyte transmigration and viral entry into the nervous system with a focus on neuroAIDS. *Journal of Neuroimmune Pharmacology, 1*, 160–181.

Carroll, F. I., Blough, B. E., Abraham, P., Mills, A. C., Holleman, J. A., Wolckenhauer, S. A., ... Forster, M. J. (2009). Synthesis and biological evaluation of bupropion analogues as potential pharmacotherapies for cocaine addiction. *Journal of Medicinal Chemistry, 52*(21), 6768–6781. doi:10.1021/jm901189z PMID:19821577

Carroll, F. I., Howard, J. L., Howell, L. L., Fox, B. S., & Kuhar, M. J. (2008). Development of the dopamine transporter selective RTI-336 as a pharmacotherapy for cocaine abuse. In R. S. Papaka & W. Sadee (Eds.), *Drug Addiction* (pp. 179–191). Springer. doi:10.1007/978-0-387-76678-2_12

Chang, L., Wang, G. J., Volkow, N. D., Ernst, T., Telang, F., Logan, J., & Fowler, J. S. (2008). Decreased brain dopamine transporters are related to cognitive deficits in HIV patients with or without cocaine abuse. *NeuroImage, 42*(2), 869–878. doi:10.1016/j.neuroimage.2008.05.011 PMID:18579413

Chang, L., Wang, G. J., Volkow, N. D., Ernst, T., Telang, F., Logan, J., & Fowler, J. S. (2008). Decreased brain dopamine transporters are related to cognitive deficits in HIV patients with or without cocaine abuse. *NeuroImage, 42*(2), 869–878. doi:10.1016/j.neuroimage.2008.05.011 PMID:18579413

Chen, R., Tilley, M. R., Wei, H., Zhou, F., Zhou, F. M., Ching, S., ... Gu, H. H. (2006). Abolished cocaine reward in mice with a cocaine-insensitive dopamine transporter. *Proceedings of the National Academy of Sciences of the United States of America, 103*(24), 9333–9338. doi:10.1073/pnas.0600905103 PMID:16754872

Claxton, D. P., Quick, M., Shi, L., de Carvalho, F. D., Weinstein, H., Javitch, J. A., & McHaourab, H. S. (2010). Ion/substrate-dependent conformational dynamics of a bacterial homolog of neurotransmitter: Sodium symporters. *Nature Structural & Molecular Biology, 17*(7), 822–829. doi:10.1038/nsmb.1854 PMID:20562855

Dahal, R. A., Pramod, A. B., Sharma, B., Krout, D., Foster, J. D., Cha, J. H., & Henry, L. K. (2014). Computational and biochemical docking of the irreversible cocaine analog RTI 82 directly demonstrates ligand positioning in the dopamine transporter central substrate-binding site. *The Journal of Biological Chemistry*, *289*(43), 29712–29727. doi:10.1074/jbc.M114.571521 PMID:25179220

Davis, L. E., Hjelle, B. L., Miller, V. E., Palmer, D. L., Llewellyn, A. L., & Merlin, T. L. (1992) Early viral brain invasion in iatrogenic human immunodeficiency virus infection. *Neurology*, 42.

Del Valle, L., Croul, S., Morgello, S., Amini, S., Rappaport, J., & Khalili, K. (2000). Detection of HIV-1 Tat and JCV capsid protein, VP1, in AIDS brain with progressive multifocal leukoencephalopathy. *Journal of Neurovirology*, *6*(3), 221–228. doi:10.3109/13550280009015824 PMID:10878711

Del Valle, L., Croul, S., Morgello, S., Amini, S., Rappaport, J., & Khalili, K. (2000). Detection of HIV-1 Tat and JCV capsid protein, VP1, in AIDS brain with progressive multifocal leukoencephalopathy. *Journal of Neurovirology*, *6*(3), 221–228. doi:10.3109/13550280009015824 PMID:10878711

Ernst, T., Jiang, C. S., Nakama, H., Buchthal, S., & Chang, L. (2010). Lower brain glutamate is associated with cognitive deficits in HIV patients: A new mechanism for HIV-associated neurocognitive disorder. Journal of magnetic resonance imaging. *Journal of Magnetic Resonance Imaging*, *32*(5), 1045–1053. doi:10.1002/jmri.22366 PMID:21031507

Ernst, T., Yakupov, R., Nakama, H., Crocket, G., Cole, M., Watters, M., ... Chang, L. (2009). Declined neural efficiency in cognitively stable human immunodeficiency virus patients. *Annals of Neurology*, *65*(3), 316–325. doi:10.1002/ana.21594 PMID:19334060

Everitt, B. J., & Robbins, T. W. (2005). Neural systems of reinforcement for drug addiction: From actions to habits to compulsion. *Nature Neuroscience*, *8*(11), 1481–1489. doi:10.1038/nn1579 PMID:16251991

Fabbiani, M., Ciccarelli, N., Tana, M., Farina, S., Baldonero, E., Di Cristo, V., ... Di Giambenedetto, S. (2013). Cardiovascular risk factors and carotid intima-media thickness are associated with lower cognitive performance in HIV-infected patients. *HIV Medicine*, *14*(3), 136–144. doi:10.1111/j.1468-1293.2012.01044.x PMID:22994586

Fazeli, P. L., Crowe, M., Ross, L. A., Wadley, V., Ball, K., & Vance, D. E. (2015). Cognitive functioning in adults aging with HIV: A cross-sectional analysis of cognitive subtypes and influential factors. *Journal of Clinical Research in HIV AIDS and Prevention*, *1*, 155–169. PMID:25386565

Ferrarese, C., Aliprandi, A., Tremolizzo, L., Stanzani, L., De Micheli, A., Dolara, A., & Frattola, L. (2001). Increased glutamate in CSF and plasma of patients with HIV dementia. *Neurology*, *57*(4), 671–675. doi:10.1212/WNL.57.4.671 PMID:11524477

Ferris, M. J., Frederick-Duus, D., Fadel, J., Mactutus, C. F., & Booze, R. M. (2009). The human immunodeficiency virus-1-associated protein, Tat1–86, impairs dopamine transporters and interacts with cocaine to reduce nerve terminal function: A no-net-flux microdialysis study. *Neuroscience*, *159*(4), 1292–1299. doi:10.1016/j.neuroscience.2009.01.024 PMID:19344635

Ferris, M. J., Frederick-Duus, D., Fadel, J., Mactutus, C. F., & Booze, R. M. (2010). Hyperdopaminergic tone in HIV-1 protein treated rat and cocaine sensitization. *Journal of Neurochemistry*, *115*(4), 885–896. doi:10.1111/j.1471-4159.2010.06968.x PMID:20796175

Ferris, M. J., Frederick-Duus, D., Fadel, J., Mactutus, C. F., & Booze, R. M. (2010). Hyperdopaminergic tone in HIV-1 protein treated rats and cocaine sensitization. *Journal of Neurochemistry*, *115*(4), 885–896. doi:10.1111/j.1471-4159.2010.06968.x PMID:20796175

Ferris, M. J., Mactutus, C. F., & Booze, R. M. (2008). Neurotoxic profiles of HIV, psychostimulant drugs of abuse, and their concerted effect on the brain: Current status of dopamine system vulnerability in NeuroAIDS. *Neuroscience and Biobehavioral Reviews*, *32*(5), 883–909. doi:10.1016/j.neubiorev.2008.01.004 PMID:18430470

Ferris, M. J., Mactutus, C. F., & Booze, R. M. (2008). Neurotoxic profiles of HIV, psychostimulant drugs of abuse, and their concerted effect on the brain: Current status of dopamine system vulnerability in NeuroAIDS. *Neuroscience and Biobehavioral Reviews*, *32*(5), 883–909. doi:10.1016/j.neubiorev.2008.01.004 PMID:18430470

Fois, F., & Brew, B. J. (2015). The potential of the CNS as a reservoir for HIV-1 infection: Implications for HIV eradication. *Current HIV/AIDS Reports*, *12*(2), 299–303. doi:10.1007/s11904-015-0257-9 PMID:25869939

Forrest, L. R., Zhang, Y. W., Jacobs, M. T., Gesmonde, J., Xie, L., Honig, B. H., & Rudnick, G. (2008). Mechanism for alternating access in neurotransmitter transporters. *Proceedings of the National Academy of Sciences of the United States of America*, *105*(30), 10338–10343. doi:10.1073/pnas.0804659105 PMID:18647834

Froimowitz, M., Gu, Y., Dakin, L. A., Nagafuji, P. M., Kelley, C. J., Parrish, D., ... Janowsky, A. (2007). Slow-onset, long-duration, alkyl analogues of methylphenidate with enhanced selectivity for the dopamine transporter. *Journal of Medicinal Chemistry*, *50*(2), 219–232. doi:10.1021/jm0608614 PMID:17228864

Gaskill, P. J., Calderon, T. M., Luers, A. J., Eugenin, E. A., Javitch, J. A., & Berman, J. W. (2009). Human immunodeficiency virus (HIV) infection of human macrophages is increased by dopamine: A bridge between HIV-associated neurologic disorders and drug abuse. *American Journal of Pathology*, *175*(3), 1148–1159. doi:10.2353/ajpath.2009.081067 PMID:19661443

Gedeon, P. C., Indarte, M., Surratt, C. K., & Madura, J. D. (2010). Molecular dynamics of leucine and dopamine transporter proteins in a model cell membrane lipid bilayer. *Proteins*, *78*(4), 797–811. doi:10.1002/prot.22601 PMID:19899168

Gelman, B. B., Lisinicchia, J. G., Chen, T., Johnson, K. M., Jennings, K., Freeman, D. H., & Soukup, V. M. (2012). Prefrontal Dopaminergic and Enkephalinergic Synaptic Accommodation in HIV-associated Neurocognitive Disorders and Encephalitis. *Journal of Neuroimmune Pharmacology*, *7*(3), 686–700. doi:10.1007/s11481-012-9345-4 PMID:22391864

Gelman, B. B., Lisinicchia, J. G., Chen, T., Johnson, K. M., Jennings, K., Freeman, D. H., & Soukup, V. M. (2012). Prefrontal dopaminergic and enkephalinergic synaptic accommodation in HIV-associated neurocognitive disorders and encephalitis. *Journal of Neuroimmune Pharmacology*, *7*(3), 686–700. doi:10.1007/s11481-012-9345-4 PMID:22391864

Grouleff, J., Ladefoged, L. K., Koldsø, H., & Schiøtt, B. (2015). Monoamine transporters: Insights from molecular dynamics simulations. *Frontiers in Pharmacology*, *6*, 235. doi:10.3389/fphar.2015.00235 PMID:26528185

Guptaroy, B., Zhang, M., Bowton, E., Binda, F., Shi, L., Weinstein, H., ... Gnegy, M. E. (2009). A juxtamembrane mutation in the N terminus of the dopamine transporter induces preference for an inward-facing conformation. *Molecular Pharmacology*, *75*(3), 514–524. doi:10.1124/mol.108.048744 PMID:19098122

Heaton, R., Franklin, D., Letendre, S., Ellis, R., & Fennema-Notestine, C, Vaida. F, Smith D,... ..., Grant, I. (2012). Aging amplifies HIV neurocognitive impairment: The effects may be related to vascular and metabolic factors. *Journal of Neurovirology*, *18*, S46.

Heaton, R. K., Clifford, D. B., Franklin, D. R., Woods, S. P., Ake, C., Vaida, F., ... Grant, I. (2010a). HIV-associated neurocognitive disorders (HAND) persist in the era of potent antiretroviral therapy: The CHARTER Study. *Neurology*, *75*(23), 2087–2096. doi:10.1212/WNL.0b013e318200d727 PMID:21135382

Heaton, R. K., Clifford, D. B., Franklin, D. R., Woods, S. P., Ake, C., Vaida, F., ... Grant, I. (2010b). HIV-associated neurocognitive disorders persist in the era of potent antiretroviral therapy: CHARTER Study. *Neurology*, *75*(23), 2087–2096. doi:10.1212/WNL.0b013e318200d727 PMID:21135382

Heaton, R. K., Clifford, D. B., Franklin, D. R., Woods, S. P., Ake, C., Vaida, F., ... Grant, I. (2010c). HIV-associated neurocognitive disorders persist in the era of potent antiretroviral therapy: CHARTER Study. *Neurology*, *75*(23), 2087–2096. doi:10.1212/WNL.0b013e318200d727 PMID:21135382

Heaton, R. K., Franklin, D. R., Ellis, R. J., McCutchan, J. A., Letendre, S. L., Leblanc, S., ... Grant, I. (2011). HIV-associated neurocognitive disorders before and during the era of combination antiretroviral therapy: Differences in rates, nature, and predictors. *Journal of Neurovirology*, *17*(1), 3–16. doi:10.1007/s13365-010-0006-1 PMID:21174240

Heaton, R. K., Velin, R. A., McCutchan, J. A., Gulevich, S. J., Atkinson, J. H., Wallace, M. R., ... Grant, I. (1994). Neuropsychological impairment in human immunodeficiency virus-infection: Implications for employment. HNRC Group HIV Neurobehavioral Research Center. *Psychosomatic Medicine*, *56*(1), 8–17. doi:10.1097/00006842-199401000-00001 PMID:8197319

Henry, L.K., Iwamoto, H., Field, J.R., Kaufmann, K., Dawson, E.S., & Jacobs, M.T., … Blakely, R.D. (2011). A conserved asparagine residue in TM1 of the serotonin transporter dictates chloride-coupled neurotransmitter transport. *The Journal of Biological Chemistry*, *286*(35), 30823–30836. doi:10.1074/jbc.M111.250308 PMID:21730057

Huang, X., Gu, H. H., & Zhan, C.-G. (2009). Mechanism for cocaine blocking the transport of dopamine: Insights from molecular modeling and dynamics simulations. *The Journal of Physical Chemistry B*, *113*(45), 15057–15066. doi:10.1021/jp900963n PMID:19831380

Huang, X., & Zhan, C. G. (2007). How dopamine transporter interacts with dopamine: Insights from molecular modeling and simulation. *Biophysical Journal*, *93*(10), 3627–3639. doi:10.1529/biophysj.107.110924 PMID:17704152

Huang, X., & Zhan, C. G. (2007). How dopamine transporter interacts with dopamine: Insights from molecular modeling and simulation. *Biophysical Journal*, *93*(10), 3627–3639. doi:10.1529/biophysj.107.110924 PMID:17704152

Hudson, L., Liu, J., Nath, A., Jones, M., Raghavan, R., Narayan, O., ... Everall, I. (2000). Detection of the human immunodeficiency virus regulatory protein tat in CNS tissues. *Journal of Neurovirology*, *6*(2), 145–155. doi:10.3109/13550280009013158 PMID:10822328

Hudson, L., Liu, J., Nath, A., Jones, M., Raghavan, R., Narayan, O., ... Everall, I. (2000). Detection of the human immunodeficiency virus regulatory protein tat in CNS tissues. *Journal of Neurovirology*, *6*(2), 145–155. doi:10.3109/13550280009013158 PMID:10822328

Jacobs, M. M., Murray, J., Byrd, D. A., Hurd, Y. L., & Morgello, S. (2013). HIV-related cognitive impairment shows bi-directional association with dopamine receptor DRD1 and DRD2 polymorphisms in substance-dependent and substance-independent populations. *Journal of Neurovirology*, *19*(5), 495–504. doi:10.1007/s13365-013-0204-8 PMID:24078558

Janssen, R. S., Nwanyanwu, O. C., Selik, R. M., & Stehr-Green, J. K. (1992). Epidemiology of human immunodeficiency virus encephalopathy in the United States. *Neurology*, *42*(8), 1472–1476. doi:10.1212/WNL.42.8.1472 PMID:1641138

Joska, J. A., Westgarth-Taylor, J., Hoare, J., Thomas, K. G., Paul, R., Myer, L., & Stein, D. J. (2012). Neuropsychological outcomes in adults commencing highly active anti-retroviral treatment in South Africa: A prospective study. *BMC Infectious Diseases*, *12*(1), 39. doi:10.1186/1471-2334-12-39 PMID:22335937

Joska, J. A., Westgarth-Taylor, J., Myer, L., Hoare, J., Thomas, K. G., Combrinck, M., ... Flisher, A. J. (2011). Characterization of HIV-associated neurocognitive disorders among individuals starting antiretroviral therapy in South Africa. *AIDS and Behavior*, *15*(6), 1197–1203. doi:10.1007/s10461-010-9744-6 PMID:20614176

Kim, J., Yoon, J.-H., & Kim, Y.-S. (2013). HIV-1 Tat interacts with and regulates the localization and processing of amyloid precursor protein. *PLoS One*, *8*(11), e77972. doi:10.1371/journal.pone.0077972 PMID:24312169

Kimmel, H. L., Oconnor, J. A. A., Carroll, F. I., & Howell, L. L. (2007). Faster onset and dopamine transporter selectivity predict stimulant and reinforcing effects of cocaine analogs in squirrel monkeys. *Pharmacology, Biochemistry, and Behavior*, *86*(1), 45–54. doi:10.1016/j.pbb.2006.12.006 PMID:17258302

Koldsø, H., Christiansen, A. B., Sinning, S., & Schiøtt, B. (2012). Comparative modeling of the human monoamine transporters: Similarities in substrate binding. *ACS Chemical Neuroscience*, *4*(2), 295–309. doi:10.1021/cn300148r PMID:23421681

Koldsø, H., Grouleff, J., & Schiøtt, B. (2015). Insights to ligand binding to the monoamine transporters – from homology modeling to LeuBAT and dDAT. *Frontiers in Pharmacology*, *6*, 208. doi:10.3389/fphar.2015.00208 PMID:26441663

Koldsø, H., Noer, P., Grouleff, J., Autzen, H. E., Sinning, S., & Schiøtt, B. (2011). Unbiased simulations reveal the inward-facing conformation of the human serotonin transporter and Na+ ion release. *PLoS Computational Biology*, *7*(10), e1002246. doi:10.1371/journal.pcbi.1002246 PMID:22046120

Koutsilieri, E., Czub, S., Scheller, C., Sopper, S., Tatschner, T., Stahl-Hennig, C., ... Riederer, P. (2000). Brain choline acetyltransferase reduction in SIV infection. An index of early dementia? *Neuroreport*, *11*(11), 2391–2393. doi:10.1097/00001756-200008030-00011 PMID:10943691

Koutsilieri, E., Meulen, V., & Riederer, P. (2001). Neurotransmission in HIV associated dementia: A short review. *Journal of Neural Transmission (Vienna, Austria)*, *108*(6), 767–775. doi:10.1007/s007020170051 PMID:11478426

Koutsilieri, E., Sopper, S., Scheller, C., ter Meulen, V., & Riederer, P. (2002). Involvement of dopamine in the progression of AIDS Dementia Complex. *Journal of Neural Transmission (Vienna, Austria)*, *109*(3), 399–410. doi:10.1007/s007020200032 PMID:11956960

Krishnamurthy, H., & Gouaux, E. (2012). X-ray structures of LeuT in substrate-free outward-open and apo inward-open states. *Nature*, *481*(7382), 469–474. doi:10.1038/nature10737 PMID:22230955

Krishnamurthy, H., Piscitelli, C. L., & Gouaux, E. (2009). Unlocking the molecular secrets of sodium-coupled transporters. *Nature*, *459*(7245), 347–355. doi:10.1038/nature08143 PMID:19458710

Kristensen, A. S., Andersen, J., Jørgensen, T. N., Sørensen, L., Eriksen, J., Loland, C. J., ... Gether, U. (2011). SLC6 neurotransmitter transporters: Structure, function, and regulation. *Pharmacological Reviews*, *63*(3), 585–640. doi:10.1124/pr.108.000869 PMID:21752877

Kumar, A. M., Fernandez, J. B., Singer, E. J., Commins, D., Waldrop-Valverde, D., Ownby, R. L., & Kumar, M. (2009). Human immunodeficiency virus type 1 in the central nervous system leads to decreased dopamine in different regions of postmortem human brains. *Journal of Neurovirology*, *15*(3), 257–274. doi:10.1080/13550280902973952 PMID:19499455

Kumar, A. M., Ownby, R. L., Waldrop-Valverde, D., Fernandez, B., & Kumar, M. (2011). Human immunodeficiency virus infection in the CNS and decreased dopamine availability: Relationship with neuropsychological performance. *Journal of Neurovirology*, *17*(1), 26–40. doi:10.1007/s13365-010-0003-4 PMID:21165787

Kumar, A. M., Ownby, R. L., Waldrop-Valverde, D., Fernandez, B., & Kumar, M. (2011). Human immunodeficiency virus infection in the CNS and decreased dopamine availability: Relationship with neuropsychological performance. *Journal of Neurovirology*, *17*(1), 26–40. doi:10.1007/s13365-010-0003-4 PMID:21165787

Lamers, S. L., Salemi, M., Galligan, D. C., Morris, A., Gray, R., Fogel, G., ... McGrath, M. S. (2010). Human immunodeficiency virus-1 evolutionary patterns associated with pathogenic processes in the brain. *Journal of Neurovirology*, *16*(3), 230–241. doi:10.3109/13550281003735709 PMID:20367240

Lamers, S. L., Salemi, M., Galligan, D. C., Morris, A., Gray, R., Fogel, G., ... McGrath, M. S. (2010). Human immunodeficiency virus-1 evolutionary patterns associated with pathogenic processes in the brain. *Journal of Neurovirology*, *16*(3), 230–241. doi:10.3109/13550281003735709 PMID:20367240

Liu, S., & Molino, B. F. (2007). Recent developments in monoamine reuptake inhibitors. *Annual Reports in Medicinal Chemistry*, *42*, 13–26. doi:10.1016/S0065-7743(07)42002-4

Loland, C. J. (2014). The use of LeuT as a model in elucidating binding sites for substrates and inhibitors in neurotransmitter transporters. *Biochimica et Biophysica Acta*, *1850*(3), 500–510. doi:10.1016/j.bbagen.2014.04.011 PMID:24769398

Loland, C. J., Norgaard-Nielsen, K., & Gether, U. (2003). Probing dopamine transporter structure and function by Zn2+-site engineering. *European Journal of Pharmacology*, *479*(1–3), 187–197. doi:10.1016/j.ejphar.2003.08.068 PMID:14612149

Lüdemann, S. K., Lounnas, V., & Wade, R. C. (2000). How do substrates enter and products exit the buried active site of cytochrome P450cam? 1. Random expulsion molecular dynamics investigation of ligand access channels and mechanisms. *Journal of Molecular Biology, 303*(5), 797–811. doi:10.1006/jmbi.2000.4154 PMID:11061976

Manepalli, S., Surratt, C. K., Madura, J. D., & Nolan, T. L. (2012). Monoamine transporter structure, function, dynamics, and drug discovery: A computational perspective. *The AAPS Journal, 14*(4), 820–831. doi:10.1208/s12248-012-9391-0 PMID:22918625

Marquine, M. J., Umlauf, A., Rooney, A. S., Fazeli, P. L., Gouaux, B. D., Paul Woods, S., ... Moore, D. J. (2014). The veterans aging cohort study index is associated with concurrent risk for neurocognitive impairment. *JAIDS Journal of Acquired Immune Deficiency Syndromes, 65*(2), 190–197. doi:10.1097/QAI.0000000000000008 PMID:24442225

Mattson, M. P., Haughey, N. J., & Nath, A. (2005). Cell death in HIV dementia. *Cell Death and Differentiation, 12*(S1), 893–904. doi:10.1038/sj.cdd.4401577 PMID:15761472

McArthur, J. C., Steiner, J., Sacktor, N., & Nath, A. (2010). Human immunodeficiency virus-associated neurocognitive disorders: Mind the gap. *Annals of Neurology, 67*, 699–714. PMID:20517932

McCutchan, J. A., Marquie-Beck, J. A., Fitzsimons, C. A., Letendre, S. L., Ellis, R. J., Heaton, R. K., ... Grant, I. (2012). Role of obesity, metabolic variables, and diabetes in HIV-associated neurocognitive disorder. *Neurology, 78*(7), 485–492. doi:10.1212/WNL.0b013e3182478d64 PMID:22330412

Meade, C. S., Conn, N. A., Skalski, L. M., & Safren, S. A. (2011a). Neurocognitive impairment and medication adherence in HIV patients with and without cocaine dependence. *Journal of Behavioral Medicine, 34*(2), 128–138. doi:10.1007/s10865-010-9293-5 PMID:20857187

Meade, C. S., Lowen, S. B., MacLean, R. R., Key, M. D., & Lukas, S. E. (2011). MRI brain activation during a delay discounting task in HIV positive adults with and without cocaine dependence. *Psychiatry Research, 192*(3), 167–175. doi:10.1016/j.pscychresns.2010.12.011 PMID:21546221

Meade, C. S., Lowen, S. B., MacLean, R. R., Key, M. D., & Lukas, S. E. (2011b). fMRI brain activation during a delay discounting task in HIV-positive adults with and without cocaine dependence. *Psychiatry Research, 192*(3), 167–175. doi:10.1016/j.pscychresns.2010.12.011 PMID:21546221

Midde, N. M., Gomez, A. M., & Zhu, J. (2012). HIV-1 Tat protein decreases dopamine transporter cell surface expression and vesicular monoamine transporter-2 function in Rat striatal synaptosomes. *Journal of Neuroimmune Pharmacology*, *7*(3), 629–639. doi:10.1007/s11481-012-9369-9 PMID:22570010

Midde, N. M., Gomez, A. M., & Zhu, J. (2012). HIV-1 Tat protein decreases dopamine transporter cell surface expression and vesicular monoamine transporter-2 function in rat striatal synaptosomes. *Journal of Neuroimmune Pharmacology*, *7*(3), 629–639. doi:10.1007/s11481-012-9369-9 PMID:22570010

Midde, N. M., Huang, X., Gomez, A. M., Booze, R. M., Zhan, C. G., & Zhu, J. (2013). Mutation of tyrosine 470 of human dopamine transporter is critical for HIV-1 Tat-induced inhibition of dopamine transport and transporter conformational transitions. *Journal of Neuroimmune Pharmacology*, *8*(4), 975–987. doi:10.1007/s11481-013-9464-6 PMID:23645138

Midde, N. M., Yuan, Y., Quizon, P. M., Sun, W. L., Huang, X., Zhan, C. G., & Zhu, J. (2015). Mutations at tyrosine 88, lysine 92 and tyrosine 470 of human dopamine transporter result in an attenuation of HIV-1 Tat-induced inhibition of dopamine transport. *Journal of Neuroimmune Pharmacology*, *10*(1), 122–135. doi:10.1007/s11481-015-9583-3 PMID:25604666

Nair, M. P. N., & Samikkannu, T. (2012). Differential regulation of neurotoxin in HIV clades: Role of cocaine and methamphetamine. *Current HIV Research*, *10*, 429–434. doi:10.2174/157016212802138742 PMID:22591367

Nath, A., Anderson, C., Jones, M., Maragos, W., Booze, R., Mactutus, C., ... Mattson, M. (2000b). Neurotoxicity and dysfunction of dopaminergic systems associated with AIDS dementia. *Journal of Psychopharmacology (Oxford, England)*, *14*(3), 222–227. doi:10.1177/026988110001400305 PMID:11106300

Nath, A., & Clements, J. E. (2011). Eradication of HIV from the brain: Reasons for pause. *AIDS (London, England)*, *25*(5), 577–580. doi:10.1097/QAD.0b013e3283437d2f PMID:21160414

Nath, A., Jankovic, J., & Pettigrew, L. C. (1987). Movement disorders and AIDS. *Neurology*, *37*(1), 37–41. doi:10.1212/WNL.37.1.37 PMID:3796836

Nath, A., Maragos, W. F., Avison, M. J., Schmitt, F. A., & Berger, J. R. (2001). Acceleration of HIV dementia with methamphetamine and cocaine. *Journal of Neurovirology*, *7*(1), 66–71. doi:10.1080/135502801300069737 PMID:11519485

Nayeem, A., Sitkoff, D., & Krystek, S. (2006). A comparative study of available software for high-accuracy homology modeling: From sequence alignments to structural models. *Protein Science*, *15*(4), 808–824. doi:10.1110/ps.051892906 PMID:16600967

Norregaard, L., Frederiksen, D., Nielsen, E. Ø., & Gether, U. (1998). Delineation of an endogenous zinc-binding site in the human dopamine transporter. *The EMBO Journal*, *17*(15), 4266–4273. doi:10.1093/emboj/17.15.4266 PMID:9687495

Papakostas, G. I. (2006). Dopaminergic-based pharmacotherapies for depression. *European Neuropsychopharmacology*, *16*(6), 391–402. doi:10.1016/j.euroneuro.2005.12.002 PMID:16413172

Pei, J., Tang, M., & Grishin, N. V. (2008). PROMALS3D web server for accurate multiple protein sequence and structure alignments. *Nucleic Acids Research*, *36*(Web ServerSuppl. 2), W30–W34. doi:10.1093/nar/gkn322 PMID:18503087

Penmatsa, A., Wang, K. H., & Gouaux, E. (2013). X-ray structure of dopamine transporter elucidates antidepressant mechanism. *Nature*, *503*(7474), 85–90. doi:10.1038/nature12533 PMID:24037379

Penmatsa, A., Wang, K. H., & Gouaux, E. (2015). X-ray structures of drosophila dopamine transporter in complex with nisoxetine and reboxetine. *Nature Structural & Molecular Biology*, *22*(6), 506–508. doi:10.1038/nsmb.3029 PMID:25961798

Purohit, V., Rapaka, R., & Shurtleff, D. (2011). Drugs of abuse, dopamine, and HIV-associated neurocognitive disorders/HIV-associated dementia. *Molecular Neurobiology*, *44*(1), 102–110. doi:10.1007/s12035-011-8195-z PMID:21717292

Purohit, V., Rapaka, R., & Shurtleff, D. (2011). Drugs of Abuse, Dopamine, and HIV-Associated Neurocognitive Disorders/HIV-Associated Dementia. *Molecular Neurobiology*, *44*(1), 102–110. doi:10.1007/s12035-011-8195-z PMID:21717292

Purohit, V., Rapaka, R., & Shurtleff, D. (2011). Drugs of abuse, dopamine, and HIV-associated neurocognitive disorders/ HIV-associated dementia. *Molecular Neurobiology*, *44*(1), 102–110. doi:10.1007/s12035-011-8195-z PMID:21717292

Purohit, V., Rapaka, R., & Shurtleff, D. (2011). Drugs of abuse, dopamine, and HIV-associated neurocognitive disorders/HIV-associated dementia. *Molecular Neurobiology*, *44*(1), 102–110. doi:10.1007/s12035-011-8195-z PMID:21717292

Quizon, P. M., Sun, W. L., Yuan, Y., Midde, N. M., Zhan, C. G., & Zhu, J. (2016). Molecular mechanism: The human dopamine transporter histidine 547 regulates basal and HIV-1 Tat protein-inhibited dopamine transport. *Scientific Reports*, *6*(39048), 1–14. PMID:27966610

Ragin, A. B., Wu, Y., Gao, Y., Keating, S., Du, H., Sammet, C., ... Epstein, L. G. (2015). Brain alterations within the first 100 days of HIV infection. *Annals of Clinical and Translational Neurology*, *2*(1), 12–21. doi:10.1002/acn3.136 PMID:25642430

Richard, B. R., John, S. P., Saini, S. K. O., Moukha, C. V., Michael, H., & Baumann, S. A. (2015). Identification of novel allosteric dopamine transporter ligands with nanomolar potency. *Drug and Alcohol Dependence*, *156*, e193–e194. doi:10.1016/j.drugalcdep.2015.07.521

Robertson, K. R., Smurzynski, M., Parsons, T. D., Wu, K., Bosch, R. J., Wu, J., ... Ellis, R. J. (2007). The prevalence and incidence of neurocognitive impairment in the HAART era. *AIDS (London, England)*, *21*(14), 1915–1921. doi:10.1097/QAD.0b013e32828e4e27 PMID:17721099

Runyon, S. P., & Carroll, F. (2006). Dopamine transporter ligands: Recent developments and therapeutic potential. *Current Topics in Medicinal Chemistry*, *6*(17), 1825–1843. doi:10.2174/156802606778249775 PMID:17017960

Šali, A., Potterton, L., Yuan, F., Van Vlijmen, H., & Karplus, M. (1995). Evaluation of comparative protein modeling by MODELLER. *Proteins*, *23*(3), 318–326. doi:10.1002/prot.340230306 PMID:8710825

Sardar, A. M., Czudek, C., & Reynolds, G. P. (1996). Dopamine deficits in the brain: The neurochemical basis of parkinsonian symptoms in AIDS. *Neuroreport*, *7*(4), 910–912. doi:10.1097/00001756-199603220-00015 PMID:8724671

Scheller, C., Arendt, G., Nolting, T., Antke, C., Sopper, S., Maschke, M., ... Koutsilieri, E. (2010). Increased dopaminergic neurotransmission in therapy-naive asymptomatic HIV patients is not associated with adaptive changes at the dopaminergic synapses. *Journal of Neural Transmission (Vienna, Austria)*, *117*(6), 699–705. doi:10.1007/s00702-010-0415-6 PMID:20454983

Scheller, C., Arendt, G., Nolting, T., Antke, C., Sopper, S., Maschke, M., ... Koutsilieri, E. (2010). Increased dopaminergic neurotransmission in therapy-naive asymptomatic HIV patients is not associated with adaptive changes at the dopaminergic synapses. *Journal of Neural Transmission (Vienna, Austria)*, *117*(6), 699–705. doi:10.1007/s00702-010-0415-6 PMID:20454983

Schmitt, K. C., & Reith, M. E. (2011). The atypical stimulant and nootropic modafinil interacts with the dopamine transporter in a different manner than classical cocaine-like inhibitors. *PLoS One*, *6*(10), e25790. doi:10.1371/journal.pone.0025790 PMID:22043293

Seddik, A., Holy, M., Weissensteiner, R., Zdrazil, B., Sitte, H. H., & Ecker, G. F. (2013). Probing the selectivity of monoamine transporter substrates by means of molecular modeling. *Molecular Informatics*, *32*(5-6), 409–413. doi:10.1002/minf.201300013 PMID:23956802

Severinsen, K., Kraft, J. F., Koldsø, H., Vinberg, K. A., Rothman, R. B., Partilla, J. S., ... Sinning, S. (2012). Binding of the amphetamine-like 1-phenyl-piperazine to monoamine transporters. *ACS Chemical Neuroscience*, *3*(9), 693–705. doi:10.1021/cn300040f PMID:23019496

Shan, J., Javitch, J. A., Shi, L., & Weinstein, H. (2011). The substrate driven transition to an inward-facing conformation in the functional mechanism of the dopamine transporter. *PLoS One*, *6*(1), e16350. doi:10.1371/journal.pone.0016350 PMID:21298009

Silverstein, P., Shah, A., Weemhoff, J., Kumar, S. P., Singh, D., & Kumar, A. (2012). HIV-1 gp120 and drugs of abuse: Interactions in the central nervous system. *Current HIV Research*, *10*, 369–383. doi:10.2174/157016212802138724 PMID:22591361

Singh, S. K., Piscitelli, C. L., Yamashita, A., & Gouaux, E. (2008). A competitive inhibitor traps LeuT in an open-to-out conformation. *Science*, *322*(5908), 1655–1661. doi:10.1126/science.1166777 PMID:19074341

Stockner, T., Montgomery, T. R., Kudlacek, O., Weissensteiner, R., Ecker, G. F., Freissmuth, M., & Sitte, H. H. (2013). Mutational analysis of the high-affinity Zinc binding site validates a refined human dopamine transporter homology model. *PLoS Computational Biology*, *9*(2), e1002909. doi:10.1371/journal.pcbi.1002909 PMID:23436987

Sucic, S., Dallinger, S., Zdrazil, B., Weissensteiner, R., Jørgensen, T. N., Holy, M., ... Sitte, H. H. (2010). The N terminus of monoamine transporters is a lever required for the action of amphetamines. *The Journal of Biological Chemistry*, *285*(14), 10924–10938. doi:10.1074/jbc.M109.083154 PMID:20118234

Sulzer, D. (2011). How addictive drugs disrupt presynaptic dopamine neurotransmission. *Neuron, 69*(4), 628–649. doi:10.1016/j.neuron.2011.02.010 PMID:21338876

Torres, G. E., Gainetdinov, R., & Caron, M. G. (2003). Plasma membrane monoamine transporters: structure, regulation and function. *Nat. Rev. ci., 4*(1), 13–25.

Tozzi, V., Balestra, P., Bellagamba, R., Corpolongo, A., Salvatori, M. F., Visco-Comandini, U., ... Narciso, P. (2007). Persistence of neuropsychologic deficits despite long-term highly active antiretroviral therapy in patients with HIV-related neurocognitive impairment: Prevalence and risk factors. *JAIDS Journal of Acquired Immune Deficiency Syndromes, 45*(2), 174–182. doi:10.1097/QAI.0b013e318042e1ee PMID:17356465

Uhl, G. R. (2003). Dopamine transporter: Basic science and human variation of a key molecule for dopaminergic function, locomotion, and parkinsonism. *Movement Disorders, 18*(S7), S71–S80. doi:10.1002/mds.10578 PMID:14531049

UNICEF. (2016). Global report: UNAIDS report on the global AIDS epidemic 2016. Geneva: UNAIDS.

Valcour, V., Shikuma, C., Shiramizu, B., Watters, M., Poff, P., Selnes, O., ... Sacktor, N. (2004). Higher frequency of dementia in older HIV-1 individuals: The Hawaii Aging with HIV-1 Cohort. *Neurology, 63*(5), 822–827. doi:10.1212/01.WNL.0000134665.58343.8D PMID:15365130

Vivithanaporn, P., Nelles, K., DeBlock, L., Newman, S. C., Gill, M. J., & Power, C. (2012). Hepatitis C virus co-infection increases neurocognitive impairment severity and risk of death in treated HIV/AIDS. *Journal of the Neurological Sciences, 312*(1-2), 45–51. doi:10.1016/j.jns.2011.08.025 PMID:21925684

Vo, Q. T., Cox, C., Li, X., Jacobson, L. P., McKaig, R., Sacktor, N., ... Miller, E. N. (2013). Neuropsychological test performance before and after HIV-1 seroconversion: The Multicenter AIDS Cohort Study. *Journal of Neurovirology, 19*(1), 24–31. doi:10.1007/s13365-012-0136-8 PMID:23229349

Wang, C. I., & Lewis, R. J. (2010). Emerging structure–function relationships defining monoamine NSS transporter substrate and ligand affinity. ochem. *Pharmacol., 79*(8), 1083–1091. PMID:19954741

Wang, G. J., Chang, L., Volkow, N. D., Telang, F., Logan, J., ... Fowler, J. S. (2004). Decreased brain dopaminergic transporters in HIV-associated dementia patients. *Brain, 1*(27), 2452–2458. doi:10.1093/brain/awh269 PMID:15319273

Wang, K. H., Penmatsa, A., & Gouaux, E. (2015). Neurotransmitter and psychostimulant recognition by the dopamine transporter. *Nature*, *521*(7552), 322–327. doi:10.1038/nature14431 PMID:25970245

Westendorp, M. O., Frank, R., Ochsenbauer, C., Stricker, K., Dhein, J., Walczak, H., ... Krammer, P. H. (1995). Sensitization of T cells to CD95-mediated apoptosis by HIV-1 Tat and gp120. *Nature*, *375*(6531), 497–500. doi:10.1038/375497a0 PMID:7539892

Williams, D. W., Calderon, T. M., Lopez, L., Carvallo-Torres, L., Gaskill, P. J., Eugenin, E. A., ... Berman, J. W. (2013). Mechanisms of HIV entry into the CNS: Increased sensitivity of HIV infected CD14+CD16+ monocytes to CCL2 and key roles of CCR2, JAM-A, and ALCAM in diapedesis. *PLoS One*, *8*(7), e69270. doi:10.1371/journal.pone.0069270 PMID:23922698

Wise, R. A., & Bozarth, M. A. (1987). A psychomotor stimulant theory of addiction. *Psychological Review*, *94*(4), 469–492. doi:10.1037/0033-295X.94.4.469 PMID:3317472

Xiao, H., Neuveut, C., Tiffany, H. L., Benkirane, M., Rich, E. A., Murphy, P. M., & Jeang, K. T. (2000). Selective CXCR4 antagonism by Tat: Implications for in vivo expansion of coreceptor use by HIV-1. *Proceedings of the National Academy of Sciences of the United States of America*, *97*(21), 11466–11471. doi:10.1073/pnas.97.21.11466 PMID:11027346

Yamashita, A., Singh, S. K., Kawate, T., Jin, Y., & Gouaux, E. (2005). Crystal structure of a bacterial homologue of Na+/Cl-dependent neurotransmitter transporters. *Nature*, *437*(7056), 215–223. doi:10.1038/nature03978 PMID:16041361

Yohn, S. E., Gogoj, A., Haque, A., Lopez-Cruz, L., Haley, A., Huxley, P., ... Salamone, J. D. (2016). Evaulation of the effortrelated motivational effects of the novel dopamine uptake inhibitor Prx-14040. *Pharmacology, Biochemistry, and Behavior*, *148*, 84–91. doi:10.1016/j.pbb.2016.06.004 PMID:27296079

Yuan, Y., Huang, X., Midde, N. M., Quizon, P. M., Sun, W. L., Zhu, J., & Zhan, C. G. (2015). Molecular mechanism of HIV-1 Tat interacting with human dopamine transporter. *ACS Chemical Neuroscience*, *6*(4), 658–665. doi:10.1021/acschemneuro.5b00001 PMID:25695767

Yuan, Y., Quizon, P. M., Sun, W. L., Yao, J., Zhu, J., & Zhan, C. G. (2016). Role of histidine 547 of human dopamine transporter in molecular interaction with HIV-1 Tat and dopamine uptake. *Scientific Reports*, *6*(1), 27314. doi:10.1038/srep27314 PMID:27250920

Zhu, J., Mactutus, C. F., Wallace, D. R., & Booze, R. M. (2009). HIV-1 Tat protein-induced rapid and reversible decrease in [3H]dopamine uptake: Dissociation of [3H] dopamine uptake and [3H]2beta-carbomethoxy-3-beta-(4-fluorophenyl)tropane (WIN 35,428) binding in rat striatal synaptosomes. *The Journal of Pharmacology and Experimental Therapeutics*, *329*(3), 1071–1083. doi:10.1124/jpet.108.150144 PMID:19325033

Zhu, J., Mactutus, C. F., Wallace, D. R., & Booze, R. M. (2009). HIV-1 Tat protein-induced rapid and reversible decrease in [3H] dopamine uptake: Dissociation of [3H] dopamine uptake and [3H]2beta-carbomethoxy-3-beta-(4-fluorophenyl) tropane (WIN 35,428) binding in rat striatal synaptosomes. *The Journal of Pharmacology and Experimental Therapeutics*, *329*(3), 1071–1083. doi:10.1124/jpet.108.150144 PMID:19325033

Zhu, J., & Reith, M. E. (2008). Role of dopamine transporter in the action of psychostimulants, nicotine, and other drugs of abuse. *CNS & Neurological Disorders - Drug Targets*, *7*(5), 393–409. doi:10.2174/187152708786927877 PMID:19128199

Related References

To continue our tradition of advancing medicine, healthcare, and life sciences research, we have compiled a list of recommended IGI Global readings. These references will provide additional information and guidance to further enrich your knowledge and assist you with your own research and future publications.

Abu-Faraj, Z. O. (2012). Bioengineering/biomedical engineering education. In Z. Abu-Faraj (Ed.), *Handbook of research on biomedical engineering education and advanced bioengineering learning: Interdisciplinary concepts* (pp. 1–59). Hershey, PA: IGI Global. doi:10.4018/978-1-4666-0122-2.ch001

Achehboune, A., & Driouchi, A. (2014). Potential skilled labor migration, internationalization of education with focus on medical education: The case of Arab countries. In A. Driouchi (Ed.), *Labor and health economics in the Mediterranean region: Migration and mobility of medical doctors* (pp. 83–122). Hershey, PA: IGI Global. doi:10.4018/978-1-4666-4723-7.ch004

Adomi, E. E., Egbaivwie, E., & Ogugua, J. C. (2013). Use of the internet by medical practitioners in private hospitals in Warri, Delta State, Nigeria. In A. Cartelli (Ed.), *Fostering 21st century digital literacy and technical competency* (pp. 213–221). Hershey, PA: IGI Global. doi:10.4018/978-1-4666-2943-1.ch015

Afolabi, M. O., Babalola, O. O., & Ola-Olorun, O. J. (2012). Counselling in pharmacy practice: Exploring the use of online counselling interactions to improve medicine use among people living with HIV/AIDS (PLWHA). In B. Popoola & O. Adebowale (Eds.), *Online guidance and counseling: Toward effectively applying technology* (pp. 91–103). Hershey, PA: IGI Global. doi:10.4018/978-1-61350-204-4.ch007

Ahmad, Y. J., Raghavan, V. V., & Martz, W. B. Jr. (2011). Adoption of electronic health records. In *Clinical technologies: Concepts, methodologies, tools and applications* (pp. 132–146). Hershey, PA: IGI Global. doi:10.4018/978-1-60960-561-2.ch109

Al-Dossary, S., Al-Dulaijan, N., Al-Mansour, S., Al-Zahrani, S., Al-Fridan, M., & Househ, M. (2013). Organ donation and transplantation: Processes, registries, consent, and restrictions in Saudi Arabia. In M. Cruz-Cunha, I. Miranda, & P. Gonçalves (Eds.), *Handbook of research on ICTs for human-centered healthcare and social care services* (pp. 511–528). Hershey, PA: IGI Global. doi:10.4018/978-1-4666-3986-7.ch027

Al-Khudairy, S. (2014). Caring for our aging population: Using CPOE and telehomecare systems as a response to health policy concerns. In C. El Morr (Ed.), *Research perspectives on the role of informatics in health policy and management* (pp. 153–166). Hershey, PA: IGI Global. doi:10.4018/978-1-4666-4321-5.ch010

Albert, A., Serrano, A. J., Soria, E., & Jiménez, N. V. (2010). Clinical decision support system to prevent toxicity in patients treated with Digoxin. In A. Shukla & R. Tiwari (Eds.), *Intelligent medical technologies and biomedical engineering: Tools and applications* (pp. 1–21). Hershey, PA: IGI Global. doi:10.4018/978-1-61520-977-4.ch001

Alexandrou, D. A., & Pardalis, K. V. (2014). SEMantic PATHways: Modeling, executing, and monitoring intra-organizational healthcare business processes towards personalized treatment. In *Software design and development: Concepts, methodologies, tools, and applications* (pp. 1036–1062). Hershey, PA: IGI Global. doi:10.4018/978-1-4666-4301-7.ch050

Alhaqbani, B., & Fidge, C. (2013). A medical data trustworthiness assessment model. In *User-driven healthcare: Concepts, methodologies, tools, and applications* (pp. 1425–1445). Hershey, PA: IGI Global. doi:10.4018/978-1-4666-2770-3.ch071

Ali, S., Abbadeni, N., & Batouche, M. (2012). *Multidisciplinary computational intelligence techniques: Applications in business, engineering, and medicine* (pp. 1–365). Hershey, PA: IGI Global. doi:10.4018/978-1-4666-1830-5

Alonso, J. M., Castiello, C., Lucarelli, M., & Mencar, C. (2013). Modeling interpretable fuzzy rule-based classifiers for medical decision support. In *Data mining: Concepts, methodologies, tools, and applications* (pp. 1064–1081). Hershey, PA: IGI Global. doi:10.4018/978-1-4666-2455-9.ch054

Alonso-Barba, J. I., Nielsen, J. D., de la Ossa, L., & Puerta, J. M. (2012). Learning probabilistic graphical models: A review of techniques and applications in medicine. In R. Magdalena-Benedito, E. Soria-Olivas, J. Martínez, J. Gómez-Sanchis, & A. Serrano-López (Eds.), *Medical applications of intelligent data analysis: Research advancements* (pp. 223–236). Hershey, PA: IGI Global. doi:10.4018/978-1-4666-1803-9.ch015

Anderson, J. G. (2010). Improving patient safety with information technology. In K. Khoumbati, Y. Dwivedi, A. Srivastava, & B. Lal (Eds.), *Handbook of research on advances in health informatics and electronic healthcare applications: Global adoption and impact of information communication technologies* (pp. 144–152). Hershey, PA: IGI Global. doi:10.4018/978-1-60566-030-1.ch009

Anderson, J. G. (2011). Regional patient safety initiatives. In *Clinical technologies: Concepts, methodologies, tools and applications* (pp. 1491–1503). Hershey, PA: IGI Global. doi:10.4018/978-1-60960-561-2.ch506

Andonegui, J., Serrano, L., & Eguzkiza, A. (2010). E-health applications in ophthalmic diseases: Ongoing developments. In M. Cruz-Cunha, A. Tavares, & R. Simoes (Eds.), *Handbook of research on developments in e-health and telemedicine: Technological and social perspectives* (pp. 1088–1115). Hershey, PA: IGI Global. doi:10.4018/978-1-61520-670-4.ch052

Andrés, A. R. (2014). Understanding the migration of medical doctors in the context of Europe. In A. Driouchi (Ed.), *Labor and health economics in the Mediterranean region: Migration and mobility of medical doctors* (pp. 139–157). Hershey, PA: IGI Global. doi:10.4018/978-1-4666-4723-7.ch006

Ann, O. C., & Theng, L. B. (2014). A facial expression mediated natural user interface communication model for children with motor impairments. In G. Kouroupetroglou (Ed.), *Assistive technologies and computer access for motor disabilities* (pp. 254–284). Hershey, PA: IGI Global. doi:10.4018/978-1-4666-4438-0.ch009

Anselma, L., Bottrighi, A., Molino, G., Montani, S., Terenziani, P., & Torchio, M. (2011). Supporting knowledge-based decision making in the medical context: The GLARE approach. *International Journal of Knowledge-Based Organizations*, *1*(1), 42–60. doi:10.4018/ijkbo.2011010103

Apostolakis, I., Valsamos, P., & Varlamis, I. (2011). Quality assurance in evidence-based medicine. In A. Moumtzoglou & A. Kastania (Eds.), *E-health systems quality and reliability: Models and standards* (pp. 86–99). Hershey, PA: IGI Global. doi:10.4018/978-1-61692-843-8.ch008

Archibald, D., MacDonald, C. J., Hogue, R., & Mercer, J. (2013). Accessing knowledge from the bedside: Introducing the tablet computer to clinical teaching. In C. Rückemann (Ed.), *Integrated information and computing systems for natural, spatial, and social sciences* (pp. 96–109). Hershey, PA: IGI Global. doi:10.4018/978-1-4666-2190-9.ch005

Aspradaki, A. A. (2013). Deliberative democracy and nanotechnologies in health. *International Journal of Technoethics*, *4*(2), 1–14. doi:10.4018/jte.2013070101

Assis-Hassid, S., Reychav, I., Pliskin, J. S., & Heart, T. H. (2013). The effects of electronic medical record (EMR) use in primary care on the physician-patient relationship. In M. Cruz-Cunha, I. Miranda, & P. Gonçalves (Eds.), *Handbook of research on ICTs for human-centered healthcare and social care services* (pp. 130–150). Hershey, PA: IGI Global. doi:10.4018/978-1-4666-3986-7.ch007

Atanasov, A. (2011). Quality and reliability aspects in evidence based e-medicine. In A. Moumtzoglou & A. Kastania (Eds.), *E-health systems quality and reliability: Models and standards* (pp. 100–117). Hershey, PA: IGI Global. doi:10.4018/978-1-61692-843-8.ch009

Attalla, D. S. (2011). Health hazards of mobile information communication technologies. In A. Abdel-Wahab & A. El-Masry (Eds.), *Mobile information communication technologies adoption in developing countries: Effects and implications* (pp. 237–251). Hershey, PA: IGI Global. doi:10.4018/978-1-61692-818-6.ch016

Au, S., & Gupta, A. (2011). Gastrointestinal motility online educational endeavor. In A. Moumtzoglou & A. Kastania (Eds.), *E-health systems quality and reliability: Models and standards* (pp. 163–182). Hershey, PA: IGI Global. doi:10.4018/978-1-61692-843-8.ch014

Azar, A. T. (2013). Overview of biomedical engineering. In Bioinformatics: Concepts, methodologies, tools, and applications (pp. 1-28). Hershey, PA: IGI Global. doi:10.4018/978-1-4666-3604-0.ch001

Azar, A. T., & Eljamel, M. S. (2014). Medical robotics. In Robotics: Concepts, methodologies, tools, and applications (pp. 1116-1147). Hershey, PA: IGI Global. doi:10.4018/978-1-4666-4607-0.ch054

Bagheri, F. B. (2013). eSelf or computerized self network: A tool for individual empowerment & implementation of optimal healthcare. *International Journal of User-Driven Healthcare*, *3*(2), 20–32. doi:10.4018/ijudh.2013040103

Baharadwaj, N., Wadhwa, S., Goel, P., Sethi, I., Arora, C. S., Goel, A., ... Parthasarathy, H. (2014). De-noising, clustering, classification, and representation of microarray data for disease diagnostics. In R. Srivastava, S. Singh, & K. Shukla (Eds.), *Research developments in computer vision and image processing: Methodologies and applications* (pp. 149–174). Hershey, PA: IGI Global. doi:10.4018/978-1-4666-4558-5.ch009

Baijou, A. (2014). A descriptive overview of the emigration of medical doctors from MENA to EU. In A. Driouchi (Ed.), *Labor and health economics in the Mediterranean region: Migration and mobility of medical doctors* (pp. 192–218). Hershey, PA: IGI Global. doi:10.4018/978-1-4666-4723-7.ch008

Bauer, K. (2010). Healthcare ethics in the information age. In J. Rodrigues (Ed.), *Health information systems: Concepts, methodologies, tools, and applications* (pp. 1761–1776). Hershey, PA: IGI Global. doi:10.4018/978-1-60566-988-5.ch114

Bauer, K. A. (2013). Caught in the web: The internet and the demise of medical privacy. In *User-driven healthcare: Concepts, methodologies, tools, and applications* (pp. 1252–1272). Hershey, PA: IGI Global. doi:10.4018/978-1-4666-2770-3.ch063

Bayona, S., Espadero, J. M., Fernández, J. M., Pastor, L., & Rodríguez, Á. (2011). Implementing virtual reality in the healthcare sector. In N. Rao (Ed.), *Virtual technologies for business and industrial applications: Innovative and synergistic approaches* (pp. 138–163). Hershey, PA: IGI Global. doi:10.4018/978-1-61520-631-5.ch009

Begg, M., Dewhurst, D., & Ross, M. (2010). Game informed virtual patients: Catalysts for online learning communities and professional development of medical teachers. In J. Lindberg & A. Olofsson (Eds.), *Online learning communities and teacher professional development: Methods for improved education delivery* (pp. 190–208). Hershey, PA: IGI Global. doi:10.4018/978-1-60566-780-5.ch011

Bennett, E. E., Blanchard, R. D., & Fernandez, G. L. (2012). Knowledge sharing in academic medical centers: Examining the nexus of higher education and workforce development. In V. Wang (Ed.), *Encyclopedia of e-leadership, counseling and training* (pp. 212–232). Hershey, PA: IGI Global. doi:10.4018/978-1-61350-068-2.ch016

Bera, T. K., & Nagaraju, J. (2014). Electrical impedance tomography (EIT): A harmless medical imaging modality. In R. Srivastava, S. Singh, & K. Shukla (Eds.), *Research developments in computer vision and image processing: Methodologies and applications* (pp. 235–273). Hershey, PA: IGI Global. doi:10.4018/978-1-4666-4558-5.ch013

Berler, A., & Apostolakis, I. (2014). Normalizing cross-border healthcare in europe via new e-prescription paradigms. In C. El Morr (Ed.), *Research perspectives on the role of informatics in health policy and management* (pp. 168–208). Hershey, PA: IGI Global. doi:10.4018/978-1-4666-4321-5.ch011

Beswetherick, J. (2012). Health care information systems and the risk of privacy issues for the disabled. In *Cyber crime: Concepts, methodologies, tools and applications* (pp. 870–890). Hershey, PA: IGI Global. doi:10.4018/978-1-61350-323-2.ch411

Bhattacharya, P., Asanga, A. P., & Biswas, R. (2011). Stomodeum to proctodeum: Email narratives on clinical problem solving in gastroenterology. In R. Biswas & C. Martin (Eds.), *User-driven healthcare and narrative medicine: Utilizing collaborative social networks and technologies* (pp. 34–53). Hershey, PA: IGI Global. doi:10.4018/978-1-60960-097-6.ch003

Biswas, R., & Martin, C. M. (2011). *User-driven healthcare and narrative medicine: Utilizing collaborative social networks and technologies*. Hershey, PA: IGI Global. doi:10.4018/978-1-60960-097-6

Biswas, R., Martin, C. M., Sturmberg, J., Mukherji, K., Lee, E. W., & Umakanth, S. (2011). Social cognitive ontology and user driven healthcare. In *Clinical technologies: Concepts, methodologies, tools and applications* (pp. 1996–2012). Hershey, PA: IGI Global. doi:10.4018/978-1-60960-561-2.ch710

Biswas, R., Sturmberg, J., Martin, C. M., Ganesh, A. U., Umakanth, S., & Lee, E. W. (2011). Persistent clinical encounters in user driven e-health care. In *Clinical technologies: Concepts, methodologies, tools and applications* (pp. 1030–1046). Hershey, PA: IGI Global. doi:10.4018/978-1-60960-561-2.ch403

Black, N. P., Fromme, H. B., Maniscalco, J., Ferrell, C., Myers, J., & Augustine, E. ... Blankenburg, R. (2013). Innovation in patient care and medical resident education: Using blended instruction to transform nighttime patient care from a service model into an educational model. In A. Ritzhaupt, & S. Kumar (Eds.) Cases on educational technology implementation for facilitating learning (pp. 161-176). Hershey, PA: IGI Global. doi:10.4018/978-1-4666-3676-7.ch010

Blatt, A. J. (2013). Geospatial applications in disease surveillance: Solutions for the future. *International Journal of Applied Geospatial Research*, *4*(2), 1–8. doi:10.4018/jagr.2013040101

Boaduo, N. A., & Boaduo, N. K. (2012). ICTs for enhanced use of indigenous medicinal plants by the Ashante speaking people of Ghana. In R. Lekoko & L. Semali (Eds.), *Cases on developing countries and ICT integration: Rural community development* (pp. 16–24). Hershey, PA: IGI Global. doi:10.4018/978-1-60960-117-1.ch002

Boboc, C., & Titan, E. (2014). Inputs from the new economics of migration of medical doctors in eastern and central Europe. In A. Driouchi (Ed.), *Labor and health economics in the Mediterranean region: Migration and mobility of medical doctors* (pp. 241–266). Hershey, PA: IGI Global. doi:10.4018/978-1-4666-4723-7.ch010

Boboc, C., & Ţiţan, E. (2014). Migration of medical doctors, health, medical education, and employment in eastern and central Europe. In A. Driouchi (Ed.), *Labor and health economics in the Mediterranean region: Migration and mobility of medical doctors* (pp. 158–191). Hershey, PA: IGI Global. doi:10.4018/978-1-4666-4723-7.ch007

Bolsin, S., & Colson, M. (2010). IT benefits in healthcare performance and safety. In J. Rodrigues (Ed.), *Health information systems: Concepts, methodologies, tools, and applications* (pp. 71–88). Hershey, PA: IGI Global. doi:10.4018/978-1-60566-988-5.ch006

Bongers, B., & Smith, S. (2014). Interactivating rehabilitation through active multimodal feedback and guidance. In *Assistive technologies: Concepts, methodologies, tools, and applications* (pp. 1650–1674). Hershey, PA: IGI Global. doi:10.4018/978-1-4666-4422-9.ch087

Borges, A. P., & Laranjeira, E. (2013). Why and how did health economics appear? Who were the main authors? What is the role of ITCs in its development? In M. Cruz-Cunha, I. Miranda, & P. Gonçalves (Eds.), *Handbook of research on ICTs and management systems for improving efficiency in healthcare and social care* (pp. 971–987). Hershey, PA: IGI Global. doi:10.4018/978-1-4666-3990-4.ch051

Bourgeois, S., & Yaylacicegi, U. (2012). Electronic health records: Improving patient safety and quality of care in Texas acute care hospitals. In J. Tan (Ed.), *Advancing technologies and intelligence in healthcare and clinical environments breakthroughs* (pp. 18–32). Hershey, PA: IGI Global. doi:10.4018/978-1-4666-1755-1.ch002

Brandt, R., & Rice, R. (2012). Dermatological telemedicine diagnoses and andragogical training using web 2.0 mobile medicine video conferencing. In V. Dennen & J. Myers (Eds.), *Virtual professional development and informal learning via social networks* (pp. 276–293). Hershey, PA: IGI Global. doi:10.4018/978-1-4666-1815-2.ch016

Brzezinski, J., Kosiedowski, M., Mazurek, C., Slowinski, K., Slowinski, R., Stroinski, M., & Weglarz, J. (2013). Towards telemedical centers: Digitization of inter-professional communication in healthcare. In M. Cruz-Cunha, I. Miranda, & P. Gonçalves (Eds.), *Handbook of research on ICTs and management systems for improving efficiency in healthcare and social care* (pp. 805–829). Hershey, PA: IGI Global. doi:10.4018/978-1-4666-3990-4.ch042

Carlén, U., & Lindström, B. (2012). Informed design of educational activities in online learning communities. In A. Olofsson & J. Lindberg (Eds.), *Informed design of educational technologies in higher education: Enhanced learning and teaching* (pp. 118–134). Hershey, PA: IGI Global. doi:10.4018/978-1-61350-080-4.ch007

Carrigan, E., Ugaz, A., Moberly, H. K., Page, J., Alpi, K. M., & Vreeland, C. (2013). Veterinary medicine: All collections great and small. In S. Holder (Ed.), *Library collection development for professional programs: Trends and best practices* (pp. 248–268). Hershey, PA: IGI Global. doi:10.4018/978-1-4666-1897-8.ch015

Caruana, C. J. (2012). The ongoing crisis in medical device education for healthcare professionals: Breaking the vicious circle through online learning. *International Journal of Reliable and Quality E-Healthcare, 1*(2), 29–40. doi:10.4018/ijrqeh.2012040103

Catapano, G., & Verkerke, G. J. (2012). Artificial organs. In Z. Abu-Faraj (Ed.), *Handbook of research on biomedical engineering education and advanced bioengineering learning: Interdisciplinary concepts* (pp. 60–95). Hershey, PA: IGI Global. doi:10.4018/978-1-4666-0122-2.ch002

Chandra, S., Shah, N. K., & Sriganesh, V. (2011). The cochrane students journal club and creating a secondary learning resource for gathering and appraising evidence: An example of rational use of medicines to prevent malaria relapse. *International Journal of User-Driven Healthcare, 1*(4), 31–41. doi:10.4018/ijudh.2011100103

Chang, A. Y., Littman-Quinn, R., Ketshogileng, D., Chandra, A., Rijken, T., Ghose, S., ... Kovarik, C. L. (2012). Smartphone-based mobile learning with physician trainees in Botswana. *International Journal of Mobile and Blended Learning, 4*(2), 1–14. doi:10.4018/jmbl.2012040101

Charissis, G., Melas, C., Moustakis, V., & Zampetakis, L. (2010). Organizational implementation of healthcare information systems. In M. Cruz-Cunha, A. Tavares, & R. Simoes (Eds.), *Handbook of research on developments in e-health and telemedicine: Technological and social perspectives* (pp. 419–450). Hershey, PA: IGI Global. doi:10.4018/978-1-61520-670-4.ch020

Chaudhuri, A., Young, J., Martin, C. M., Sturmberg, J. P., & Biswas, R. (2011). Hematology: The river within. In R. Biswas & C. Martin (Eds.), *User-driven healthcare and narrative medicine: Utilizing collaborative social networks and technologies* (pp. 16–33). Hershey, PA: IGI Global. doi:10.4018/978-1-60960-097-6.ch002

Chen, J. Y., Xu, H., Shi, P., Culbertson, A., & Meslin, E. M. (2013). Ethics and privacy considerations for systems biology applications in predictive and personalized medicine. In Bioinformatics: Concepts, methodologies, tools, and applications (pp. 1378-1404). Hershey, PA: IGI Global. doi:10.4018/978-1-4666-3604-0.ch071

Cherian, E. J., & Ryan, T. W. (2014). Incongruent needs: Why differences in the iron-triangle of priorities make health information technology adoption and use difficult. In C. El Morr (Ed.), *Research perspectives on the role of informatics in health policy and management* (pp. 209–221). Hershey, PA: IGI Global. doi:10.4018/978-1-4666-4321-5.ch012

Chetioui, Y. (2014). Perception by Moroccan physicians of factors affecting their migration decisions. In A. Driouchi (Ed.), *Labor and health economics in the mediterranean region: Migration and mobility of medical doctors* (pp. 337–375). Hershey, PA: IGI Global. doi:10.4018/978-1-4666-4723-7.ch014

Chorbev, I., & Joksimoski, B. (2011). An integrated system for e-medicine (e-health, telemedicine and medical expert systems). In *Clinical technologies: Concepts, methodologies, tools and applications* (pp. 486–507). Hershey, PA: IGI Global. doi:10.4018/978-1-60960-561-2.ch218

Ciufudean, C., Ciufudean, O., & Filote, C. (2013). New models for ICT-based medical diagnosis. In M. Cruz-Cunha, I. Miranda, & P. Gonçalves (Eds.), *Handbook of research on ICTs and management systems for improving efficiency in healthcare and social care* (pp. 892–911). Hershey, PA: IGI Global. doi:10.4018/978-1-4666-3990-4.ch046

Clark, J. M. (2014). Implementation of electronic records in a medical practice setting. In J. Krueger (Ed.), *Cases on electronic records and resource management implementation in diverse environments* (pp. 211–225). Hershey, PA: IGI Global. doi:10.4018/978-1-4666-4466-3.ch013

Clark, T. (2011). Health and health care grid services and delivery integrating eHealth and telemedicine. In E. Kldiashvili (Ed.), *Grid technologies for e-health: Applications for telemedicine services and delivery* (pp. 36–64). Hershey, PA: IGI Global. doi:10.4018/978-1-61692-010-4.ch003

Claster, W., Ghotbi, N., & Shanmuganathan, S. (2010). Data-mining techniques for an analysis of non-conventional methodologies: Deciphering of alternative medicine. In W. Pease, M. Cooper, & R. Gururajan (Eds.), *Biomedical knowledge management: Infrastructures and processes for e-health systems* (pp. 82–91). Hershey, PA: IGI Global. doi:10.4018/978-1-60566-266-4.ch006

Condaris, C. (2012). Scales to scalpels: Doctors who practice the healing arts of music and medicine. *International Journal of User-Driven Healthcare*, *2*(3), 84–84. doi:10.4018/ijudh.2012070109

Corrigan, D., Hederman, L., Khan, H., Taweel, A., Kostopoulou, O., & Delaney, B. (2013). An ontology-driven approach to clinical evidence modelling implementing clinical prediction rules. In A. Moumtzoglou & A. Kastania (Eds.), *E-health technologies and improving patient safety: Exploring organizational factors* (pp. 257–284). Hershey, PA: IGI Global. doi:10.4018/978-1-4666-2657-7.ch016

Crisóstomo-Acevedo, M. J., & Aurelio Medina-Garrido, J. (2010). Difficulties in accepting telemedicine. In J. Rodrigues (Ed.), *Health information systems: Concepts, methodologies, tools, and applications* (pp. 1628–1639). Hershey, PA: IGI Global. doi:10.4018/978-1-60566-988-5.ch104

Danforth, D. R. (2010). Development of an interactive virtual 3-D model of the human testis using the second life platform. *International Journal of Virtual and Personal Learning Environments*, *1*(2), 45–58. doi:10.4018/jvple.2010040104

Daniel, V. M. (2011). Genomics and genetic engineering: Playing god? In S. Hongladarom (Ed.), *Genomics and bioethics: Interdisciplinary perspectives, technologies and advancements* (pp. 111–129). Hershey, PA: IGI Global. doi:10.4018/978-1-61692-883-4.ch008

Daskalaki, A. (2010). *Informatics in oral medicine: Advanced techniques in clinical and diagnostic technologies*. Hershey, PA: IGI Global. doi:10.4018/978-1-60566-733-1

Davis, S. A. (2013). Global telemedicine and eHealth: Advances for future healthcare – Using a systems approach to integrate healthcare functions. In V. Gulla, A. Mori, F. Gabbrielli, & P. Lanzafame (Eds.), *Telehealth networks for hospital services: New methodologies* (pp. 15–32). Hershey, PA: IGI Global. doi:10.4018/978-1-4666-2979-0.ch002

de Leeuw, E. (2012). The politics of medical curriculum accreditation: Thoughts, not facts? *International Journal of User-Driven Healthcare*, *2*(1), 53–69. doi:10.4018/ijudh.2012010108

De Luca, S., & Memo, E. (2010). Better knowledge for better health services: Discovering guideline compliance. In J. Rodrigues (Ed.), *Health information systems: Concepts, methodologies, tools, and applications* (pp. 233–255). Hershey, PA: IGI Global. doi:10.4018/978-1-60566-988-5.ch017

DeSimio, T., & Chrisagis, X. (2012). Medical e-reference: A benchmark for e-reference publishing in other disciplines. In S. Polanka (Ed.), *E-reference context and discoverability in libraries: Issues and concepts* (pp. 116–125). Hershey, PA: IGI Global. doi:10.4018/978-1-61350-308-9.ch011

Dhakal, B., & Ross, S. D. (2011). Medical student perspectives: Journey through different worlds. In R. Biswas & C. Martin (Eds.), *User-driven healthcare and narrative medicine: Utilizing collaborative social networks and technologies* (pp. 125–133). Hershey, PA: IGI Global. doi:10.4018/978-1-60960-097-6.ch009

Dong, Y., Lu, H., Gajic, O., & Pickering, B. (2012). Intensive care unit operational modeling and analysis. In A. Kolker & P. Story (Eds.), *Management engineering for effective healthcare delivery: Principles and applications* (pp. 132–147). Hershey, PA: IGI Global. doi:10.4018/978-1-60960-872-9.ch006

Doyle, D. (2011). E-medical education: An overview. In A. Shukla & R. Tiwari (Eds.), *Biomedical engineering and information systems: Technologies, tools and applications* (pp. 219–238). Hershey, PA: IGI Global. doi:10.4018/978-1-61692-004-3.ch012

Driouchi, A. (2014). Introduction to labor and health economics: Mobility of medical doctors in the Mediterranean region. In A. Driouchi (Ed.), *Labor and health economics in the Mediterranean region: Migration and mobility of medical doctors* (pp. 1–22). Hershey, PA: IGI Global. doi:10.4018/978-1-4666-4723-7.ch001

Driouchi, A. (2014). Medical knowledge, north-south cooperation, and mobility of medical doctors. In A. Driouchi (Ed.), *Labor and health economics in the Mediterranean region: Migration and mobility of medical doctors* (pp. 376–395). Hershey, PA: IGI Global. doi:10.4018/978-1-4666-4723-7.ch015

Duan, X., Wang, X., & Huang, Q. (2014). Medical manipulators for surgical applications. In Robotics: Concepts, methodologies, tools, and applications (pp. 608-618). Hershey, PA: IGI Global. doi:10.4018/978-1-4666-4607-0.ch030

Dyro, J. F. (2012). Clinical engineering. In Z. Abu-Faraj (Ed.), *Handbook of research on biomedical engineering education and advanced bioengineering learning: Interdisciplinary concepts* (pp. 521–576). Hershey, PA: IGI Global. doi:10.4018/978-1-4666-0122-2.ch012

El Morr, C., & Subercaze, J. (2010). Knowledge management in healthcare. In M. Cruz-Cunha, A. Tavares, & R. Simoes (Eds.), *Handbook of research on developments in e-health and telemedicine: Technological and social perspectives* (pp. 490–510). Hershey, PA: IGI Global. doi:10.4018/978-1-61520-670-4.ch023

Eleni, A., & Maglogiannis, I. (2010). Adoption of wearable systems in modern patient telemonitoring systems. In M. Cruz-Cunha, A. Tavares, & R. Simoes (Eds.), *Handbook of research on developments in e-health and telemedicine: Technological and social perspectives* (pp. 1004–1023). Hershey, PA: IGI Global. doi:10.4018/978-1-61520-670-4.ch048

Epstein, J. H., Goldberg, A., Krol, M., & Levine, A. (2013). Virtual tools in medical education. In Y. Kats (Ed.), *Learning management systems and instructional design: Best practices in online education* (pp. 364–380). Hershey, PA: IGI Global. doi:10.4018/978-1-4666-3930-0.ch019

Eskeland, S., & Oleshchuk, V. (2010). Information security and privacy in medical application scenario. In K. Khoumbati, Y. Dwivedi, A. Srivastava, & B. Lal (Eds.), *Handbook of research on advances in health informatics and electronic healthcare applications: Global adoption and impact of information communication technologies* (pp. 274–287). Hershey, PA: IGI Global. doi:10.4018/978-1-60566-030-1.ch017

Esposito, A. (2013). The impact of social media on scholarly practices in higher education: Online engagement and ICTs appropriation in senior, young, and doctoral researchers. In B. Pătruţ, M. Pătruţ, & C. Cmeciu (Eds.), *Social media and the new academic environment: Pedagogical challenges* (pp. 342–367). Hershey, PA: IGI Global. doi:10.4018/978-1-4666-2851-9.ch017

Facelli, J. C., Hurdle, J. F., & Mitchell, J. A. (2012). Medical informatics and bioinformatics. In Z. Abu-Faraj (Ed.), *Handbook of research on biomedical engineering education and advanced bioengineering learning: Interdisciplinary concepts* (pp. 577–604). Hershey, PA: IGI Global. doi:10.4018/978-1-4666-0122-2.ch013

Fairchild, K. D., & Moorman, J. R. (2012). Heart rate characteristics monitoring in the NICU: A new tool for clinical care and research. In W. Chen, S. Oetomo, & L. Feijs (Eds.), *Neonatal monitoring technologies: Design for integrated solutions* (pp. 175–200). Hershey, PA: IGI Global. doi:10.4018/978-1-4666-0975-4.ch008

Fakhar, A. (2014). Beyond brain drain: A case study of the benefits of cooperation on medical immigration. In A. Driouchi (Ed.), *Labor and health economics in the Mediterranean region: Migration and mobility of medical doctors* (pp. 294–313). Hershey, PA: IGI Global. doi:10.4018/978-1-4666-4723-7.ch012

Farrell, M. (2011). Use of handheld computers in nursing education. In *Clinical technologies: Concepts, methodologies, tools and applications* (pp. 1504–1517). Hershey, PA: IGI Global. doi:10.4018/978-1-60960-561-2.ch507

Ferrer-Roca, O. (2011). Standards in telemedicine. In A. Moumtzoglou & A. Kastania (Eds.), *E-health systems quality and reliability: Models and standards* (pp. 220–243). Hershey, PA: IGI Global. doi:10.4018/978-1-61692-843-8.ch017

Fiaidhi, J., Mohammed, S., & Wei, Y. (2010). Implications of web 2.0 technology on healthcare: A biomedical semantic blog case study. In S. Kabene (Ed.), *Healthcare and the effect of technology: Developments, challenges and advancements* (pp. 269–289). Hershey, PA: IGI Global. doi:10.4018/978-1-61520-733-6.ch016

Fialho, A. S., Cismondi, F., Vieira, S. M., Reti, S. R., Sousa, J. M., & Finkelstein, S. N. (2013). Challenges and opportunities of soft computing tools in health care delivery. In M. Cruz-Cunha, I. Miranda, & P. Gonçalves (Eds.), *Handbook of research on ICTs and management systems for improving efficiency in healthcare and social care* (pp. 321–340). Hershey, PA: IGI Global. doi:10.4018/978-1-4666-3990-4.ch016

Freitas, A., Brazdil, P., & Costa-Pereira, A. (2012). Cost-sensitive learning in medicine. In *Machine learning: Concepts, methodologies, tools and applications* (pp. 1625–1641). Hershey, PA: IGI Global. doi:10.4018/978-1-60960-818-7.ch607

Freitas, A., & Costa-Pereira, A. (2010). Learning cost-sensitive decision trees to support medical diagnosis. In T. Nguyen (Ed.), *Complex data warehousing and knowledge discovery for advanced retrieval development: Innovative methods and applications* (pp. 287–307). Hershey, PA: IGI Global. doi:10.4018/978-1-60566-748-5.ch013

Freitas, L., Pereira, R. T., Pereira, H. G., Martini, R., Mozzaquatro, B. A., Kasper, J., & Librelotto, G. (2013). Ontological representation and an architecture for homecare pervasive systems. In R. Martinho, R. Rijo, M. Cruz-Cunha, & J. Varajão (Eds.), *Information systems and technologies for enhancing health and social care* (pp. 215–234). Hershey, PA: IGI Global. doi:10.4018/978-1-4666-3667-5.ch015

Frigo, C. A., & Pavan, E. E. (2014). Prosthetic and orthotic devices. In *Assistive technologies: Concepts, methodologies, tools, and applications* (pp. 549–613). Hershey, PA: IGI Global. doi:10.4018/978-1-4666-4422-9.ch028

Frunza, O., & Inkpen, D. (2012). Natural language processing and machine learning techniques help achieve a better medical practice. In R. Magdalena-Benedito, E. Soria-Olivas, J. Martínez, J. Gómez-Sanchis, & A. Serrano-López (Eds.), *Medical applications of intelligent data analysis: Research advancements* (pp. 237–254). Hershey, PA: IGI Global. doi:10.4018/978-1-4666-1803-9.ch016

Fung-Kee-Fung, M., Morash, R., & Goubanova, E. (2011). Evaluating CoPs in cancer surgery. In O. Hernáez & E. Bueno Campos (Eds.), *Handbook of research on communities of practice for organizational management and networking: Methodologies for competitive advantage* (pp. 456–466). Hershey, PA: IGI Global. doi:10.4018/978-1-60566-802-4.ch025

Gabbrielli, F. (2013). Telemedicine R&D influencing incoming strategies and organization models. In V. Gulla, A. Mori, F. Gabbrielli, & P. Lanzafame (Eds.), *Telehealth networks for hospital services: New methodologies* (pp. 250–264). Hershey, PA: IGI Global. doi:10.4018/978-1-4666-2979-0.ch017

Ganz, A., Schafer, J., Yu, X., Lord, G., Burstein, J., & Ciottone, G. R. (2013). Real-time scalable resource tracking framework (DIORAMA) for mass casualty incidents. *International Journal of E-Health and Medical Communications*, *4*(2), 34–49. doi:10.4018/jehmc.2013040103

Gao, X. W., Loomes, M., & Comley, R. (2012). Bridging the abridged: The diffusion of telemedicine in Europe and China. In J. Rodrigues, I. de la Torre Díez, & B. Sainz de Abajo (Eds.), *Telemedicine and e-health services, policies, and applications: Advancements and developments* (pp. 451–495). Hershey, PA: IGI Global. doi:10.4018/978-1-4666-0888-7.ch017

Gavgani, V. Z. (2011). Ubiquitous information therapy service through social networking libraries: An operational web 2.0 service model. In R. Biswas & C. Martin (Eds.), *User-driven healthcare and narrative medicine: Utilizing collaborative social networks and technologies* (pp. 446–461). Hershey, PA: IGI Global. doi:10.4018/978-1-60960-097-6.ch030

Germaine-McDaniel, N. S. (2013). The emerging hispanic use of online health information in the United States: Cultural convergence or dissociation? In *User-driven healthcare: Concepts, methodologies, tools, and applications* (pp. 1607–1621). Hershey, PA: IGI Global. doi:10.4018/978-1-4666-2770-3.ch079

Ghalib, N. (2014). The design and implementation of paperless medical system (PMS) for offshore operating company: A structured approach. In Software design and development: Concepts, methodologies, tools, and applications (pp. 1064-1072). Hershey, PA: IGI Global. doi:10.4018/978-1-4666-4301-7.ch051

Gill, S., & Paranjape, R. (2010). A review of recent contribution in agent-based health care modeling. In J. Rodrigues (Ed.), *Health information systems: Concepts, methodologies, tools, and applications* (pp. 356–373). Hershey, PA: IGI Global. doi:10.4018/978-1-60566-988-5.ch024

Gilligan, J., & Smith, P. (2014). A formal representation system for modelling assistive technology systems. In G. Kouroupetroglou (Ed.), *Disability informatics and web accessibility for motor limitations* (pp. 1–42). Hershey, PA: IGI Global. doi:10.4018/978-1-4666-4442-7.ch001

Goldberg, E. M. (2014). Business continuity and disaster recovery considerations for healthcare technology. In *Crisis management: Concepts, methodologies, tools and applications* (pp. 1455–1462). Hershey, PA: IGI Global. doi:10.4018/978-1-4666-4707-7.ch073

Gonçalves, F., & David, G. (2013). Definition of a retrospective health information policy based on (re)use study. In M. Cruz-Cunha, I. Miranda, & P. Gonçalves (Eds.), *Handbook of research on ICTs and management systems for improving efficiency in healthcare and social care* (pp. 1130–1155). Hershey, PA: IGI Global. doi:10.4018/978-1-4666-3990-4.ch059

Gopalakrishnan, R., & Mugler, D. H. (2010). The evolution of hermite transform in biomedical applications. In A. Shukla & R. Tiwari (Eds.), *Intelligent medical technologies and biomedical engineering: Tools and applications* (pp. 260–278). Hershey, PA: IGI Global. doi:10.4018/978-1-61520-977-4.ch013

Goyal, R. K., O'Neill, M., Agostinelli, N., & Wyer, P. (2011). Critical illness and the emergency room. In R. Biswas & C. Martin (Eds.), *User-driven healthcare and narrative medicine: Utilizing collaborative social networks and technologies* (pp. 63–74). Hershey, PA: IGI Global. doi:10.4018/978-1-60960-097-6.ch005

Graham, I. W. (2011). The nature of nursing work. In A. Cashin & R. Cook (Eds.), *Evidence-based practice in nursing informatics: Concepts and applications* (pp. 51–63). Hershey, PA: IGI Global. doi:10.4018/978-1-60960-034-1.ch005

Greenshields, I., & El-Sayed, G. (2012). Aspects of visualization and the grid in a biomedical context. In *Grid and cloud computing: Concepts, methodologies, tools and applications* (pp. 1686–1701). Hershey, PA: IGI Global. doi:10.4018/978-1-4666-0879-5.ch710

Grimnes, S., & Høgetveit, J. O. (2012). Biomedical sensors. In Z. Abu-Faraj (Ed.), *Handbook of research on biomedical engineering education and advanced bioengineering learning: Interdisciplinary concepts* (pp. 356–436). Hershey, PA: IGI Global. doi:10.4018/978-1-4666-0122-2.ch009

Guedouar, R., & Zarrad, B. (2012). Forward projection for use with iterative reconstruction. In A. Malik, T. Choi, & H. Nisar (Eds.), *Depth map and 3D imaging applications: Algorithms and technologies* (pp. 27–55). Hershey, PA: IGI Global. doi:10.4018/978-1-61350-326-3.ch003

Gullà, V. (2013). Leading the technological innovation in healthcare systems: The telematic medicine approach. In V. Gulla, A. Mori, F. Gabbrielli, & P. Lanzafame (Eds.), *Telehealth networks for hospital services: New methodologies* (pp. 134–153). Hershey, PA: IGI Global. doi:10.4018/978-1-4666-2979-0.ch009

Guo, R., Wang, Y., Yan, H., Li, F., Yan, J., & Xu, Z. (2011). Pulse wave analysis of traditional chinese medicine based on hemodynamics principles. In L. Liu, D. Wei, & Y. Li (Eds.), *Interdisciplinary research and applications in bioinformatics, computational biology, and environmental sciences* (pp. 194–203). Hershey, PA: IGI Global. doi:10.4018/978-1-60960-064-8.ch017

Gupta, A., Goyal, R. K., Joiner, K. A., & Saini, S. (2010). Outsourcing in the healthcare industry: Information technology, intellectual property, and allied aspects. In M. Khosrow-Pour (Ed.), *Global, social, and organizational implications of emerging information resources management: Concepts and applications* (pp. 18–44). Hershey, PA: IGI Global. doi:10.4018/978-1-60566-962-5.ch002

Gupta, S., Mukherjee, S., & Roy, S. S. (2013). Modernization of healthcare and medical diagnosis system using multi agent system (MAS): A comparative study. In S. Bhattacharyya & P. Dutta (Eds.), *Handbook of research on computational intelligence for engineering, science, and business* (pp. 592–622). Hershey, PA: IGI Global. doi:10.4018/978-1-4666-2518-1.ch023

Ha, S. H. (2011). Medical domain knowledge and associative classification rules in diagnosis. *International Journal of Knowledge Discovery in Bioinformatics, 2*(1), 60–73. doi:10.4018/jkdb.2011010104

Haheim, L. L., & Morland, B. (2010). Health technology assessment: Development and future. In J. Rodrigues (Ed.), *Health information systems: Concepts, methodologies, tools, and applications* (pp. 26–41). Hershey, PA: IGI Global. doi:10.4018/978-1-60566-988-5.ch003

Hai-Jew, S. (2010). An elusive formula: The IT role in behavior change in public health. In T. Yuzer & G. Kurubacak (Eds.), *Transformative learning and online education: Aesthetics, dimensions and concepts* (pp. 347–373). Hershey, PA: IGI Global. doi:10.4018/978-1-61520-985-9.ch022

Haida, M. (2013). Implications of NIRS brain signals. In J. Wu (Ed.), *Biomedical engineering and cognitive neuroscience for healthcare: Interdisciplinary applications* (pp. 120–128). Hershey, PA: IGI Global. doi:10.4018/978-1-4666-2113-8.ch013

Haidegger, T. (2012). Surgical robots: System development, assessment, and clearance. In T. Sobh & X. Xiong (Eds.), *Prototyping of robotic systems: Applications of design and implementation* (pp. 288–326). Hershey, PA: IGI Global. doi:10.4018/978-1-4666-0176-5.ch010

Hajiheydari, N., Khakbaz, S. B., & Farhadi, H. (2013). Proposing a business model in healthcare industry: E-diagnosis. *International Journal of Healthcare Information Systems and Informatics*, *8*(2), 41–57. doi:10.4018/jhisi.2013040104

Hanada, E. (2013). Effective use of RFID in medicine and general healthcare. In T. Issa, P. Isaías, & P. Kommers (Eds.), *Information systems and technology for organizations in a networked society* (pp. 335–352). Hershey, PA: IGI Global. doi:10.4018/978-1-4666-4062-7.ch018

Hara, H. (2013). Women and health in Japan: The rise and obstacles of gender and sex-specific medicine. In M. Merviö (Ed.), *Healthcare management and economics: Perspectives on public and private administration* (pp. 203–207). Hershey, PA: IGI Global. doi:10.4018/978-1-4666-3982-9.ch016

Harnett, B. (2013). Patient centered medicine and technology adaptation. In *User-driven healthcare: Concepts, methodologies, tools, and applications* (pp. 77–98). Hershey, PA: IGI Global. doi:10.4018/978-1-4666-2770-3.ch005

Hatton, J. D., Schmidt, T. M., & Jelen, J. (2013). Adoption of electronic health care records: Physician heuristics and hesitancy. In R. Martinho, R. Rijo, M. Cruz-Cunha, & J. Varajão (Eds.), *Information systems and technologies for enhancing health and social care* (pp. 148–165). Hershey, PA: IGI Global. doi:10.4018/978-1-4666-3667-5.ch010

Heaberg, G. (2011). Case study: Research matchmaker, an advanced nursing practice informatics application. In A. Cashin & R. Cook (Eds.), *Evidence-based practice in nursing informatics: Concepts and applications* (pp. 217–236). Hershey, PA: IGI Global. doi:10.4018/978-1-60960-034-1.ch017

Hegde, B. (2011). Learning medicine: A personal view. In R. Biswas & C. Martin (Eds.), *User-driven healthcare and narrative medicine: Utilizing collaborative social networks and technologies* (pp. 184–190). Hershey, PA: IGI Global. doi:10.4018/978-1-60960-097-6.ch014

Heilman, J. (2012). Creating awareness for using a wiki to promote collaborative health professional education. *International Journal of User-Driven Healthcare*, *2*(1), 86–87. doi:10.4018/ijudh.2012010113

Heinzel, A., Fechete, R., Söllner, J., Perco, P., Heinze, G., Oberbauer, R., ... Mayer, B. (2012). Data graphs for linking clinical phenotype and molecular feature space. *International Journal of Systems Biology and Biomedical Technologies*, *1*(1), 11–25. doi:10.4018/ijsbbt.2012010102

Hernández-Chan, G. S., Rodríguez-González, A., & Colomo-Palacios, R. (2013). Using social networks to obtain medical diagnosis. In M. Cruz-Cunha, I. Miranda, & P. Gonçalves (Eds.), *Handbook of research on ICTs and management systems for improving efficiency in healthcare and social care* (pp. 306–320). Hershey, PA: IGI Global. doi:10.4018/978-1-4666-3990-4.ch015

Hine, M. J., Farion, K. J., Michalowski, W., & Wilk, S. (2011). Decision making by emergency room physicians and residents: Implications for the design of clinical decision support systems. In J. Tan (Ed.), *New technologies for advancing healthcare and clinical practices* (pp. 131–148). Hershey, PA: IGI Global. doi:10.4018/978-1-60960-780-7.ch008

Hoonakker, P., McGuire, K., & Carayon, P. (2011). Sociotechnical issues of tele-ICU technology. In D. Haftor & A. Mirijamdotter (Eds.), *Information and communication technologies, society and human beings: Theory and framework (festschrift in honor of Gunilla Bradley)* (pp. 225–240). Hershey, PA: IGI Global. doi:10.4018/978-1-60960-057-0.ch018

Hopper, K. B., & Johns, C. L. (2012). Educational technology in the medical industry. In *Wireless technologies: Concepts, methodologies, tools and applications* (pp. 1306–1322). Hershey, PA: IGI Global. doi:10.4018/978-1-61350-101-6.ch511

Hsu, P., Tsai, W., & Tsai, C. (2013). Patient safety concerns among emergency medical staff and patients. *International Journal of Privacy and Health Information Management*, *1*(1), 29–52. doi:10.4018/ijphim.2013010103

Huang, K., Geller, J., Halper, M., Elhanan, G., & Perl, Y. (2011). Scalability of piecewise synonym identification in integration of SNOMED into the UMLS. *International Journal of Computational Models and Algorithms in Medicine*, *2*(3), 26–45. doi:10.4018/jcmam.2011070103

Hughes, B. (2012). Managing e-health in the age of web 2.0: The impact on e-health evaluation. In E-marketing: Concepts, methodologies, tools, and applications (pp. 1268-1288). Hershey, PA: IGI Global. doi:10.4018/978-1-4666-1598-4.ch074

Hyde, A., Nee, J., Butler, M., Drennan, J., & Howlett, E. (2011). Preferred types of menopause service delivery: A qualitative study of menopausal women's perceptions. *International Journal of Healthcare Delivery Reform Initiatives*, *3*(1), 1–12. doi:10.4018/jhdri.2011010101

Ilie, V., Van Slyke, C., Courtney, J. F., & Styne, P. (2011). Challenges associated with physicians' usage of electronic medical records. In J. Tan (Ed.), *New technologies for advancing healthcare and clinical practices* (pp. 234–251). Hershey, PA: IGI Global. doi:10.4018/978-1-60960-780-7.ch014

Inomata, C., & Nitta, S. (2013). Nursing in integrative medicine and nurses' engagement in caring-healing: A discussion based on the practice and study of music therapy and nursing care for patients with neurodegenerative disorders. In J. Wu (Ed.), *Technological advancements in biomedicine for healthcare applications* (pp. 235–239). Hershey, PA: IGI Global. doi:10.4018/978-1-4666-2196-1.ch025

Inthiran, A., Alhashmi, S. M., & Ahmed, P. K. (2012). Medical information retrieval strategies: An exploratory study on the information retrieval behaviors of non-medical professionals. *International Journal of Healthcare Information Systems and Informatics*, *7*(1), 31–45. doi:10.4018/jhisi.2012010103

Isern, D., & Moreno, A. (2010). HeCaSe2: A multi-agent system that automates the application of clinical guidelines. In R. Paranjape & A. Sadanand (Eds.), *Multi-agent systems for healthcare simulation and modeling: Applications for system improvement* (pp. 113–136). Hershey, PA: IGI Global. doi:10.4018/978-1-60566-772-0.ch007

Ishaq, G. M., Hussain, P. T., Iqbal, M. J., & Mushtaq, M. B. (2013). Risk-benefit analysis of combination vs. unopposed HRT in post-menopausal women. In Bioinformatics: Concepts, methodologies, tools, and applications (pp. 1424-1440). Hershey, PA: IGI Global. doi:10.4018/978-1-4666-3604-0.ch073

Iwaki, S. (2013). Multimodal neuroimaging to visualize human visual processing. In J. Wu (Ed.), *Biomedical engineering and cognitive neuroscience for healthcare: Interdisciplinary applications* (pp. 274–282). Hershey, PA: IGI Global. doi:10.4018/978-1-4666-2113-8.ch028

James, R. (2011). Practical pointers in medicine over seven decades: Reflections of an individual physician. In R. Biswas & C. Martin (Eds.), *User-driven healthcare and narrative medicine: Utilizing collaborative social networks and technologies* (pp. 173–183). Hershey, PA: IGI Global. doi:10.4018/978-1-60960-097-6.ch013

Janczewski, M. (2010). Healthcare transformation in a net-centric environment. In S. Ghosh (Ed.), *Net centricity and technological interoperability in organizations: Perspectives and strategies* (pp. 99–114). Hershey, PA: IGI Global. doi:10.4018/978-1-60566-854-3.ch007

Jesus, Â., & Gomes, M. J. (2013). Web 2.0 tools in biomedical education: Limitations and possibilities. In Y. Kats (Ed.), *Learning management systems and instructional design: Best practices in online education* (pp. 208–231). Hershey, PA: IGI Global. doi:10.4018/978-1-4666-3930-0.ch011

Ji, Z., Sugi, T., Goto, S., Wang, X., & Nakamura, M. (2013). Multi-channel template extraction for automatic EEG spike detection. In J. Wu (Ed.), *Biomedical engineering and cognitive neuroscience for healthcare: Interdisciplinary applications* (pp. 255–265). Hershey, PA: IGI Global. doi:10.4018/978-1-4666-2113-8.ch026

Jifa, G., Wuqi, S., Zhengxiang, Z., Rui, G., & Yijun, L. (2012). Expert mining and traditional Chinese medicine knowledge. In W. Lee (Ed.), *Systems approaches to knowledge management, transfer, and resource development* (pp. 239–251). Hershey, PA: IGI Global. doi:10.4018/978-1-4666-1782-7.ch016

Johnson, D. E. (2012). Electronic medical records (EMR): Issues and implementation perspectives. In A. Kolker & P. Story (Eds.), *Management engineering for effective healthcare delivery: Principles and applications* (pp. 333–351). Hershey, PA: IGI Global. doi:10.4018/978-1-60960-872-9.ch016

Johnson, K., & Tashiro, J. (2013). Interprofessional care and health care complexity: Factors shaping human resources effectiveness in health information management. In *User-driven healthcare: Concepts, methodologies, tools, and applications* (pp. 1273–1302). Hershey, PA: IGI Global. doi:10.4018/978-1-4666-2770-3.ch064

Jose, J. (2012). Pharmacovigilance: Basic concepts and applications of pharmacoinformatics. In T. Gasmelseid (Ed.), *Pharmacoinformatics and drug discovery technologies: Theories and applications* (pp. 322–343). Hershey, PA: IGI Global. doi:10.4018/978-1-4666-0309-7.ch020

Juzoji, H. (2012). Legal bases for medical supervision via mobile telecommunications in Japan. *International Journal of E-Health and Medical Communications*, *3*(1), 33–45. doi:10.4018/jehmc.2012010103

Juzwishin, D. W. (2010). Enabling technologies and challenges for the future of ubiquitous health the interoperability framework. In S. Mohammed & J. Fiaidhi (Eds.), *Ubiquitous health and medical informatics: The ubiquity 2.0 trend and beyond* (pp. 596–622). Hershey, PA: IGI Global. doi:10.4018/978-1-61520-777-0.ch028

Kabene, S., & Wolfe, M. (2011). Risks and benefits of technology in health care. In *Clinical technologies: Concepts, methodologies, tools and applications* (pp. 13–24). Hershey, PA: IGI Global. doi:10.4018/978-1-60960-561-2.ch102

Kabene, S. M., Wolfe, M., & Leduc, R. (2012). Recruitment and retention of healthcare professionals for the changing demographics, culture, and access in Canada. In *Human resources management: Concepts, methodologies, tools, and applications* (pp. 276–290). Hershey, PA: IGI Global. doi:10.4018/978-1-4666-1601-1.ch017

Kadiri, M., & Zouag, N. (2014). The new economics of skilled labor migration: The case of medical doctors in MENA. In A. Driouchi (Ed.), *Labor and health economics in the Mediterranean region: Migration and mobility of medical doctors* (pp. 267–292). Hershey, PA: IGI Global. doi:10.4018/978-1-4666-4723-7.ch011

Kalantri, S. P. (2012). On being a patient. *International Journal of User-Driven Healthcare*, *2*(4), 1–4. doi:10.4018/ijudh.2012100101 PMID:29090137

Kaldoudi, E., Konstantinidis, S., & Bamidis, P. D. (2010). Web 2.0 approaches for active, collaborative learning in medicine and health. In S. Mohammed & J. Fiaidhi (Eds.), *Ubiquitous health and medical informatics: The ubiquity 2.0 trend and beyond* (pp. 127–149). Hershey, PA: IGI Global. doi:10.4018/978-1-61520-777-0.ch007

Kannry, J. L. (2011). Operationalizing the science. In *Clinical technologies: Concepts, methodologies, tools and applications* (pp. 1600–1622). Hershey, PA: IGI Global. doi:10.4018/978-1-60960-561-2.ch601

Karayanni, D. (2010). A cluster analysis of physician's values, prescribing behaviour and attitudes towards firms' marketing communications. *International Journal of Customer Relationship Marketing and Management*, *1*(4), 62–79. doi:10.4018/jcrmm.2010100104

Kastania, A., & Moumtzoglou, A. (2012). Quality implications of the medical applications for 4G mobile phones. *International Journal of Reliable and Quality E-Healthcare*, *1*(1), 58–67. doi:10.4018/ijrqeh.2012010106

Kastania, A. N. (2013). Evaluation considerations for e-health systems. In *User-driven healthcare: Concepts, methodologies, tools, and applications* (pp. 1126–1140). Hershey, PA: IGI Global. doi:10.4018/978-1-4666-2770-3.ch057

Kaufman, D. (2010). Simulation in health professional education. In D. Kaufman & L. Sauvé (Eds.), *Educational gameplay and simulation environments: Case studies and lessons learned* (pp. 51–67). Hershey, PA: IGI Global. doi:10.4018/978-1-61520-731-2.ch003

Kazandjian, V. A. (2013). Learning to accept uncertainty as a quality of care dimension. In A. Moumtzoglou & A. Kastania (Eds.), *E-health technologies and improving patient safety: Exploring organizational factors* (pp. 1–12). Hershey, PA: IGI Global. doi:10.4018/978-1-4666-2657-7.ch001

Kearns, W. D., Fozard, J. L., & Lamm, R. S. (2011). How knowing who, where and when can change health care delivery. In C. Röcker & M. Ziefle (Eds.), *E-health, assistive technologies and applications for assisted living: Challenges and solutions* (pp. 139–160). Hershey, PA: IGI Global. doi:10.4018/978-1-60960-469-1.ch007

Khan, T. (2013). Transformation of a reluctant patient to a proactive health advocate. *International Journal of User-Driven Healthcare, 3*(1), 71–74. doi:10.4018/ijudh.2013010109

Khetarpal, A., & Singh, S. (2012). Disability studies in medical education. *International Journal of User-Driven Healthcare, 2*(2), 44–51. doi:10.4018/ijudh.2012040105

Kim, J. (2011). The development and implementation of patient safety information systems (PSIS). In Clinical technologies: Concepts, methodologies, tools and applications (pp. 2054-2072). Hershey, PA: IGI Global. doi:10.4018/978-1-60960-561-2.ch804

Kldiashvili, E. (2011). The application of virtual organization technology for eHealth. In E. Kldiashvili (Ed.), *Grid technologies for e-health: Applications for telemedicine services and delivery* (pp. 1–17). Hershey, PA: IGI Global. doi:10.4018/978-1-61692-010-4.ch001

Kldiashvili, E. (2012). The cloud computing as the tool for implementation of virtual organization technology for eHealth. *Journal of Information Technology Research, 5*(1), 18–34. doi:10.4018/jitr.2012010102

Kldiashvili, E. (2013). Implementation of telecytology in Georgia. In V. Gulla, A. Mori, F. Gabbrielli, & P. Lanzafame (Eds.), *Telehealth networks for hospital services: New methodologies* (pp. 341–361). Hershey, PA: IGI Global. doi:10.4018/978-1-4666-2979-0.ch022

Klemer, D. P. (2010). Advances in biosensors for in vitro diagnostics. In A. Lazakidou (Ed.), *Biocomputation and biomedical informatics: Case studies and applications* (pp. 178–186). Hershey, PA: IGI Global. doi:10.4018/978-1-60566-768-3.ch011

Kotwani, A. (2013). Transparency and accountability in public procurement of essential medicines in developing countries. In *Supply chain management: Concepts, methodologies, tools, and applications* (pp. 1437–1452). Hershey, PA: IGI Global. doi:10.4018/978-1-4666-2625-6.ch085

Kuehler, M., Schimke, N., & Hale, J. (2012). Privacy considerations for electronic health records. In G. Yee (Ed.), *Privacy protection measures and technologies in business organizations: Aspects and standards* (pp. 210–226). Hershey, PA: IGI Global. doi:10.4018/978-1-61350-501-4.ch008

Kukar, M., Kononenko, I., & Grošelj, C. (2013). Automated diagnostics of coronary artery disease: Long-term results and recent advancements. In *Data mining: Concepts, methodologies, tools, and applications* (pp. 1043–1063). Hershey, PA: IGI Global. doi:10.4018/978-1-4666-2455-9.ch053

Kumalasari, C. D., Caplow, J. A., & Fearing, N. (2013). Simulation followed by a reflection and feedback session in medical education. In L. Tomei (Ed.), *Learning tools and teaching approaches through ICT advancements* (pp. 68–81). Hershey, PA: IGI Global. doi:10.4018/978-1-4666-2017-9.ch007

Kumar, R., & Srivastava, R. (2014). Detection of cancer from microscopic biopsy images using image processing tools. In R. Srivastava, S. Singh, & K. Shukla (Eds.), *Research developments in computer vision and image processing: Methodologies and applications* (pp. 175–194). Hershey, PA: IGI Global. doi:10.4018/978-1-4666-4558-5.ch010

Kuruvilla, A., & Alexander, S. M. (2010). Predicting ambulance diverson. *International Journal of Information Systems in the Service Sector*, *2*(1), 1–10. doi:10.4018/jisss.2010093001

Kyriazis, D., Menychtas, A., Tserpes, K., Athanaileas, T., & Varvarigou, T. (2010). High performance computing in biomedicine. In A. Lazakidou (Ed.), *Biocomputation and biomedical informatics: Case studies and applications* (pp. 106–118). Hershey, PA: IGI Global. doi:10.4018/978-1-60566-768-3.ch006

LaBrunda, M., & LaBrunda, A. (2010). Fuzzy logic in medicine. In M. Khosrow-Pour (Ed.), *Breakthrough discoveries in information technology research: Advancing trends* (pp. 218–224). Hershey, PA: IGI Global. doi:10.4018/978-1-60566-966-3.ch017

Lagares-Lemos, Á. M., Lagares-Lemos, M., Colomo-Palacios, R., García-Crespo, Á., & Gómez-Berbís, J. M. (2011). DISMON. In *Clinical technologies: Concepts, methodologies, tools and applications* (pp. 995–1007). Hershey, PA: IGI Global. doi:10.4018/978-1-60960-561-2.ch324

Lagares-Lemos, Á. M., Lagares-Lemos, M., Colomo-Palacios, R., García-Crespo, Á., & Gómez-Berbís, J. M. (2013). DISMON: Using social web and semantic technologies to monitor diseases in limited environments. In M. Khosrow-Pour (Ed.), *Interdisciplinary advances in information technology research* (pp. 48–59). Hershey, PA: IGI Global. doi:10.4018/978-1-4666-3625-5.ch004

Lappas, K. (2014). Functional assessment of persons with motor limitations: Methods and tools. In G. Kouroupetroglou (Ed.), *Disability informatics and web accessibility for motor limitations* (pp. 43–74). Hershey, PA: IGI Global. doi:10.4018/978-1-4666-4442-7.ch002

Lazakidou, A., & Daskalaki, A. (2012). *Quality assurance in healthcare service delivery, nursing and personalized medicine: Technologies and processes*. Hershey, PA: IGI Global. doi:10.4018/978-1-61350-120-7

Leal, S., Suarez, C., Framinan, J. M., Parra, C. L., & Gómez, T. (2010). Virtual reality for supporting surgical planning. In M. Cruz-Cunha, A. Tavares, & R. Simoes (Eds.), *Handbook of research on developments in e-health and telemedicine: Technological and social perspectives* (pp. 614–635). Hershey, PA: IGI Global. doi:10.4018/978-1-61520-670-4.ch029

Lemma, F., Denko, M. K., Tan, J. K., & Kassegne, S. K. (2011). Envisioning a national e-medicine network architecture in a developing country: A case study. In J. Tan (Ed.), *Developments in healthcare information systems and technologies: Models and methods* (pp. 35–53). Hershey, PA: IGI Global. doi:10.4018/978-1-61692-002-9.ch003

Li, G., You, M., Xu, L., & Huang, S. (2012). Personalized experience sharing of Cai's TCM gynecology. In A. Lazakidou & A. Daskalaki (Eds.), *Quality assurance in healthcare service delivery, nursing and personalized medicine: Technologies and processes* (pp. 26–47). Hershey, PA: IGI Global. doi:10.4018/978-1-61350-120-7.ch002

Lim, V. K. (2012). The process of medical curriculum development in Malaysia. *International Journal of User-Driven Healthcare*, *2*(1), 33–39. doi:10.4018/ijudh.2012010105

Lin, H. (2013). Cultivating chan as proactive therapy for social wellness. In M. Cruz-Cunha, I. Miranda, & P. Gonçalves (Eds.), *Handbook of research on ICTs for human-centered healthcare and social care services* (pp. 151–170). Hershey, PA: IGI Global. doi:10.4018/978-1-4666-3986-7.ch008

Liu, Q., Poon, C. C., & Zhang, Y. T. (2012). Wearable technologies for neonatal monitoring. In W. Chen, S. Oetomo, & L. Feijs (Eds.), *Neonatal monitoring technologies: Design for integrated solutions* (pp. 12–40). Hershey, PA: IGI Global. doi:10.4018/978-1-4666-0975-4.ch002

Llobet, H., Llobet, P., & LaBrunda, M. (2011). Imaging advances of the cardiopulmonary system. In *Clinical technologies: Concepts, methodologies, tools and applications* (pp. 2183–2190). Hershey, PA: IGI Global. doi:10.4018/978-1-60960-561-2.ch812

Logeswaran, R. (2010). Neural networks in medicine: improving difficult automated detection of cancer in the bile ducts. In R. Chiong (Ed.), *Nature-inspired informatics for intelligent applications and knowledge discovery: Implications in business, science, and engineering* (pp. 144–165). Hershey, PA: IGI Global. doi:10.4018/978-1-60566-705-8.ch006

Logeswaran, R. (2011). Neural networks in medicine. In *Clinical technologies: Concepts, methodologies, tools and applications* (pp. 744–765). Hershey, PA: IGI Global. doi:10.4018/978-1-60960-561-2.ch308

Long, L. R., Antani, S., Thoma, G. R., & Deserno, T. M. (2011). Content-based image retrieval for advancing medical diagnostics, treatment and education. In J. Tan (Ed.), *New technologies for advancing healthcare and clinical practices* (pp. 1–17). Hershey, PA: IGI Global. doi:10.4018/978-1-60960-780-7.ch001

Lueth, T. C., D'Angelo, L. T., & Czabke, A. (2010). TUM-AgeTech: A new framework for pervasive medical devices. In A. Coronato & G. De Pietro (Eds.), *Pervasive and smart technologies for healthcare: Ubiquitous methodologies and tools* (pp. 295–321). Hershey, PA: IGI Global. doi:10.4018/978-1-61520-765-7.ch014

Lui, K. (2013). The health informatics professional. In *User-driven healthcare: Concepts, methodologies, tools, and applications* (pp. 120–141). Hershey, PA: IGI Global. doi:10.4018/978-1-4666-2770-3.ch007

Lui, T., & Goel, L. (2012). A framework for conceptualizing the current role and future trends of information systems in medical training. *International Journal of Healthcare Information Systems and Informatics*, *7*(1), 1–12. doi:10.4018/jhisi.2012010101

MacDonald, C. J., McKeen, M., Leith-Gudbranson, D., Montpetit, M., Archibald, D., & Rivet, C. … Hirsh, M. (2013). University of Ottawa department of family medicine faculty development curriculum framework. In K. Patel, & S. Vij (Eds.) Enterprise resource planning models for the education sector: Applications and methodologies (pp. 197-215). Hershey, PA: IGI Global. doi:10.4018/978-1-4666-2193-0.ch014

MacGregor, R. C., Hyland, P. N., & Harvie, C. (2010). Associations between driving forces to adopt ICT and benefits derived from that adoption in medical practices in Australia. In M. Cruz-Cunha, A. Tavares, & R. Simoes (Eds.), *Handbook of research on developments in e-health and telemedicine: Technological and social perspectives* (pp. 652–668). Hershey, PA: IGI Global. doi:10.4018/978-1-61520-670-4.ch031

Mackert, M., Whitten, P., & Holtz, B. (2010). Health infonomics: Intelligent applications of information technology. In J. Rodrigues (Ed.), *Health information systems: Concepts, methodologies, tools, and applications* (pp. 117–132). Hershey, PA: IGI Global. doi:10.4018/978-1-60566-988-5.ch008

Malik, A. S., & Malik, R. H. (2012). Adolescent medicine curriculum at faculty of medicine, Universiti Teknologi MARA, Malaysia. *International Journal of User-Driven Healthcare, 2*(1), 40–48. doi:10.4018/ijudh.2012010106

Martin, C. M., Biswas, R., Sturmberg, J. P., Topps, D., Ellaway, R., & Smith, K. (2011). Patient journey record systems (PaJR) for preventing ambulatory care sensitive conditions: A developmental framework. In R. Biswas & C. Martin (Eds.), *User-driven healthcare and narrative medicine: Utilizing collaborative social networks and technologies* (pp. 93–112). Hershey, PA: IGI Global. doi:10.4018/978-1-60960-097-6.ch007

Masayuki, K., Eiji, K., Tetsuo, T., & Nozomu, M. (2013). Evaluation of olfactory impairment in Parkinson's disease using near-infrared spectroscopy. In J. Wu (Ed.), *Biomedical engineering and cognitive neuroscience for healthcare: Interdisciplinary applications* (pp. 293–302). Hershey, PA: IGI Global. doi:10.4018/978-1-4666-2113-8.ch030

Mazzanti, I., Maolo, A., & Antonicelli, R. (2014). E-health and telemedicine in the elderly: State of the art. In *Assistive technologies: Concepts, methodologies, tools, and applications* (pp. 693–704). Hershey, PA: IGI Global. doi:10.4018/978-1-4666-4422-9.ch034

Medhekar, A., Wong, H. Y., & Hall, J. (2014). Innovation in medical tourism service marketing: A case of India. In A. Goyal (Ed.), *Innovations in services marketing and management: Strategies for emerging economies* (pp. 49–66). Hershey, PA: IGI Global. doi:10.4018/978-1-4666-4671-1.ch003

Medhekar, A., Wong, H. Y., & Hall, J. (2014). Medical tourism: A conceptual framework for an innovation in global healthcare provision. In A. Goyal (Ed.), *Innovations in services marketing and management: Strategies for emerging economies* (pp. 148–169). Hershey, PA: IGI Global. doi:10.4018/978-1-4666-4671-1.ch009

Memmola, M., Palumbo, G., & Rossini, M. (2010). Web & RFID technology: New frontiers in costing and process management for rehabilitation medicine. In J. Symonds (Ed.), *Ubiquitous and pervasive computing: Concepts, methodologies, tools, and applications* (pp. 623–647). Hershey, PA: IGI Global. doi:10.4018/978-1-60566-960-1.ch039

Menciassi, A., & Laschi, C. (2014). Biorobotics. In Robotics: Concepts, methodologies, tools, and applications (pp. 1613-1643). Hershey, PA: IGI Global. doi:10.4018/978-1-4666-4607-0.ch079

Mika, K. (2010). Cybermedicine, telemedicine, and data protection in the United States. In J. Rodrigues (Ed.), *Health information systems: Concepts, methodologies, tools, and applications* (pp. 274–296). Hershey, PA: IGI Global. doi:10.4018/978-1-60566-988-5.ch019

Mirbagheri, A., Baniasad, M. A., Farahmand, F., Behzadipour, S., & Ahmadian, A. (2013). Medical robotics: State-of-the-art applications and research challenges. *International Journal of Healthcare Information Systems and Informatics*, *8*(2), 1–14. doi:10.4018/jhisi.2013040101

Miscione, G. (2013). Telemedicine and development: Situating information technologies in the Amazon. In J. Abdelnour-Nocera (Ed.), *Knowledge and technological development effects on organizational and social structures* (pp. 132–145). Hershey, PA: IGI Global. doi:10.4018/978-1-4666-2151-0.ch009

Mobasheri, A. (2013). Regeneration of articular cartilage: Opportunities, challenges, and perspectives. In A. Daskalaki (Ed.), *Medical advancements in aging and regenerative technologies: Clinical tools and applications* (pp. 137–168). Hershey, PA: IGI Global. doi:10.4018/978-1-4666-2506-8.ch007

Monzon, J. E. (2012). Bioethics. In Z. Abu-Faraj (Ed.), *Handbook of research on biomedical engineering education and advanced bioengineering learning: Interdisciplinary concepts* (pp. 198–237). Hershey, PA: IGI Global. doi:10.4018/978-1-4666-0122-2.ch005

Morais da Costa, G. J., Araújo da Silva Nuno, M., & Alves da Silva Nuno, S. (2010). The human centred approach to bionanotechnology in telemedicine: Ethical considerations. In M. Cruz-Cunha, A. Tavares, & R. Simoes (Eds.), *Handbook of research on developments in e-health and telemedicine: Technological and social perspectives* (pp. 311–335). Hershey, PA: IGI Global. doi:10.4018/978-1-61520-670-4.ch015

Morgade, A. T., Martínez-Romero, M., Vázquez-Naya, J. M., Loureiro, M. P., Albo, Á. G., & Loureiro, J. P. (2011). Development of a knowledge based system for an intensive care environment using ontologies. *Journal of Information Technology Research*, *4*(1), 21–33. doi:10.4018/jitr.2011010102

Morita, A. (2013). The quantitative EEG change in Parkinson's disease. In J. Wu (Ed.), *Biomedical engineering and cognitive neuroscience for healthcare: Interdisciplinary applications* (pp. 225–234). Hershey, PA: IGI Global. doi:10.4018/978-1-4666-2113-8.ch023

Moumtzoglou, A. (2011). E-health as the realm of healthcare quality: A mental image of the future. In A. Moumtzoglou & A. Kastania (Eds.), *E-health systems quality and reliability: Models and standards* (pp. 291–310). Hershey, PA: IGI Global. doi:10.4018/978-1-61692-843-8.ch022

Moumtzoglou, A. (2011). E-health as the realm of healthcare quality. In *Clinical technologies: Concepts, methodologies, tools and applications* (pp. 73–92). Hershey, PA: IGI Global. doi:10.4018/978-1-60960-561-2.ch105

Moumtzoglou, A. (2011). E-health: A bridge to people-centered health care. In A. Moumtzoglou & A. Kastania (Eds.), *E-health systems quality and reliability: Models and standards* (pp. 47–63). Hershey, PA: IGI Global. doi:10.4018/978-1-61692-843-8.ch005

Moumtzoglou, A. (2013). Health 2.0 and medicine 2.0: Safety, ownership and privacy issues. In User-driven healthcare: Concepts, methodologies, tools, and applications (pp. 1508-1522). Hershey, PA: IGI Global. doi:10.4018/978-1-4666-2770-3.ch075

Moumtzoglou, A. (2013). Risk perception as a patient safety dimension. In A. Moumtzoglou & A. Kastania (Eds.), *E-health technologies and improving patient safety: Exploring organizational factors* (pp. 285–299). Hershey, PA: IGI Global. doi:10.4018/978-1-4666-2657-7.ch017

Mourtzikou, A., Stamouli, M., & Athanasiadi, E. (2013). Improvement of clinical laboratory services through quality. *International Journal of Reliable and Quality E-Healthcare*, *2*(2), 38–46. doi:10.4018/ijrqeh.2013040103

Muriithi, M. K., & Mwabu, G. (2014). Demand for health care in Kenya: The effects of information about quality. In P. Schaeffer & E. Kouassi (Eds.), *Econometric methods for analyzing economic development* (pp. 102–110). Hershey, PA: IGI Global. doi:10.4018/978-1-4666-4329-1.ch007

Murugan, B. O., & Sornam, S. A. (2013). Internet and online medical journal access skills of the medical practitioners of Tamilnadu: A study. In S. Thanuskodi (Ed.), *Challenges of academic library management in developing countries* (pp. 75–82). Hershey, PA: IGI Global. doi:10.4018/978-1-4666-4070-2.ch006

Nadathur, S. G. (2010). Bayesian networks in the health domain. In A. Ali & Y. Xiang (Eds.), *Dynamic and advanced data mining for progressing technological development: Innovations and systemic approaches* (pp. 342–376). Hershey, PA: IGI Global. doi:10.4018/978-1-60566-908-3.ch014

Naidoo, V., & Naidoo, Y. (2014). Home telecare, medical implant, and mobile technology: Evolutions in geriatric care. In C. El Morr (Ed.), *Research Perspectives on the role of informatics in health policy and management* (pp. 222–237). Hershey, PA: IGI Global. doi:10.4018/978-1-4666-4321-5.ch013

Najarian, S., & Afshari, E. (2010). Applications of robots in surgery. In A. Shukla & R. Tiwari (Eds.), *Intelligent medical technologies and biomedical engineering: Tools and applications* (pp. 241–259). Hershey, PA: IGI Global. doi:10.4018/978-1-61520-977-4.ch012

Nakajima, I. (2012). Cross-border medical care and telemedicine. *International Journal of E-Health and Medical Communications*, *3*(1), 46–61. doi:10.4018/jehmc.2012010104

Nakayasu, K., & Sato, C. (2012). Liability for telemedicine. *International Journal of E-Health and Medical Communications*, *3*(1), 1–21. doi:10.4018/jehmc.2012010101

Narasimhalu, D. (2010). Redefining medical tourism. In S. Becker & R. Niebuhr (Eds.), *Cases on technology innovation: Entrepreneurial successes and pitfalls* (pp. 267–285). Hershey, PA: IGI Global. doi:10.4018/978-1-61520-609-4.ch014

Naulaers, G., Caicedo, A., & Van Huffel, S. (2012). Use of near-infrared spectroscopy in the neonatal intensive care unit. In W. Chen, S. Oetomo, & L. Feijs (Eds.), *Neonatal monitoring technologies: Design for integrated solutions* (pp. 56–83). Hershey, PA: IGI Global. doi:10.4018/978-1-4666-0975-4.ch004

Nokata, M. (2014). Small medical robot. In I. Management Association (Ed.), Robotics: Concepts, methodologies, tools, and applications (pp. 638-646). Hershey, PA: IGI Global. doi:10.4018/978-1-4666-4607-0.ch032

Noteboom, C. (2013). Physician interaction with EHR: The importance of stakeholder identification and change management. In S. Sarnikar, D. Bennett, & M. Gaynor (Eds.), *Cases on healthcare information technology for patient care management* (pp. 95–112). Hershey, PA: IGI Global. doi:10.4018/978-1-4666-2671-3.ch005

Noury, N., Bourquard, K., Bergognon, D., & Schroeder, J. (2013). Regulations initiatives in France for the interoperability of communicating medical devices. *International Journal of E-Health and Medical Communications*, *4*(2), 50–64. doi:10.4018/jehmc.2013040104

O'Hanlon, S. (2013). Avoiding adverse consequences of e-health. In A. Moumtzoglou & A. Kastania (Eds.), *E-health technologies and improving patient safety: Exploring organizational factors* (pp. 13–26). Hershey, PA: IGI Global. doi:10.4018/978-1-4666-2657-7.ch002

O'Leary, D. E. (2012). An activity theory analysis of RFID in hospitals. In Z. Luo (Ed.), *Innovations in logistics and supply chain management technologies for dynamic economies* (pp. 148–166). Hershey, PA: IGI Global. doi:10.4018/978-1-4666-0267-0.ch010

O'Neill, L., Talbert, J., & Klepack, W. (2010). Physician characteristics associated with early adoption of electronic medical records in smaller group practices. In J. Rodrigues (Ed.), *Health information systems: Concepts, methodologies, tools, and applications* (pp. 1503–1512). Hershey, PA: IGI Global. doi:10.4018/978-1-60566-988-5.ch096

Ogawa, T., Ikeda, M., Suzuki, M., & Araki, K. (2014). Medical practical knowledge circulation based on purpose-oriented service modeling. In M. Kosaka & K. Shirahada (Eds.), *Progressive trends in knowledge and system-based science for service innovation* (pp. 400–424). Hershey, PA: IGI Global. doi:10.4018/978-1-4666-4663-6.ch022

Oliveira, T. C., Oliveira, M. D., & Peña, T. (2013). Towards a post-implementation evaluation framework of outpatient electronic drug prescribing. In M. Cruz-Cunha, I. Miranda, & P. Gonçalves (Eds.), *Handbook of research on ICTs and management systems for improving efficiency in healthcare and social care* (pp. 133–155). Hershey, PA: IGI Global. doi:10.4018/978-1-4666-3990-4.ch007

Orizio, G., & Gelatti, U. (2012). Human behaviors in online pharmacies. In Z. Yan (Ed.), *Encyclopedia of cyber behavior* (pp. 661–670). Hershey, PA: IGI Global. doi:10.4018/978-1-4666-0315-8.ch056

Otero, A., Félix, P., & Barro, S. (2010). Current state of critical patient monitoring and outstanding challenges. In M. Cruz-Cunha, A. Tavares, & R. Simoes (Eds.), *Handbook of research on developments in e-health and telemedicine: Technological and social perspectives* (pp. 981–1003). Hershey, PA: IGI Global. doi:10.4018/978-1-61520-670-4.ch047

Ozturk, Y., & Sharma, J. (2013). mVITAL: A standards compliant vital sign monitor. In IT policy and ethics: Concepts, methodologies, tools, and applications (pp. 515-538). Hershey, PA: IGI Global. doi:10.4018/978-1-4666-2919-6.ch024

Pal, K., Ghosh, G., & Bhattacharya, M. (2014). Biomedical watermarking: An emerging and secure tool for data security and better tele-diagnosis in modern health care system. In R. Srivastava, S. Singh, & K. Shukla (Eds.), *Research developments in computer vision and image processing: Methodologies and applications* (pp. 208–234). Hershey, PA: IGI Global. doi:10.4018/978-1-4666-4558-5.ch012

Paolucci, F., Ergas, H., Hannan, T., & Aarts, J. (2011). The effectiveness of health informatics. In *Clinical technologies: Concepts, methodologies, tools and applications* (pp. 25–49). Hershey, PA: IGI Global. doi:10.4018/978-1-60960-561-2.ch103

Parasher, A., Goldschmidt-Clermont, P. J., & Tien, J. M. (2012). Healthcare delivery as a service system: Barriers to co-production and implications of healthcare reform. In A. Kolker & P. Story (Eds.), *Management engineering for effective healthcare delivery: Principles and applications* (pp. 191–214). Hershey, PA: IGI Global. doi:10.4018/978-1-60960-872-9.ch009

Parry, D. (2010). Coding and messaging systems for women's health informatics. In J. Rodrigues (Ed.), *Health information systems: Concepts, methodologies, tools, and applications* (pp. 2192–2205). Hershey, PA: IGI Global. doi:10.4018/978-1-60566-988-5.ch139

Parry, D. (2012). Computerised decision support for women's health informatics. In *Machine learning: Concepts, methodologies, tools and applications* (pp. 1404–1416). Hershey, PA: IGI Global. doi:10.4018/978-1-60960-818-7.ch513

Payne, G. W. (2011). The role of blended learning in 21st century medical education: Current trends and future directions. In A. Kitchenham (Ed.), *Blended learning across disciplines: Models for implementation* (pp. 132–146). Hershey, PA: IGI Global. doi:10.4018/978-1-60960-479-0.ch008

Penchovsky, R. (2013). Engineering gene control circuits with allosteric ribozymes in human cells as a medicine of the future. In Bioinformatics: Concepts, methodologies, tools, and applications (pp. 860-883). Hershey, PA: IGI Global. doi:10.4018/978-1-4666-3604-0.ch047

Pestana, O. (2014). Information value and quality for the health sector: A case study of search strategies for optimal information retrieval. In G. Jamil, A. Malheiro, & F. Ribeiro (Eds.), *Rethinking the conceptual base for new practical applications in information value and quality* (pp. 116–133). Hershey, PA: IGI Global. doi:10.4018/978-1-4666-4562-2.ch006

Peterson, C., & Willis, E. (2011). Social construction of chronic disease: Narratives on the experience of chronic illness. In R. Biswas & C. Martin (Eds.), *User-driven healthcare and narrative medicine: Utilizing collaborative social networks and technologies* (pp. 395–409). Hershey, PA: IGI Global. doi:10.4018/978-1-60960-097-6.ch027

Petoukhov, S., & He, M. (2010). Biological evolution of dialects of the genetic code. In S. Petoukhov & M. He (Eds.), *Symmetrical analysis techniques for genetic systems and bioinformatics: Advanced patterns and applications* (pp. 50–64). Hershey, PA: IGI Global. doi:10.4018/978-1-60566-124-7.ch003

Petty, G. C., & Joyner, D. H. (2012). The efficacy of continuing education technology for public health physicians practicing in remote areas. In V. Wang (Ed.), *Encyclopedia of e-leadership, counseling and training* (pp. 453–467). Hershey, PA: IGI Global. doi:10.4018/978-1-61350-068-2.ch033

Phua, C., Roy, P. C., Aloulou, H., Biswas, J., Tolstikov, A., & Foo, V. S. … Xu, D. (2014). State-of-the-art assistive technology for people with dementia. In Assistive technologies: Concepts, methodologies, tools, and applications (pp. 1606-1625). Hershey, PA: IGI Global. doi:10.4018/978-1-4666-4422-9.ch085

Portela, F., Cabral, A., Abelha, A., Salazar, M., Quintas, C., Machado, J., … Santos, M. F. (2013). Knowledge acquisition process for intelligent decision support in critical health care. In R. Martinho, R. Rijo, M. Cruz-Cunha, & J. Varajão (Eds.) Information systems and technologies for enhancing health and social care (pp. 55-68). Hershey, PA: IGI Global. doi:10.4018/978-1-4666-3667-5.ch004

Postolache, O., Girão, P., & Postolache, G. (2013). Seismocardiogram and ballistocardiogram sensing. In A. Lay-Ekuakille (Ed.), *Advanced instrument engineering: Measurement, calibration, and design* (pp. 223–246). Hershey, PA: IGI Global. doi:10.4018/978-1-4666-4165-5.ch017

Premkumar, K. (2011). Mobile learning in medicine. In A. Kitchenham (Ed.), *Models for interdisciplinary mobile learning: Delivering information to students* (pp. 137–153). Hershey, PA: IGI Global. doi:10.4018/978-1-60960-511-7.ch008

Price, M. (2011). A bio-psycho-social review of usability methods and their applications in healthcare. In *Clinical technologies: Concepts, methodologies, tools and applications* (pp. 1874–1899). Hershey, PA: IGI Global. doi:10.4018/978-1-60960-561-2.ch704

Prigione, A. (2012). Stem cell-based personalized medicine: From disease modeling to clinical applications. In *Computer engineering: Concepts, methodologies, tools and applications* (pp. 1855–1866). Hershey, PA: IGI Global. doi:10.4018/978-1-61350-456-7.ch803

Quinaz, F., Fazendeiro, P., Castelo-Branco, M., & Araújo, P. (2013). Soft methods for automatic drug infusion in medical care environment. In M. Cruz-Cunha, I. Miranda, & P. Gonçalves (Eds.), *Handbook of research on ICTs and management systems for improving efficiency in healthcare and social care* (pp. 830–854). Hershey, PA: IGI Global. doi:10.4018/978-1-4666-3990-4.ch043

Quoniam, L., & Lima de Magalhães, J. (2014). Perception of the information value for public health: A case study for neglected diseases. In G. Jamil, A. Malheiro, & F. Ribeiro (Eds.), *Rethinking the conceptual base for new practical applications in information value and quality* (pp. 211–232). Hershey, PA: IGI Global. doi:10.4018/978-1-4666-4562-2.ch009

Raghupathi, W. (2010). Designing clinical decision support systems in health care: A systemic view. In M. Hunter (Ed.), *Strategic information systems: Concepts, methodologies, tools, and applications* (pp. 652–661). Hershey, PA: IGI Global. doi:10.4018/978-1-60566-677-8.ch043

Raghupathi, W., & Nerur, S. (2012). The intellectual structure of health and medical informatics. In J. Tan (Ed.), *Advancing technologies and intelligence in healthcare and clinical environments breakthroughs* (pp. 1–16). Hershey, PA: IGI Global. doi:10.4018/978-1-4666-1755-1.ch001

Räisänen, T., Oinas-Kukkonen, H., Leiviskä, K., Seppänen, M., & Kallio, M. (2010). Managing mobile healthcare knowledge: Physicians' perceptions on knowledge creation and reuse. In J. Rodrigues (Ed.), *Health information systems: Concepts, methodologies, tools, and applications* (pp. 733–749). Hershey, PA: IGI Global. doi:10.4018/978-1-60566-988-5.ch046

Raval, M. S. (2011). Data hiding in digitized medical images: From concepts to applications. In A. Daskalaki (Ed.), *Digital forensics for the health sciences: Applications in practice and research* (pp. 29–47). Hershey, PA: IGI Global. doi:10.4018/978-1-60960-483-7.ch003

Ravka, N. (2014). Informatics and health services: The potential benefits and challenges of electronic health records and personal electronic health records in patient care, cost control, and health research – An overview. In C. El Morr (Ed.), *Research perspectives on the role of informatics in health policy and management* (pp. 89–114). Hershey, PA: IGI Global. doi:10.4018/978-1-4666-4321-5.ch007

Reyes Álamo, J. M., Yang, H., Babbitt, R., & Wong, J. (2010). Support for medication safety and compliance in smart home environments. In J. Rodrigues (Ed.), *Health information systems: Concepts, methodologies, tools, and applications* (pp. 2091–2110). Hershey, PA: IGI Global. doi:10.4018/978-1-60566-988-5.ch133

Ribeiro, C., Monteiro, M., Corredoura, S., Candeias, F., & Pereira, J. (2013). Games in higher education: Opportunities, expectations, challenges, and results in medical education. In S. de Freitas, M. Ott, M. Popescu, & I. Stanescu (Eds.), *New pedagogical approaches in game enhanced learning: Curriculum integration* (pp. 228–247). Hershey, PA: IGI Global. doi:10.4018/978-1-4666-3950-8.ch012

Rocci, L. (2010). Biomedical technoethics. In R. Luppicini (Ed.), *Technoethics and the evolving knowledge society: Ethical issues in technological design, research, development, and innovation* (pp. 128–145). Hershey, PA: IGI Global. doi:10.4018/978-1-60566-952-6.ch007

Rockland, R., Kimmel, H., Carpinelli, J., Hirsch, L. S., & Burr-Alexander, L. (2014). Medical robotics in k-12 education. In Robotics: Concepts, methodologies, tools, and applications (pp. 1096-1115). Hershey, PA: IGI Global. doi:10.4018/978-1-4666-4607-0.ch053

Rodrigues, J. J. (2012). *Emerging communication technologies for e-health and medicine*. Hershey, PA: IGI Global. doi:10.4018/978-1-4666-0909-9

Rodrigues, J. J. (2013). *Digital advances in medicine, e-health, and communication technologies*. Hershey, PA: IGI Global. doi:10.4018/978-1-4666-2794-9

Rodrigues, J. J. (2014). *Advancing medical practice through technology: Applications for healthcare delivery, management, and quality*. Hershey, PA: IGI Global. doi:10.4018/978-1-4666-4619-3

Rodríguez-González, A., García-Crespo, Á., Colomo-Palacios, R., Gómez-Berbís, J. M., & Jiménez-Domingo, E. (2013). Using ontologies in drug prescription: The SemMed approach. In J. Wang (Ed.), *Intelligence methods and systems advancements for knowledge-based business* (pp. 247–261). Hershey, PA: IGI Global. doi:10.4018/978-1-4666-1873-2.ch014

Rojo, M. G., & Daniel, C. (2011). Digital pathology and virtual microscopy integration in e-health records. In *Clinical technologies: Concepts, methodologies, tools and applications* (pp. 1235–1262). Hershey, PA: IGI Global. doi:10.4018/978-1-60960-561-2.ch415

Rompas, A., Tsirmpas, C., Anastasiou, A., Iliopoulou, D., & Koutsouris, D. (2013). Statistical power and sample size in personalized medicine. *International Journal of Systems Biology and Biomedical Technologies, 2*(2), 72–88. doi:10.4018/ijsbbt.2013040105

Rosiek, A. B., & Leksowski, K. (2011). Quality assurance and evaluation of healthcare reform initiatives: Strategy for improving the quality of health care services in public health care units, management model that allows the providing of high quality health care and efficient brand-building. *International Journal of Healthcare Delivery Reform Initiatives, 3*(3), 42–53. doi:10.4018/jhdri.2011070104

Ross, S. (2011). A lexicon for user driven healthcare. *International Journal of User-Driven Healthcare, 1*(1), 50–54. doi:10.4018/ijudh.2011010107

Ross, S. D. (2011). Multiple paths in health care. In R. Biswas & C. Martin (Eds.), *User-driven healthcare and narrative medicine: Utilizing collaborative social networks and technologies* (pp. 113–124). Hershey, PA: IGI Global. doi:10.4018/978-1-60960-097-6.ch008

Rosu, S. M., & Dragoi, G. (2014). E-health sites development using open source software and OMT methodology as support for family doctors' activities: A Romanian case study. In M. Cruz-Cunha, F. Moreira, & J. Varajão (Eds.), *Handbook of research on enterprise 2.0: Technological, social, and organizational dimensions* (pp. 72–88). Hershey, PA: IGI Global. doi:10.4018/978-1-4666-4373-4.ch004

Ruiz-Fernandez, D., & Soriano-Paya, A. (2011). A distributed approach of a clinical decision support system based on cooperation. In *Clinical technologies: Concepts, methodologies, tools and applications* (pp. 1782–1799). Hershey, PA: IGI Global. doi:10.4018/978-1-60960-561-2.ch612

Ryan, P. (2012). Paying for performance: Key design features and the bigger picture. *International Journal of Public and Private Healthcare Management and Economics, 2*(2), 1–16. doi:10.4018/ijpphme.2012040101

Sainz de Abajo, B., & Ballestero, A. L. (2012). Overview of the most important open source software: Analysis of the benefits of OpenMRS, OpenEMR, and VistA. In J. Rodrigues, I. de la Torre Díez, & B. Sainz de Abajo (Eds.), *Telemedicine and e-health services, policies, and applications: Advancements and developments* (pp. 315–346). Hershey, PA: IGI Global. doi:10.4018/978-1-4666-0888-7.ch012

Salcido, G. J., & Delgado, E. C. (2013). Intelligent agent to identify rheumatic diseases. In M. Cruz-Cunha, I. Miranda, & P. Gonçalves (Eds.), *Handbook of research on ICTs and management systems for improving efficiency in healthcare and social care* (pp. 451–473). Hershey, PA: IGI Global. doi:10.4018/978-1-4666-3990-4.ch023

Schallenberg, S., Petzold, C., Riewaldt, J., & Kretschmer, K. (2013). Regulatory T cell-based immunotherapy: Prospects of antigen-specific tolerance induction. In A. Daskalaki (Ed.), *Medical advancements in aging and regenerative technologies: Clinical tools and applications* (pp. 112–136). Hershey, PA: IGI Global. doi:10.4018/978-1-4666-2506-8.ch006

Scheepers-Hoeks, A., Klijn, F., van der Linden, C., Grouls, R., Ackerman, E., & Minderman, N. ... Korsten, E. (2013). Clinical decision support systems for 'making it easy to do it right. In Data mining: Concepts, methodologies, tools, and applications (pp. 1461-1471). Hershey, PA: IGI Global. doi:10.4018/978-1-4666-2455-9.ch076

Seçkin, G. (2012). Cyber behaviors of self health care management. In Z. Yan (Ed.), *Encyclopedia of cyber behavior* (pp. 722–734). Hershey, PA: IGI Global. doi:10.4018/978-1-4666-0315-8.ch061

Serrano, M., Elmisery, A., Foghlú, M. Ó., Donnelly, W., Storni, C., & Fernström, M. (2013). Pervasive computing support in the transition towards personalised health systems. In J. Rodrigues (Ed.), *Digital advances in medicine, e-health, and communication technologies* (pp. 49–64). Hershey, PA: IGI Global. doi:10.4018/978-1-4666-2794-9.ch003

Shachak, A., & Reis, S. (2010). The computer-assisted patient consultation: Promises and challenges. In S. Kabene (Ed.), *Healthcare and the effect of technology: Developments, challenges and advancements* (pp. 72–83). Hershey, PA: IGI Global. doi:10.4018/978-1-61520-733-6.ch005

Shachak, A., & Reis, S. (2011). The computer-assisted patient consultation. In *Clinical technologies: Concepts, methodologies, tools and applications* (pp. 160–171). Hershey, PA: IGI Global. doi:10.4018/978-1-60960-561-2.ch111

Shankar, P. R. (2011). Medical Humanities. In R. Biswas & C. Martin (Eds.), *User-driven healthcare and narrative medicine: Utilizing collaborative social networks and technologies* (pp. 210–227). Hershey, PA: IGI Global. doi:10.4018/978-1-60960-097-6.ch016

Shanmuganathan, S. (2010). A stroke information system (SIS): Critical issues and solutions. In W. Pease, M. Cooper, & R. Gururajan (Eds.), *Biomedical knowledge management: Infrastructures and processes for e-health systems* (pp. 177–191). Hershey, PA: IGI Global. doi:10.4018/978-1-60566-266-4.ch012

Shegog, R. (2010). Application of behavioral theory in computer game design for health behavior change. In J. Cannon-Bowers & C. Bowers (Eds.), *Serious game design and development: Technologies for training and learning* (pp. 196–232). Hershey, PA: IGI Global. doi:10.4018/978-1-61520-739-8.ch011

Shendge, S., Deka, B., & Kotwani, A. (2012). A cross-sectional evaluation of illness perception about asthma among asthma patients at a referral tertiary care public chest hospital in Delhi, India. *International Journal of User-Driven Healthcare, 2*(3), 32–43. doi:10.4018/ijudh.2012070104

Shimoyama, I., Shimada, H., & Ninchoji, T. (2013). Kanji perception and brain function. In J. Wu (Ed.), *Biomedical engineering and cognitive neuroscience for healthcare: Interdisciplinary applications* (pp. 266–273). Hershey, PA: IGI Global. doi:10.4018/978-1-4666-2113-8.ch027

Shrestha, S. (2013). Clinical decision support system for diabetes prevention: An illustrative case. In S. Sarnikar, D. Bennett, & M. Gaynor (Eds.), *Cases on healthcare information technology for patient care management* (pp. 308–329). Hershey, PA: IGI Global. doi:10.4018/978-1-4666-2671-3.ch017

Shukla, A., Tiwari, R., & Rathore, C. P. (2011). Intelligent biometric system using soft computing tools. In A. Shukla & R. Tiwari (Eds.), *Biomedical engineering and information systems: Technologies, tools and applications* (pp. 259–276). Hershey, PA: IGI Global. doi:10.4018/978-1-61692-004-3.ch014

Sibinga, C. T., & Oladejo, M. A. (2013). Bridging the knowledge gap in management and operations of transfusion medicine: Planning, policy and leadership issues. *Journal of Cases on Information Technology, 15*(1), 69–82. doi:10.4018/jcit.2013010105

Slavens, B., & Harris, G. F. (2012). Biomechanics. In Z. Abu-Faraj (Ed.), *Handbook of research on biomedical engineering education and advanced bioengineering learning: Interdisciplinary concepts* (pp. 284–338). Hershey, PA: IGI Global. doi:10.4018/978-1-4666-0122-2.ch007

Sliedrecht, S., & Kotzé, E. (2013). Patients with a spinal cord injury inform and co-construct services at a spinal cord rehabilitation unit. In *User-driven healthcare: Concepts, methodologies, tools, and applications* (pp. 1054–1072). Hershey, PA: IGI Global. doi:10.4018/978-1-4666-2770-3.ch053

Sood, R., & Ananthakrishnan, N. (2012). Reforming medical curriculum in India in recent years: Conflicts of political, regulator, educationist and professional natures and strategies for their resolution. *International Journal of User-Driven Healthcare, 2*(1), 1–13. doi:10.4018/ijudh.2012010101

Springer, J. A., Beever, J., Morar, N., Sprague, J. E., & Kane, M. D. (2011). Ethics, Privacy, and the future of genetic information in healthcare information assurance and security. In M. Dark (Ed.), *Information assurance and security ethics in complex systems: Interdisciplinary perspectives* (pp. 186–205). Hershey, PA: IGI Global. doi:10.4018/978-1-61692-245-0.ch009

Srivastava, S. (2011). Medical transcription a pioneer in the healthcare informatics. In A. Shukla & R. Tiwari (Eds.), *Biomedical engineering and information systems: Technologies, tools and applications* (pp. 239–258). Hershey, PA: IGI Global. doi:10.4018/978-1-61692-004-3.ch013

Srivastava, S., Sharma, N., & Singh, S. (2014). Image analysis and understanding techniques for breast cancer detection from digital mammograms. In R. Srivastava, S. Singh, & K. Shukla (Eds.), *Research developments in computer vision and image processing: Methodologies and applications* (pp. 123–148). Hershey, PA: IGI Global. doi:10.4018/978-1-4666-4558-5.ch008

Stanescu, L., & Burdescu, D. D. (2010). Medical hybrid learning tools. In F. Wang, J. Fong, & R. Kwan (Eds.), *Handbook of research on hybrid learning models: Advanced tools, technologies, and applications* (pp. 355–370). Hershey, PA: IGI Global. doi:10.4018/978-1-60566-380-7.ch022

Staudinger, B., Ostermann, H., & Staudinger, R. (2011). IT-based virtual medical centres and structures. In *Clinical technologies: Concepts, methodologies, tools and applications* (pp. 2035–2046). Hershey, PA: IGI Global. doi:10.4018/978-1-60960-561-2.ch802

Stefaniak, J. E. (2013). Resuscitating team roles within Wayburn health system. In A. Ritzhaupt & S. Kumar (Eds.), *Cases on educational technology implementation for facilitating learning* (pp. 130–145). Hershey, PA: IGI Global. doi:10.4018/978-1-4666-3676-7.ch008

Stein, R. A. (2012). Direct-to-consumer genetic testing: Interdisciplinary crossroads. *Journal of Information Technology Research, 5*(1), 35–67. doi:10.4018/jitr.2012010103

Stergachis, A., Keene, D., & Somani, S. (2013). Informatics for medicines management systems in resource-limited settings. In *Supply chain management: Concepts, methodologies, tools, and applications* (pp. 634–645). Hershey, PA: IGI Global. doi:10.4018/978-1-4666-2625-6.ch037

Stevens, D., & Kitchenham, A. (2011). An analysis of mobile learning in education, business, and medicine. In A. Kitchenham (Ed.), *Models for interdisciplinary mobile learning: Delivering information to students* (pp. 1–25). Hershey, PA: IGI Global. doi:10.4018/978-1-60960-511-7.ch001

Stolba, N., Nguyen, T. M., & Tjoa, A. M. (2010). Data warehouse facilitating evidence-based medicine. In T. Nguyen (Ed.), *Complex data warehousing and knowledge discovery for advanced retrieval development: Innovative methods and applications* (pp. 174–207). Hershey, PA: IGI Global. doi:10.4018/978-1-60566-748-5.ch008

Sugaretty, D. (2014). Risk management in a pandemic crisis at a global non profit health care organization. In *Crisis management: Concepts, methodologies, tools and applications* (pp. 1253–1270). Hershey, PA: IGI Global. doi:10.4018/978-1-4666-4707-7.ch063

Sugi, T., Goto, K., Goto, S., Goto, Y., Yamasaki, T., & Tobimatsu, S. (2013). Topography estimation of visual evoked potentials using a combination of mathematical models. In J. Wu (Ed.), *Biomedical engineering and cognitive neuroscience for healthcare: Interdisciplinary applications* (pp. 129–141). Hershey, PA: IGI Global. doi:10.4018/978-1-4666-2113-8.ch014

Sujan, H., Borrero, S., & Cranage, D. (2014). Good treats: Eating out not just for joy but also for well-being. In A. Goyal (Ed.), *Innovations in services marketing and management: Strategies for emerging economies* (pp. 118–135). Hershey, PA: IGI Global. doi:10.4018/978-1-4666-4671-1.ch007

Swennen, M. H. (2011). The gap between what is knowable and what we do in clinical practice. In R. Biswas & C. Martin (Eds.), *User-driven healthcare and narrative medicine: Utilizing collaborative social networks and technologies* (pp. 335–356). Hershey, PA: IGI Global. doi:10.4018/978-1-60960-097-6.ch024

Szewczak, E. J., & Snodgrass, C. R. (2011). Business associates in the national health information network: Implications for medical information privacy. In I. Lee (Ed.), *E-business applications for product development and competitive growth: Emerging technologies* (pp. 186–198). Hershey, PA: IGI Global. doi:10.4018/978-1-60960-132-4.ch009

Tabrizi, N. T., Torabi, Z., Bastani, P., Mokhtarkhani, M., Madani, N., Parnian, N., & Hajebrahimi, S. (2013). Assessing the perception of pain and distress of female patients undergoing routine urethral catheterization in cesarean delivery. *International Journal of User-Driven Healthcare, 3*(2), 78–84. doi:10.4018/ijudh.2013040109

Tanaka, H., & Furutani, M. (2013). Sleep management promotes healthy lifestyle, mental health, QOL, and a healthy brain. In J. Wu (Ed.), *Biomedical engineering and cognitive neuroscience for healthcare: Interdisciplinary applications* (pp. 211–224). Hershey, PA: IGI Global. doi:10.4018/978-1-4666-2113-8.ch022

Tang, X., Gao, Y., Yang, W., Zhang, M., & Wu, J. (2013). Audiovisual integration of natural auditory and visual stimuli in the real-world situation. In J. Wu (Ed.), *Biomedical engineering and cognitive neuroscience for healthcare: Interdisciplinary applications* (pp. 337–344). Hershey, PA: IGI Global. doi:10.4018/978-1-4666-2113-8.ch035

Tashiro, M., Okamura, N., Watanuki, S., Furumoto, S., Furukawa, K., & Funaki, Y. ... Yanai, K. (2011). Quantitative analysis of amyloid ß deposition in patients with Alzheimer's disease using positron emission tomography. In J. Wu (Ed.), Early detection and rehabilitation technologies for dementia: Neuroscience and biomedical applications (pp. 220-230). Hershey, PA: IGI Global. doi:10.4018/978-1-60960-559-9.ch029

Taylor, B. W. (2014). Decision-making and decision support in acute care. In C. El Morr (Ed.), *Research perspectives on the role of informatics in health policy and management* (pp. 1–18). Hershey, PA: IGI Global. doi:10.4018/978-1-4666-4321-5.ch001

Thatcher, B. (2012). Intercultural rhetorical dimensions of health literacy and medicine. In *Intercultural rhetoric and professional communication: Technological advances and organizational behavior* (pp. 247–282). Hershey, PA: IGI Global. doi:10.4018/978-1-61350-450-5.ch009

Tiwari, S., & Srivastava, R. (2014). Research and developments in medical image reconstruction methods and its applications. In R. Srivastava, S. Singh, & K. Shukla (Eds.), *Research developments in computer vision and image processing: Methodologies and applications* (pp. 274–312). Hershey, PA: IGI Global. doi:10.4018/978-1-4666-4558-5.ch014

Toro-Troconis, M., & Partridge, M. R. (2010). Designing game-based learning activities in virtual worlds: Experiences from undergraduate medicine. In Y. Baek (Ed.), *Gaming for classroom-based learning: Digital role playing as a motivator of study* (pp. 270–280). Hershey, PA: IGI Global. doi:10.4018/978-1-61520-713-8.ch016

Trojer, T., Katt, B., Breu, R., Schabetsberger, T., & Mair, R. (2012). Managing privacy and effectiveness of patient-administered authorization policies. *International Journal of Computational Models and Algorithms in Medicine*, *3*(2), 43–62. doi:10.4018/jcmam.2012040103

Übeyli, E. D. (2010). Medical informatics: Preventive medicine applications via telemedicine. In M. Cruz-Cunha, A. Tavares, & R. Simoes (Eds.), *Handbook of research on developments in e-health and telemedicine: Technological and social perspectives* (pp. 475–489). Hershey, PA: IGI Global. doi:10.4018/978-1-61520-670-4.ch022

Übeyli, E. D. (2011). Telemedicine and biotelemetry for e-health systems. In *Clinical technologies: Concepts, methodologies, tools and applications* (pp. 676–692). Hershey, PA: IGI Global. doi:10.4018/978-1-60960-561-2.ch304

Vahe, M., Zain-Ul-Abdin, K., & Türel, Y. K. (2012). Social media as a learning tool in medical education: A situation analysis. In V. Dennen & J. Myers (Eds.), *Virtual professional development and informal learning via social networks* (pp. 168–183). Hershey, PA: IGI Global. doi:10.4018/978-1-4666-1815-2.ch010

Vivekananda-Schmidt, P. (2013). Ethics in the design of serious games for healthcare and medicine. In S. Arnab, I. Dunwell, & K. Debattista (Eds.), *Serious games for healthcare: Applications and implications* (pp. 91–106). Hershey, PA: IGI Global. doi:10.4018/978-1-4666-1903-6.ch005

von Lubitz, D. (2010). Healthcare among the people: Teams of leaders concept (ToL) and the world of technology-oriented global healthcare. In S. Kabene (Ed.), *Healthcare and the effect of technology: Developments, challenges and advancements* (pp. 145–177). Hershey, PA: IGI Global. doi:10.4018/978-1-61520-733-6.ch010

von Lubitz, D. (2011). The teams of leaders (Tol) concept: The grid, the mesh, and the people in the world of information and knowledge-based global healthcare. In E. Kldiashvili (Ed.), *Grid technologies for e-health: Applications for telemedicine services and delivery* (pp. 65–104). Hershey, PA: IGI Global. doi:10.4018/978-1-61692-010-4.ch004

Vouyioukas, D., & Maglogiannis, I. (2010). Communication issues in pervasive healthcare systems and applications. In A. Coronato & G. De Pietro (Eds.), *Pervasive and smart technologies for healthcare: Ubiquitous methodologies and tools* (pp. 197–227). Hershey, PA: IGI Global. doi:10.4018/978-1-61520-765-7.ch010

Walczak, S., Brimhall, B. B., & Lefkowitz, J. B. (2010). Nonparametric decision support systems in medical diagnosis: Modeling pulmonary embolism. In M. Hunter (Ed.), *Strategic information systems: Concepts, methodologies, tools, and applications* (pp. 1483–1500). Hershey, PA: IGI Global. doi:10.4018/978-1-60566-677-8.ch095

Walczak, S., Brimhall, B. B., & Lefkowitz, J. B. (2011). Diagnostic cost reduction using artificial neural networks. In *Clinical technologies: Concepts, methodologies, tools and applications* (pp. 1812–1830). Hershey, PA: IGI Global. doi:10.4018/978-1-60960-561-2.ch614

Wang, G., Cong, A., Gao, H., Zhang, J., Weir, V. J., Xu, X., & Bennett, J. (2012). Medical imaging. In Z. Abu-Faraj (Ed.), *Handbook of research on biomedical engineering education and advanced bioengineering learning: Interdisciplinary concepts* (pp. 634–712). Hershey, PA: IGI Global. doi:10.4018/978-1-4666-0122-2.ch015

Watanabe, Y., Tanaka, H., & Hirata, K. (2013). Evaluation of cognitive function in migraine patients: A study using event-related potentials. In J. Wu (Ed.), *Biomedical engineering and cognitive neuroscience for healthcare: Interdisciplinary applications* (pp. 303–310). Hershey, PA: IGI Global. doi:10.4018/978-1-4666-2113-8.ch031

Watfa, M. K., Majeed, H., & Salahuddin, T. (2012). Healthcare applications for clinicians. In M. Watfa (Ed.), *E-healthcare systems and wireless communications: Current and future challenges* (pp. 49–69). Hershey, PA: IGI Global. doi:10.4018/978-1-61350-123-8.ch003

Weigel, F. K., Rainer, R. K., Hazen, B. T., Cegielski, C. G., & Ford, F. N. (2012). Use of diffusion of innovations theory in medical informatics research. *International Journal of Healthcare Information Systems and Informatics*, *7*(3), 44–56. doi:10.4018/jhisi.2012070104

Whitaker, R. (2013). Securing health-effective medicine in practice: A critical perspective on user-driven healthcare. In R. Biswas (Ed.), *Clinical solutions and medical progress through user-driven healthcare* (pp. 35–50). Hershey, PA: IGI Global. doi:10.4018/978-1-4666-1876-3.ch005

Wilkowska, W., & Ziefle, M. (2011). User diversity as a challenge for the integration of medical technology into future smart home environments. In M. Ziefle & C. Röcker (Eds.), *Human-centered design of e-health technologies: Concepts, methods and applications* (pp. 95–126). Hershey, PA: IGI Global. doi:10.4018/978-1-60960-177-5.ch005

Xuan, X., & Xiaowei, Z. (2012). The dilemma and resolution: The patentability of traditional Chinese medicine. *International Journal of Asian Business and Information Management*, *3*(3), 1–8. doi:10.4018/jabim.2012070101

Yamamoto, S. (2010). IT applications for medical services in Japan. In W. Pease, M. Cooper, & R. Gururajan (Eds.), *Biomedical knowledge management: Infrastructures and processes for e-health systems* (pp. 327–336). Hershey, PA: IGI Global. doi:10.4018/978-1-60566-266-4.ch024

Yan, B., Lei, Y., Tong, L., & Chen, K. (2013). Functional neuroimaging of acupuncture: A systematic review. In J. Wu (Ed.), *Biomedical engineering and cognitive neuroscience for healthcare: Interdisciplinary applications* (pp. 142–155). Hershey, PA: IGI Global. doi:10.4018/978-1-4666-2113-8.ch015

Yang, J. (2014). Towards healthy public policy: GIS and food systems analysis. In C. El Morr (Ed.), *Research perspectives on the role of informatics in health policy and management* (pp. 135–152). Hershey, PA: IGI Global. doi:10.4018/978-1-4666-4321-5.ch009

Yang, W., Gao, Y., & Wu, J. (2013). Effects of selective and divided attention on audiovisual interaction. In J. Wu (Ed.), *Biomedical engineering and cognitive neuroscience for healthcare: Interdisciplinary applications* (pp. 311–319). Hershey, PA: IGI Global. doi:10.4018/978-1-4666-2113-8.ch032

Yap, K. Y. (2013). The evolving role of pharmacoinformatics in targeting drug-related problems in clinical oncology practice. In *User-driven healthcare: Concepts, methodologies, tools, and applications* (pp. 1541–1588). Hershey, PA: IGI Global. doi:10.4018/978-1-4666-2770-3.ch077

Young, J. W., Thapaliya, P., & Sapkota, S. (2013). Caught in the middle: The divide between conventional and alternative medicine. In R. Biswas (Ed.), *Clinical solutions and medical progress through user-driven healthcare* (pp. 26–34). Hershey, PA: IGI Global. doi:10.4018/978-1-4666-1876-3.ch004

Yu, J., Guo, C., & Kim, M. (2010). Developing a user centered model for ubiquitous healthcare system implementation: An empirical study. In J. Rodrigues (Ed.), *Health information systems: Concepts, methodologies, tools, and applications* (pp. 1243–1259). Hershey, PA: IGI Global. doi:10.4018/978-1-60566-988-5.ch077

Yu, J., Guo, C., & Kim, M. (2011). Towards a conceptual framework of adopting ubiquitous technology in chronic health care. In J. Tan (Ed.), *Developments in healthcare information systems and technologies: Models and methods* (pp. 214–231). Hershey, PA: IGI Global. doi:10.4018/978-1-61692-002-9.ch015

Zaheer, S. (2014). Implementation of evidence-based practice and the PARIHS framework. In C. El Morr (Ed.), *Research perspectives on the role of informatics in health policy and management* (pp. 19–36). Hershey, PA: IGI Global. doi:10.4018/978-1-4666-4321-5.ch002

Zhang, H. H., Meyer, R. R., Shi, L., & D'Souza, W. D. (2012). Machine learning applications in radiation therapy. In S. Kulkarni (Ed.), *Machine learning algorithms for problem solving in computational applications: Intelligent techniques* (pp. 59–84). Hershey, PA: IGI Global. doi:10.4018/978-1-4666-1833-6.ch005

Zhang, W. (2011). YinYang bipolar quantum bioeconomics for equilibrium-based biosystem simulation and regulation. In *YinYang bipolar relativity: A unifying theory of nature, agents and causality with applications in quantum computing, cognitive informatics and life sciences* (pp. 266–297). Hershey, PA: IGI Global. doi:10.4018/978-1-60960-525-4.ch009

Zhang, Z., Gao, B., Liao, G., Mu, L., & Wei, W. (2011). The study of transesophageal oxygen saturation monitoring. In *Clinical technologies: Concepts, methodologies, tools and applications* (pp. 2191–2200). Hershey, PA: IGI Global. doi:10.4018/978-1-60960-561-2.ch813

Zhao, B., Zhang, D. S., & Zhao, Y. Z. (2013). Construction competitiveness evaluation system of regional BioPharma industry and case study: Taking Shijiazhuang as an example. In T. Gao (Ed.), *Global applications of pervasive and ubiquitous computing* (pp. 80–88). Hershey, PA: IGI Global. doi:10.4018/978-1-4666-2645-4.ch009

Zheng, K., Padman, R., Johnson, M. P., & Hasan, S. (2010). Guideline representation ontologies for evidence-based medicine practice. In K. Khoumbati, Y. Dwivedi, A. Srivastava, & B. Lal (Eds.), *Handbook of research on advances in health informatics and electronic healthcare applications: Global adoption and impact of information communication technologies* (pp. 234–254). Hershey, PA: IGI Global. doi:10.4018/978-1-60566-030-1.ch015

Zhou, F., Yan, J., Wang, Y., Li, F., Xia, C., Guo, R., & Yan, H. (2011). Digital auscultation system of traditional Chinese medicine and its signals acquisition: Analysis methods. In L. Liu, D. Wei, & Y. Li (Eds.), *Interdisciplinary research and applications in bioinformatics, computational biology, and environmental sciences* (pp. 183–193). Hershey, PA: IGI Global. doi:10.4018/978-1-60960-064-8.ch016

Zijlstra, W., Becker, C., & Pfeiffer, K. (2011). Wearable systems for monitoring mobility related activities: From technology to application for healthcare services. In C. Röcker & M. Ziefle (Eds.), *E-Health, assistive technologies and applications for assisted living: Challenges and solutions* (pp. 244–267). Hershey, PA: IGI Global. doi:10.4018/978-1-60960-469-1.ch011

Zimmer, J., Degenkolbe, E., Wildemann, B., & Seemann, P. (2013). BMP signaling in regenerative medicine. In Bioinformatics: Concepts, methodologies, tools, and applications (pp. 1252-1281). Hershey, PA: IGI Global. doi:10.4018/978-1-4666-3604-0.ch064

Zouag, N. (2014). Patterns of migration of medical doctors from MENA and ECE to EU economies with descriptive analysis of relatives wages. In A. Driouchi (Ed.), *Labor and health economics in the Mediterranean region: Migration and mobility of medical doctors* (pp. 124–138). Hershey, PA: IGI Global. doi:10.4018/978-1-4666-4723-7.ch005

Zouag, N., & Driouchi, A. (2014). Trends and prospects of the moroccan health system: 2010-2030. In A. Driouchi (Ed.), *Labor and health economics in the Mediterranean region: Migration and mobility of medical doctors* (pp. 314–336). Hershey, PA: IGI Global. doi:10.4018/978-1-4666-4723-7.ch013

Zybeck, K. L. (2013). A question of degrees: Collecting in support of the allied health professions. In S. Holder (Ed.), *Library collection development for professional programs: Trends and best practices* (pp. 145–163). Hershey, PA: IGI Global. doi:10.4018/978-1-4666-1897-8.ch009

Compilation of References

Ackoff, R. L. (1989). From data to wisdom. *Journal of Applied Systems Analysis*, *15*, 3–9.

Adam, B.D., Husbands, W., Murray, J., & Maxwell, J. (2005). AIDS optimism, condom fatigue, or self-esteem? Explaining unsafe sex among gay and bisexual men. *Journal of Sex Research*, *42*, 238-48.

Aggarwal, C. C., & Reddy, C. K. (Eds.). (2013). *Data clustering: algorithms and applications*. CRC press.

Agrawal, M., Joshi, A. S., & Velez, A. F. (2017). *Best Practices in Data Management for Analytics Projects*. CTO Office, Persistent Systems Ltd.

Aksenova, M. V., Silvers, J. M., Aksenov, M. Y., Nath, A., Ray, P. D., Mactutus, C. F., & Booze, R. M. (2006). HIV-1 Tat neurotoxicity in primary cultures of rat midbrain fetal neurons: Changes in dopamine transporter binding and immunoreactivity. *Neuroscience Letters*, *395*(3), 235–239. doi:10.1016/j.neulet.2005.10.095 PMID:16356633

Aksenov, M. Y., Aksenova, M., Mactutus, C., & Booze, R. M. (2012). D1/NMDA receptors and concurrent methamphetamine+ HIV-1 Tat neurotoxicity. *Journal of Neuroimmune Pharmacology*, *7*(3), 599–608. doi:10.1007/s11481-012-9362-3 PMID:22552781

Almeida, H., Meurs, M. J., Kosseim, L., & Tsang, A. (2016). Data sampling and supervised learning for hiv literature screening. *IEEE Transactions on Nanobioscience*, *15*(4), 354–361. doi:10.1109/TNB.2016.2565481 PMID:28113721

Altman, R. B. (2013). Personal genomic measurements: The opportunity for information integration. *Clinical Pharmacology and Therapeutics*, *93*(1), 21–23. doi:10.1038/clpt.2012.203 PMID:23241835

Altschul, S. F., Madden, T. L., Schäffer, A. A., Zhang, J., Zhang, Z., Miller, W., & Lipman, D. J. (1997). Gapped BLAST and PSI-BLAST: A new generation of protein database search programs. *Nucleic Acids Research*, *25*(17), 3389–3402. doi:10.1093/nar/25.17.3389 PMID:9254694

American Statistical Association. (2015). *Discovery with Data: Leveraging Statistics with Computer Science to Transform Science and Society, Web. 3.0*. Retrieved from http://www.amstat.org/policy/pdfs/BigDataStatisticsJune2014.pdf

Anagnostopoulos, I., Zeadally, S., & Exposito, E. (2016). Handling big data: Research challenges and future directions. *The Journal of Supercomputing*, *72*(4), 1494–1516. doi:10.1007/s11227-016-1677-z

Andreu-Perez, J., Poon, C. C., Merrifield, R. D., Wong, S. T., & Yang, G. Z. (2015). Big data for health. *IEEE Journal of Biomedical and Health Informatics*, *19*(4), 1193–1208. doi:10.1109/JBHI.2015.2450362 PMID:26173222

Anelone, A. J., & Spurgeon, S. K. (2017). Prediction of the containment of HIV infection by antiretroviral therapy–a variable structure control approach. *IET Systems Biology*, *11*(1), 44–53. doi:10.1049/iet-syb.2016.0028 PMID:28303793

Antunes, D. A., Rigo, M. M., Sinigaglia, M., de Medeiros, R. M., Junqueira, D. M., Almeida, S. E., & Vieira, G. F. (2014). New insights into the in silico prediction of HIV protease resistance to nelfinavir. *PLoS One*, *9*(1), e87520. doi:10.1371/journal.pone.0087520 PMID:24498124

Anzai, Y. (2012). *Pattern recognition and machine learning*. Elsevier.

Appelt, K. (1993). Crystal structures of HIV-1 protease-inhibitor complexes. *Perspectives in Drug Discovery and Design*, *1*(1), 23–48. doi:10.1007/BF02171654

Arion, D., Kaushik, N., McCormick, S., Borkow, G., & Parniak, M. A. (1998). Phenotypic mechanism of HIV-1 resistance to 3 '-azido-3 '-deoxythymidine (AZT): Increased polymerization processivity and enhanced sensitivity to pyrophosphate of the mutant viral reverse transcriptase. *Biochemistry*, *37*(45), 15908–15917. doi:10.1021/bi981200e PMID:9843396

Asthmapolis. (2017). Available from: http://propellerhealth. com/

Ayers, J. W., Althouse, B. M., Allem, J. P., Rosenquist, J. N., & Ford, D. E. (2013). Seasonality in seeking mental health information on Google. *American Journal of Preventive Medicine*, *44*(5), 520–525. doi:10.1016/j.amepre.2013.01.012 PMID:23597817

Ayers, J. W., Ribisl, K. M., & Brownstein, J. S. (2011). Tracking the rise in popularity of electronic nicotine delivery systems (electronic cigarettes) using search query surveillance. *American Journal of Preventive Medicine*, *40*(4), 448–453. doi:10.1016/j.amepre.2010.12.007 PMID:21406279

Bagashev, A., & Sawaya, B. E. (2013). Roles and functions of HIV-1 Tat protein in the CNS: An overview. *Virology Journal*, *10*(1), 358. doi:10.1186/1743-422X-10-358 PMID:24359561

Baker, E. W. (2013). Relational Model Bases: A Technical Approach to Real-time Business Intelligence and Decision Making. CAIS, 33, 23.

Barreiro-Gomez, J., Quijano, N., & Ocampo-Martínez, C. (2015, October). Distributed resource management by using population dynamics: Wastewater treatment application. In *Automatic Control (CCAC), 2015 IEEE 2nd Colombian Conference on* (pp. 1-6). IEEE.

Barrett, M. A., Humblet, O., Hiatt, R. A., & Adler, N. E. (2013). Big data and disease prevention: From quantified self to quantified communities. *Big Data*, *1*(3), 168–175. doi:10.1089/big.2013.0027 PMID:27442198

Becker, J. T., Kingsley, L., Mullen, J., Cohen, B., Martin, E., Miller, E. N., ... Visscher, B. R. (2009). Multicenter AIDS Cohort Study.Vascular risk factors, HIV serostatus, and cognitive dysfunction in gay and bisexual men. *Neurology*, *73*(16), 1292–1299. doi:10.1212/WNL.0b013e3181bd10e7 PMID:19841381

Begoli, E., & Horey, J. (2012). Design principles for effective knowledge discovery from big data. In *Software Architecture (WICSA) and European Conference on Software Architecture (ECSA), 2012 joint working IEEE/IFIP conference on* (pp. 215-218). IEEE. doi:10.1109/WICSA-ECSA.212.32

Berger, J. R., & Arendt, G. (2000). HIV dementia: The role of the basal ganglia and dopaminergic systems. *Journal of Psychopharmacology (Oxford, England)*, *14*(3), 214–221. doi:10.1177/026988110001400304 PMID:11106299

Berkovich, S., & Liao, D. (2012). On clusterization of big data streams. In *Proceedings of the 3rd International Conference on Computing for Geospatial Research and Applications* (p. 26). ACM.

Berridge, K. C. (2007). The debate over dopamine's role in reward: The case for incentive salience. *Psychopharmacology*, *191*(3), 391–431. doi:10.1007/s00213-006-0578-x PMID:17072591

Beuming, T., Kniazeff, J., Bergmann, M. L., Shi, L., Gracia, L., Raniszewska, K., ... Loland, C. J. (2008). The binding sites for cocaine and dopamine in the dopamine transporter overlap. *Nature Neuroscience*, *11*(7), 780–789. doi:10.1038/nn.2146 PMID:18568020

Beyrer, C., Baral, S. D., van Griensven, F., Goodreau, S. M., Chariyalertsak, S., Writz, A. L., & Brookmeyer, R. (2012). Global epidemiology of HIV infection in men who have sex with men. *Lancet*, *28*(9839), 367–377. doi:10.1016/S0140-6736(12)60821-6 PMID:22819660

Bezemer, D., Cori, A., Ratmann, O., van Sighem, A., Hermanides, H. S., Dutilh, B. E., ... Fraser, C. (2015). Dispersion of the HIV-1 Epidemic in Men Who Have Sex with Men in the Netherlands: A Combined Mathematical Model and Phylogenetic Analysis. *PLoS Medicine*, *12*(11), e1001898. doi:10.1371/journal.pmed.1001898 PMID:26529093

Bhattacharyya, D. K., & Kalita, J. K. (2013). *Network anomaly detection: A machine learning perspective*. CRC Press.

Bickel, P., Gotze, F., & Van Zwet, W. (1997). Resampling fewer than n observations: Gains, losses and remedies for losses. *Statistica Sinica*, *7*, 1–31.

Big Data Solutions. (2017). *Harnessing the Power of Big Data for Trade and Competitiveness policy*. World Bank Group.

Borysiak, M. D., Bender, A. T., Boyle, D. S., & Posner, J. D. (2016, November). Point-of-care HIV-1 diagnostic with integrated nucleic acid extraction and amplification from whole blood. In *Healthcare Innovation Point-Of-Care Technologies Conference (HI-POCT)*, 2016 *IEEE* (pp. 74-77). IEEE. doi:10.1109/HIC.2016.7797737

Bosley, J. C., Zhao, N. W., Hill, S., Shofer, F. S., Asch, D. A., Becker, L. B., & Merchant, R. M. (2013). Decoding twitter: Surveillance and trends for cardiac arrest and resuscitation communication. *Resuscitation*, *84*(2), 206–212. doi:10.1016/j.resuscitation.2012.10.017 PMID:23108239

Bourne, P. E. (2014). What Big Data means to me.. *Journal of the American Medical Informatics Association*, *21*(2), 194. doi:10.1136/amiajnl-2014-002651 PMID:24509599

Boyd, D., & Crawford, K. (2012). Critical questions for big data: Provocations for a cultural, technological, and scholarly phenomenon. *Information Communication and Society*, *15*(5), 662–679. doi:10.1080/1369118X.2012.678878

Boyer, P. L., Sarafianos, S. G., Arnold, E., & Hughes, S. H. (2001). Selective excision of aztmp by drug-resistant human immunodeficiency virus reverse transcriptase. *Journal of Virology*, *75*(10), 4832–4842. doi:10.1128/JVI.75.10.4832-4842.2001 PMID:11312355

Branson, B. M., Handsfield, H. H., Lampe, M. A., Janssen, R. S., Taylor, A. W., & Lyss, S. B. (2006). Revised recommendations for HIV testing of adults, adolescents, and pregnant women in health-care settings. *MMWR. Recommendations and Reports*, *55*(RR-14), 1–17. PMID:16988643

Brown, B., Bughin, J., Byers, A. H., Chui, M., Dobbs, R., Manyika, J., & Roxburgh, C. (2011). *Big data: the next frontier for innovation, competition, and productivity*. McKinsey Global Institute.

Brynjolfsson, E., & McAfee, A. (2011). *Race Against the Machine: How the Digital Revolution is Accelerating Innovation, Driving Productivity, and Irreversibly Transforming Employment and the Economy*. Lexington, MA: Digital Frontier Press.

Buch, S., Yao, H., Guo, M, Mori, T., Su, T.P., & Wang, J (2011). Cocaine and HIV-1 interplay: molecular mechanisms of action and addiction. *Journal of Neuroimmune Pharmacology, 6*, 503-515.

Buckner, C.M., Luers, A.J., Calderon, T.M., Eugenin, E.A., & Berman, J.W. (2006). Neuroimmunity and the blood-brain barrier: molecular regulation of leukocyte transmigration and viral entry into the nervous system with a focus on neuroAIDS. *Journal of Neuroimmune Pharmacology, 1*, 160–181.

Burghard, C. (2012). Big data and analytics key to accountable care success. *IDC Health Insights*.

Bushman, F. D., Barton, S., Bailey, A., Greig, C., Malani, N., Bandyopadhyay, S., ... Krogan, N. (2013). Bringing it all together: Big data and HIV research. *AIDS (London, England)*, *27*(5), 835–838. doi:10.1097/QAD.0b013e32835cb785 PMID:23719353

Carroll, F. I., Blough, B. E., Abraham, P., Mills, A. C., Holleman, J. A., Wolckenhauer, S. A., ... Forster, M. J. (2009). Synthesis and biological evaluation of bupropion analogues as potential pharmacotherapies for cocaine addiction. *Journal of Medicinal Chemistry*, *52*(21), 6768–6781. doi:10.1021/jm901189z PMID:19821577

Carroll, F. I., Howard, J. L., Howell, L. L., Fox, B. S., & Kuhar, M. J. (2008). Development of the dopamine transporter selective RTI-336 as a pharmacotherapy for cocaine abuse. In R. S. Papaka & W. Sadee (Eds.), *Drug Addiction* (pp. 179–191). Springer. doi:10.1007/978-0-387-76678-2_12

Carter, M. C., Burley, V. J., Nykjaer, C., & Cade, J. E. (2013). Adherence to a smartphone application for weight loss compared to website and paper diary: Pilot randomized controlled trial. *Journal of Medical Internet Research*, *15*(4), e32. doi:10.2196/jmir.2283 PMID:23587561

Cate, F. H., & Mayer-Schönberger, V. (2013). Notice and consent in a world of Big Data. *International Data Privacy Law*, *3*(2), 67–73. doi:10.1093/idpl/ipt005

Cerin, E., Lee, K. Y., Barnett, A., Sit, C. H., Cheung, M. C., & Chan, W. M. (2013). Objectively-measured neighborhood environments and leisure-time physical activity in Chinese urban elders. *Preventive Medicine*, *56*(1), 86–89. doi:10.1016/j.ypmed.2012.10.024 PMID:23137445

Chamberlin, D. D., & Boyce, R. F. (1974, April). SEQUEL: A structured English query language. *Proc. 1974 ACM SIGFIDET Workshop*, 249-264.

Chandrasekaran, V., & Jordan, M. (2013). Computational and statistical tradeoffs via convex relaxation. *Proceedings of the National Academy of Sciences of the United States of America*, *13*(13), 1181–1190. doi:10.1073/pnas.1302293110 PMID:23479655

Chan, E. H., Sahai, V., Conrad, C., & Brownstein, J. S. (2011). Using web search query data to monitor dengue epidemics: A new model for neglected tropical disease surveillance. *PLoS Neglected Tropical Diseases*, *5*(5), e1206. doi:10.1371/journal.pntd.0001206 PMID:21647308

Chang, H., Moog, C., & Astolfi, A. (2016). Occurrence of HIV eradication for preexposure prophylaxis treatment with a deterministic HIV model. *IET Systems Biology*, *10*(6), 137–243. doi:10.1049/iet-syb.2016.0008 PMID:27879478

Chang, L., Wang, G. J., Volkow, N. D., Ernst, T., Telang, F., Logan, J., & Fowler, J. S. (2008). Decreased brain dopamine transporters are related to cognitive deficits in HIV patients with or without cocaine abuse. *NeuroImage*, *42*(2), 869–878. doi:10.1016/j.neuroimage.2008.05.011 PMID:18579413

Chaorasiya, V., & Shrivastava, A. (2015). A survey on Big Data: Techniques and Technologies. *International Journal of Research and Development in Applied Science and Engineering*, *8*(1), 1–4.

Che, D., Safran, M., & Peng, Z. (2013). From big data to big data mining: challenges, issues, and opportunities. In *International Conference on Database Systems for Advanced Applications* (pp. 1-15). Springer. doi:10.1007/978-3-642-40270-8_1

Cheng, Y., & Church, G. M. (2000). Biclustering of expression data. ISMB, 8, 93-103.

Chen, M., Rhodes, P. H., Hall, I. H., Kilmarx, P. H., Branson, B. M., & Valleroy, L. A. (2012). Prevalence of undiagnosed HIV infection among persons aged≥ 13 years—National HIV Surveillance System, United States, 2005–2008. *MMWR. Morbidity and Mortality Weekly Report*, *61*(02), 57–64. PMID:22695465

Chen, R., Tilley, M. R., Wei, H., Zhou, F., Zhou, F. M., Ching, S., ... Gu, H. H. (2006). Abolished cocaine reward in mice with a cocaine-insensitive dopamine transporter. *Proceedings of the National Academy of Sciences of the United States of America*, *103*(24), 9333–9338. doi:10.1073/pnas.0600905103 PMID:16754872

Chen, X., Wang, S., Dong, Y., & Wang, X. (2015). Big Data Storage Architecture Design in Cloud Computing. In *National Conference on Big Data Technology and Applications* (pp. 7-14). Springer.

Chew, C., & Eysenbach, G. (2010). Pandemics in the age of Twitter: Content analysis of Tweets during the 2009 H1N1 outbreak. *PLoS One*, *5*(11), e14118. doi:10.1371/journal.pone.0014118 PMID:21124761

Chua, S. (2012). *Notes from the quantified self 2012 conference*. Available from: http://sachachua.com/blog/p/23723/

Chunara, R., Andrews, J. R., & Brownstein, J. S. (2012). Social and news media enable estimation of epidemiological patterns early in the 2010 Haitian cholera outbreak. *The American Journal of Tropical Medicine and Hygiene*, *86*(1), 39–45. doi:10.4269/ajtmh.2012.11-0597 PMID:22232449

Claxton, D. P., Quick, M., Shi, L., de Carvalho, F. D., Weinstein, H., Javitch, J. A., & McHaourab, H. S. (2010). Ion/substrate-dependent conformational dynamics of a bacterial homolog of neurotransmitter: Sodium symporters. *Nature Structural & Molecular Biology*, *17*(7), 822–829. doi:10.1038/nsmb.1854 PMID:20562855

Cleveland, H. (1982, December). Information as Resource. *The Futurist*, 34–39.

Codd, E. F. (1970, June). A relational model of data for large shared data banks. *Communications of the ACM*, *13*(6), 377–387.

Code, U. S. (1999). *Gramm-Leach-Bliley Act. Gramm-Leach-Bliley Act/AHIMA*. American Health Information Management Association.

Collins, J. R., Burt, S. K., & Erickson, J. W. (1995). Flap opening in HIV-1 protease simulated by 'activated' molecular dynamics. *Nature Structural & Molecular Biology*, *2*(4), 334–338. doi:10.1038/nsb0495-334 PMID:7796268

Connolly, S., Wooledge, S., & Aster, T. (2013). *Harnessing the value of big data analytics*. Academic Press.

Cottle, M., Hoover, W., Kanwal, S., Kohn, M., Strome, T., & Treister, N. (2013). Transforming Health Care Through Big Data Strategies for leveraging big data in the health care industry. *Institute for Health Technology Transformation*. Retrieved from http://ihealthtran.com/big-data-in-healthcare

Courtney, M. (2012). Puzzling out big data. *Engineering & Technology*, *7*(12), 56–60. doi:10.1049/et.2012.1215

Cozzi-Lepri, A., Ruiz, L., Loveday, C., Phillips, A. N., Clotet, B., Reiss, P., …, , & Lundgren, J.D. (2005). Thymidine analogue mutation profiles: Factors associated with acquiring specific profiles and their impact on the virological response to therapy. *Antiviral Therapy*, *10*(7), 791. PMID:16312176

Cukier, K., & Mayer-Schoenberger, V. (2013b). The Rise of Big Data. *Foreign Affairs*, *92*(3), 28–40.

Cukier, K., & Mayer-Schonberger, V. (2013a). *Big Data: A Revolution That Will Transform How We Live, Work and Think*. Boston, MA: Houghton Mifflin Harcourt.

Curry, L. (2005). The Future of the Public's Health in the 21st Century. *Generations (San Francisco, Calif.)*, *29*(2), 82.

Dahal, R. A., Pramod, A. B., Sharma, B., Krout, D., Foster, J. D., Cha, J. H., & Henry, L. K. (2014). Computational and biochemical docking of the irreversible cocaine analog RTI 82 directly demonstrates ligand positioning in the dopamine transporter central substrate-binding site. *The Journal of Biological Chemistry*, *289*(43), 29712–29727. doi:10.1074/jbc.M114.571521 PMID:25179220

Dapaah, J. M., & Senah, K. A. (2016). HIV/AIDS clients, privacy and confidentiality; the case of two health centres in the Ashanti Region of Ghana. *BMC Medical Ethics*, *17*(1), 41. doi:10.1186/s12910-016-0123-3 PMID:27422295

Davis, L. E., Hjelle, B. L., Miller, V. E., Palmer, D. L., Llewellyn, A. L., & Merlin, T. L. (1992) Early viral brain invasion in iatrogenic human immunodeficiency virus infection. *Neurology*, 42.

Dayer, L., Heldenbrand, S., Anderson, P., Gubbins, P. O., & Martin, B. C. (2013). Smartphone medication adherence apps: Potential benefits to patients and providers. *Journal of the American Pharmacists Association: JAPhA*, *53*(2), 172–181. doi:10.1331/JAPhA.2013.12202 PMID:23571625

De Choudhury, M., Counts, S., & Horvitz, E. (2013). Predicting postpartum changes in emotion and behavior via social media. In *Proceedings of the SIGCHI Conference on Human Factors in Computing Systems* (pp. 3267-3276). ACM. doi:10.1145/2470654.2466447

Del Valle, L., Croul, S., Morgello, S., Amini, S., Rappaport, J., & Khalili, K. (2000). Detection of HIV-1 Tat and JCV capsid protein, VP1, in AIDS brain with progressive multifocal leukoencephalopathy. *Journal of Neurovirology*, *6*(3), 221–228. doi:10.3109/13550280009015824 PMID:10878711

Deo, A. (2017). *Without Data Security and Privacy Laws, Medical Records in India Are Highly Vulnerable.* Retrieved April 20, 2017, from https://thewire.in/102349/without-data-security-and-privacy-laws-medical-records-in-india-are-highly-vulnerable/

DeRoos, D., Zikopoulos, P., Brown, B., Coss, R., & Melnyk, R. B. (2014). *Hadoop for Dummies*. John Wiley & Sons, Incorporated.

Djuric, N. (2013). *Big data algorithms for visualization and supervised learning*. Temple University.

Donald, C. G., & Sanders, A. K. (2011). The Genetic Information Nondiscrimination Act of 2008. *Journal of Diversity Management*, *3*(4), 33–46. doi:10.19030/jdm.v3i4.5000

Durairaj, M., &Ranjani, V. (2013). Data mining applications in healthcare sector: A study. *International Journal of Scientific & Technology Research, 2*(10), 29-35.

Edmunds, M., Thorpe, L., Sepulveda, M., Bezold, C., & Ross, D. A. (2014). The future of public health informatics: Alternative scenarios and recommended strategies. *EGEMS (Washington, DC)*, *2*(4), 3. doi:10.13063/2327-9214.1156 PMID:25848630

Efron, B. (1979). Bootstrap methods: Another look at the jackknife. *Annals of Statistics*, *7*(1), 1–26. doi:10.1214/aos/1176344552

Ekbia, H., Mattioli, M., Kouper, I., Arave, G., Ghazinejad, A., Bowman, T., ... Sugimoto, C. R. (2015). Big data, bigger dilemmas: A critical review. *Journal of the Association for Information Science and Technology*, *66*(8), 1523–1545. doi:10.1002/asi.23294

Eliot, T. S. (1934). *The rock*. Faber & Faber. Available at: http://www.wisdomportal.com/Technology/TSEliot-TheRock.html

Erdman, A. G., Keefe, D. F., & Schiestl, R. (2013). Grand challenge: Applying regulatory science and big data to improve medical device innovation. *IEEE Transactions on Biomedical Engineering*, *60*(3), 700–706. doi:10.1109/TBME.2013.2244600 PMID:23380845

Erickson, J. W., & Burt, S. K. (1996). Structural mechanisms of HIV drug resistance. *Annual Review of Pharmacology and Toxicology*, *36*(1), 545–571. doi:10.1146/annurev.pa.36.040196.002553 PMID:8725401

Erickson, J. W., Gulnik, S. V., & Markowitz, M. (1999). Protease inhibitors: Resistance, cross resistance, fitness and the choice of initial and salvage therapies. *AIDS (London, England)*, *13*(Suppl A), S189–S204. PMID:10885776

Ernst, T., Jiang, C. S., Nakama, H., Buchthal, S., & Chang, L. (2010). Lower brain glutamate is associated with cognitive deficits in HIV patients: A new mechanism for HIV-associated neurocognitive disorder. Journal of magnetic resonance imaging. *Journal of Magnetic Resonance Imaging*, *32*(5), 1045–1053. doi:10.1002/jmri.22366 PMID:21031507

Ernst, T., Yakupov, R., Nakama, H., Crocket, G., Cole, M., Watters, M., ... Chang, L. (2009). Declined neural efficiency in cognitively stable human immunodeficiency virus patients. *Annals of Neurology*, *65*(3), 316–325. doi:10.1002/ana.21594 PMID:19334060

Everitt, B. J., & Robbins, T. W. (2005). Neural systems of reinforcement for drug addiction: From actions to habits to compulsion. *Nature Neuroscience*, *8*(11), 1481–1489. doi:10.1038/nn1579 PMID:16251991

Fabbiani, M., Ciccarelli, N., Tana, M., Farina, S., Baldonero, E., Di Cristo, V., ... Di Giambenedetto, S. (2013). Cardiovascular risk factors and carotid intima-media thickness are associated with lower cognitive performance in HIV-infected patients. *HIV Medicine*, *14*(3), 136–144. doi:10.1111/j.1468-1293.2012.01044.x PMID:22994586

Fan, W., &Bifet, A. (2013). Mining big data: current status, and forecast to the future. *ACM SIGKDD Explorations Newsletter, 14*(2), 1-5.

Fan, J., Han, F., & Liu, H. (2014). Challenges of Big Data analysis. *National Science Review*, *1*(2), 293–314. doi:10.1093/nsr/nwt032 PMID:25419469

Fan, J., & Liu, H. (2013). Statistical analysis of big data on pharmacogenomics. *Advanced Drug Delivery Reviews*, *65*(7), 987–1000. doi:10.1016/j.addr.2013.04.008 PMID:23602905

Fazeli, P. L., Crowe, M., Ross, L. A., Wadley, V., Ball, K., & Vance, D. E. (2015). Cognitive functioning in adults aging with HIV: A cross-sectional analysis of cognitive subtypes and influential factors. *Journal of Clinical Research in HIV AIDS and Prevention*, *1*, 155–169. PMID:25386565

Ferrarese, C., Aliprandi, A., Tremolizzo, L., Stanzani, L., De Micheli, A., Dolara, A., & Frattola, L. (2001). Increased glutamate in CSF and plasma of patients with HIV dementia. *Neurology*, *57*(4), 671–675. doi:10.1212/WNL.57.4.671 PMID:11524477

Ferris, M. J., Frederick-Duus, D., Fadel, J., Mactutus, C. F., & Booze, R. M. (2009). The human immunodeficiency virus-1-associated protein, Tat1–86, impairs dopamine transporters and interacts with cocaine to reduce nerve terminal function: A no-net-flux microdialysis study. *Neuroscience*, *159*(4), 1292–1299. doi:10.1016/j.neuroscience.2009.01.024 PMID:19344635

Ferris, M. J., Frederick-Duus, D., Fadel, J., Mactutus, C. F., & Booze, R. M. (2010). Hyperdopaminergic tone in HIV-1 protein treated rat and cocaine sensitization. *Journal of Neurochemistry*, *115*(4), 885–896. doi:10.1111/j.1471-4159.2010.06968.x PMID:20796175

Ferris, M. J., Mactutus, C. F., & Booze, R. M. (2008). Neurotoxic profiles of HIV, psychostimulant drugs of abuse, and their concerted effect on the brain: Current status of dopamine system vulnerability in NeuroAIDS. *Neuroscience and Biobehavioral Reviews*, *32*(5), 883–909. doi:10.1016/j.neubiorev.2008.01.004 PMID:18430470

File, I. (2012). *Proposal for a Regulation of the European Parliament and of the Council on the Protection of Individuals with Regard to the Processing of Personal Data and on the Free movement of Such Data*. General Data Protection Regulation.

Fitzgerald, P. M. D., & Springer, J. P. (1991). Structure and function of retroviral proteases. *Annual Review of Biophysics and Biophysical Chemistry*, *20*(1), 299–320. doi:10.1146/annurev.bb.20.060191.001503 PMID:1651087

Floridi, L. (2012). Big data and their epistemological challenge. *Philosophy & Technology*, *25*(4), 435–437. doi:10.1007/s13347-012-0093-4

Fois, F., & Brew, B. J. (2015). The potential of the CNS as a reservoir for HIV-1 infection: Implications for HIV eradication. *Current HIV/AIDS Reports*, *12*(2), 299–303. doi:10.1007/s11904-015-0257-9 PMID:25869939

Fokoue, E. (2015). *A taxonomy of Big Data for optimal predictive machine learning and data mining*. arXiv preprint arXiv:1501.00604

Forrest, L. R., Zhang, Y. W., Jacobs, M. T., Gesmonde, J., Xie, L., Honig, B. H., & Rudnick, G. (2008). Mechanism for alternating access in neurotransmitter transporters. *Proceedings of the National Academy of Sciences of the United States of America*, *105*(30), 10338–10343. doi:10.1073/pnas.0804659105 PMID:18647834

Forsyth, C. (2012). *For big data analytics there's no such thing as too big*. The compelling economics and technology of big data computing. White Paper.

Foster, I., Ghani, R., Jarmin, R. S., Kreuer, F., & Lane, J. (2017). *Big Data and Social Science*. Boca Raton, FL: CRC Press.

Froimowitz, M., Gu, Y., Dakin, L. A., Nagafuji, P. M., Kelley, C. J., Parrish, D., ... Janowsky, A. (2007). Slow-onset, long-duration, alkyl analogues of methylphenidate with enhanced selectivity for the dopamine transporter. *Journal of Medicinal Chemistry*, *50*(2), 219–232. doi:10.1021/jm0608614 PMID:17228864

Fujimaki, R., & Morinaga, S. (2012). The Most Advanced Data Mining of the Big Data Era. *Advanced Technologies to Support Big Data Processing, 7*(2).

Gaskill, P. J., Calderon, T. M., Luers, A. J., Eugenin, E. A., Javitch, J. A., & Berman, J. W. (2009). Human immunodeficiency virus (HIV) infection of human macrophages is increased by dopamine: A bridge between HIV-associated neurologic disorders and drug abuse. *American Journal of Pathology*, *175*(3), 1148–1159. doi:10.2353/ajpath.2009.081067 PMID:19661443

Gedeon, P. C., Indarte, M., Surratt, C. K., & Madura, J. D. (2010). Molecular dynamics of leucine and dopamine transporter proteins in a model cell membrane lipid bilayer. *Proteins*, *78*(4), 797–811. doi:10.1002/prot.22601 PMID:19899168

Gelman, B. B., Lisinicchia, J. G., Chen, T., Johnson, K. M., Jennings, K., Freeman, D. H., & Soukup, V. M. (2012). Prefrontal Dopaminergic and Enkephalinergic Synaptic Accommodation in HIV-associated Neurocognitive Disorders and Encephalitis. *Journal of Neuroimmune Pharmacology*, *7*(3), 686–700. doi:10.1007/s11481-012-9345-4 PMID:22391864

A. Geoff, & O. Jillian (Eds.). (2015). *Dementia Research and Care Can Big Data Help? Can Big Data Help?* OECD Publishing.

Ghoting, A., Kambadur, P., Pednault, E., & Kannan, R. (2011).NIMBLE: a toolkit for the implementation of parallel data mining and machine learning algorithms on mapreduce. In *Proceedings of the 17th ACM SIGKDD international conference on Knowledge discovery and data mining* (pp. 334-342). ACM. doi:10.1145/2020408.2020464

Glooko. (2017). Available from: http://www.glooko.com/

Goodreau, S. M., Goicochea, L. P., & Sanchez, J. (2005). Sexual role and transmission of HIV Type 1 among men who have sex with men, in Peru. *The Journal of Infectious Diseases*, *191*(s1), S147–S158. doi:10.1086/425268 PMID:15627225

Gostin, L. O. (2001). National health information privacy: Regulations under the Health Insurance Portability and Accountability Act. *Journal of the American Medical Association*, *285*(23), 3015–3021. doi:10.1001/jama.285.23.3015 PMID:11410101

Green, D. P., & Holger, L. K. (2012). Modeling Heterogeneous Treatment Effects in Survey Experiments with Bayesian Additive Regression Trees. *Public Opinion Quarterly*, *76*(3), 491–511. doi:10.1093/poq/nfs036

Grouleff, J., Ladefoged, L. K., Koldsø, H., & Schiøtt, B. (2015). Monoamine transporters: Insights from molecular dynamics simulations. *Frontiers in Pharmacology*, *6*, 235. doi:10.3389/fphar.2015.00235 PMID:26528185

Groves, P., Kayyali, B., Knott, D., & Kuiken, S. V. (2016). *The'bigdata'revolution in healthcare: Accelerating value and innovation*. McKinsey& Company.

Guha, S. K., & Haldar, S. N. (2012). Drug Resistance in HIV. Medicine Update, 84–88.

Gupta, S., Kumar, D., & Sharma, A. (2011). Performance analysis of various data mining classification techniques on healthcare data. *International Journal of Computer Science & Information Technology, 3*(4).

Guptaroy, B., Zhang, M., Bowton, E., Binda, F., Shi, L., Weinstein, H., ... Gnegy, M. E. (2009). A juxtamembrane mutation in the N terminus of the dopamine transporter induces preference for an inward-facing conformation. *Molecular Pharmacology*, *75*(3), 514–524. doi:10.1124/mol.108.048744 PMID:19098122

Halevi, G., & Moed, H. (2012). The evolution of big data as a research and scientific topic: Overview of the literature. *Research Trends*, *30*(1), 3–6.

Haller, S., Badoud, S., Nguyen, D., Garibotto, V., Lovblad, K. O., & Burkhard, P. R. (2012). Individual detection of patients with Parkinson disease using support vector machine analysis of diffusion tensor imaging data: Initial results. *American Journal of Neuroradiology*, *33*(11), 2123–2128. doi:10.3174/ajnr.A3126 PMID:22653326

Hammer, S. M., Eron, J. J., Reiss, P., Schooley, R. T., Thompson, M. A., Walmsley, S., ... Jacobsen, D. M. (2008). Antiretroviral treatment of adult HIV infection: 2008 recommendations of the International AIDS Society–USA panel. *Journal of the American Medical Association*, *300*(5), 555–570. doi:10.1001/jama.300.5.555 PMID:18677028

Harford, T. (2014). Big Data: A Big Mistake. *Significance*, *11*(5), 14–19. doi:10.1111/j.1740-9713.2014.00778.x

Harrison, V., Proudfoot, J., Wee, P. P., Parker, G., Pavlovic, D. H., & Manicavasagar, V. (2011). Mobile mental health: Review of the emerging field and proof of concept study. *Journal of Mental Health (Abingdon, England)*, *20*(6), 509–524. doi:10.3109/09638237.2011.608746 PMID:21988230

Hash, J. (2005). *An introductory resource guide for implementing the health insurance portability and accountability act (HIPAA) security rule* (Doctoral dissertation). National Institute of Standards and Technology.

Haussleiter, I. S., Brüne, M., & Juckel, G. (2009). Psychopathology in multiple sclerosis: Diagnosis, prevalence and treatment. *Therapeutic Advances in Neurological Disorders*, *2*(1), 13–29. doi:10.1177/1756285608100325 PMID:21180640

Hay, S. I., George, D. B., Moyes, C. L., & Brownstein, J. S. (2013). Big data opportunities for global infectious disease surveillance. *PLoS Medicine*, *10*(4), e1001413. doi:10.1371/journal.pmed.1001413 PMID:23565065

Health informatics – Information security management in health using ISO/IEC 27002 (2016)

HealthMap. (2017). Available from: http://healthmap.org/

Heaton, R. K., Clifford, D. B., Franklin, D. R., Woods, S. P., Ake, C., Vaida, F., ... Grant, I. (2010a). HIV-associated neurocognitive disorders (HAND) persist in the era of potent antiretroviral therapy: The CHARTER Study. *Neurology*, *75*(23), 2087–2096. doi:10.1212/WNL.0b013e318200d727 PMID:21135382

Heaton, R. K., Franklin, D. R., Ellis, R. J., McCutchan, J. A., Letendre, S. L., Leblanc, S., ... Grant, I. (2011). HIV-associated neurocognitive disorders before and during the era of combination antiretroviral therapy: Differences in rates, nature, and predictors. *Journal of Neurovirology*, *17*(1), 3–16. doi:10.1007/s13365-010-0006-1 PMID:21174240

Heaton, R. K., Velin, R. A., McCutchan, J. A., Gulevich, S. J., Atkinson, J. H., Wallace, M. R., ... Grant, I. (1994). Neuropsychological impairment in human immunodeficiency virus-infection: Implications for employment. HNRC Group HIV Neurobehavioral Research Center. *Psychosomatic Medicine*, *56*(1), 8–17. doi:10.1097/00006842-199401000-00001 PMID:8197319

Heaton, R., Franklin, D., Letendre, S., Ellis, R., & Fennema-Notestine, C, Vaida. F, Smith D,… ..., Grant, I. (2012). Aging amplifies HIV neurocognitive impairment: The effects may be related to vascular and metabolic factors. *Journal of Neurovirology*, *18*, S46.

Helwig, N. E., & Ma, P. (2016). Smoothing spline ANOVA for super-large samples: Scalable computation via rounding parameters. *Statistics and Its Interface*, *9*(4), 433–444. doi:10.4310/SII.2016.v9.n4.a3

Henry, L.K., Iwamoto, H., Field, J.R., Kaufmann, K., Dawson, E.S., & Jacobs, M.T., … Blakely, R.D. (2011). A conserved asparagine residue in TM1 of the serotonin transporter dictates chloride-coupled neurotransmitter transport. *The Journal of Biological Chemistry*, *286*(35), 30823–30836. doi:10.1074/jbc.M111.250308 PMID:21730057

Hill, S., Merchant, R., & Ungar, L. (2013). Lessons learned about public health from online crowd surveillance. *Big Data*, *1*(3), 160–167. doi:10.1089/big.2013.0020 PMID:25045598

Hinton, G., Deng, L., Yu, D., Dahl, G. E., Mohamed, A. R., Jaitly, N., & Kingsbury, B. (2012). Deep neural networks for acoustic modeling in speech recognition: The shared views of four research groups. *IEEE Signal Processing Magazine*, *29*(6), 82–97. doi:10.1109/MSP.2012.2205597

Hotez, P. J., Molyneux, D. H., Fenwick, A., Ottesen, E., Sachs, S. E., & Sachs, J. D. (2006). Incorporating a rapid-impact package for neglected tropical diseases with programs for HIV/AIDS, tuberculosis, and malaria. *PLoS Medicine*, *3*(5), e102. doi:10.1371/journal.pmed.0030102 PMID:16435908

Howell, D. R. (2014). *An examination of motor and cognitive recovery following concussion* (Doctoral dissertation). University of Oregon.

HR 1, The American Recovery and Reinvestment Act of 2009 (ARRA). HITECH Provisions section 1301 et seq. Amends 42 USC section 201 et seq (Public Health Service Act (PHSA)) by adding Title XXX section 3000 et seq.

Hsieh, C. J., Si, S., & Dhillon, I. (2014). A divide-and-conquer solver for kernel support vector machines. *International Conference on Machine Learning*, 566-574.

Huang, H., Chopra, R., Verdine, G. L., & Harrison, S. C. (1998). Structure of a covalently trapped catalytic complex of HIV-1 reverse transcriptase: Implications for drug resistance. *Science*, *282*(5394), 1669–1675. doi:10.1126/science.282.5394.1669 PMID:9831551

Huang, X., Gu, H. H., & Zhan, C.-G. (2009). Mechanism for cocaine blocking the transport of dopamine: Insights from molecular modeling and dynamics simulations. *The Journal of Physical Chemistry B*, *113*(45), 15057–15066. doi:10.1021/jp900963n PMID:19831380

Huang, X., & Zhan, C. G. (2007). How dopamine transporter interacts with dopamine: Insights from molecular modeling and simulation. *Biophysical Journal*, *93*(10), 3627–3639. doi:10.1529/biophysj.107.110924 PMID:17704152

Hudson, L., Liu, J., Nath, A., Jones, M., Raghavan, R., Narayan, O., ... Everall, I. (2000). Detection of the human immunodeficiency virus regulatory protein tat in CNS tissues. *Journal of Neurovirology*, *6*(2), 145–155. doi:10.3109/13550280009013158 PMID:10822328

IDC. (2011). *World's data will grow by 50X in next decade*. IDC Study.

Imai, K., & Ratkovic, M. (2013). Estimating Treatment Effect Heterogeneity, *Randomized Program Evaluation. The Annals of Applied Statistics*, *7*(1), 443–470. doi:10.1214/12-AOAS593

Institute of Medicine. (2003). *Committee on data standards for patient safety: board of health care services. Key capabilities of an electronic health record system: letter report*. The National Academy of Sciences.

IOM (Institute of Medicine). (2009). *Beyond the HIPAA Privacy Rule: Enhancing Privacy, Improving Health Through Research*. Washington, DC: The National Academies Press.

IOM (Institute of Medicine). (2012). *Monitoring HIV Care in the United States: Indicators and Data Systems*. Washington, DC: The National Academies Press.

Jacobs, M. M., Murray, J., Byrd, D. A., Hurd, Y. L., & Morgello, S. (2013). HIV-related cognitive impairment shows bi-directional association with dopamine receptor DRD1 and DRD2 polymorphisms in substance-dependent and substance-independent populations. *Journal of Neurovirology*, *19*(5), 495–504. doi:10.1007/s13365-013-0204-8 PMID:24078558

Jagadish, S. V. K., Septiningsih, E. M., Kohli, A., Thomson, M. J., Ye, C., Redoña, E., ... Singh, R. K. (2012). Genetic advances in adapting rice to a rapidly changing climate. *Journal Agronomy & Crop Science*, *198*(5), 360–373. doi:10.1111/j.1439-037X.2012.00525.x

James, G., Witten, D., Hastie, T., & Tibshirani, R. (2014). *An introduction to statistical learning with applications in R*. New York: Springer.

Janger, E. J., & Schwartz, P. M. (2001). The Gramm-Leach-Bliley Act, Information Privacy, and the Limits of Default Rules. *Minnesota Law Review*, *86*, 1219.

Janssen, R. S., Nwanyanwu, O. C., Selik, R. M., & Stehr-Green, J. K. (1992). Epidemiology of human immunodeficiency virus encephalopathy in the United States. *Neurology*, *42*(8), 1472–1476. doi:10.1212/WNL.42.8.1472 PMID:1641138

JawboneUp. (2017). Available from: https://jawbone.com/up

Jewell, D., Barros, R. D., Diederichs, S., Duijvestijn, L. M., Hammersley, M., Hazra, A., & Portilla, I. (2014). *Performance and capacity implications for big data*. IBM Redbooks.

Jokonya, O. (2014). Towards a Big Data Framework for the prevention and control of HIV/AIDS, TB and Silicosis in the mining industry. *Procedia Technology*, *16*, 1533–1541. doi:10.1016/j.protcy.2014.10.175

Jones, G., Willett, P., & Glen, R. C. (1995). Molecular recognition of receptor sites using a genetic algorithm with a description of desolvation. *Journal of Molecular Biology*, *245*(1), 43–53. doi:10.1016/S0022-2836(95)80037-9 PMID:7823319

Joseph, S., Vargas, M., Johnson, J., & Timpte, C. (2013). The Genetic Information Nondiscrimination Act. BIOL, 4700, 03.

Joska, J. A., Westgarth-Taylor, J., Hoare, J., Thomas, K. G., Paul, R., Myer, L., & Stein, D. J. (2012). Neuropsychological outcomes in adults commencing highly active anti-retroviral treatment in South Africa: A prospective study. *BMC Infectious Diseases*, *12*(1), 39. doi:10.1186/1471-2334-12-39 PMID:22335937

Joska, J. A., Westgarth-Taylor, J., Myer, L., Hoare, J., Thomas, K. G., Combrinck, M., ... Flisher, A. J. (2011). Characterization of HIV-associated neurocognitive disorders among individuals starting antiretroviral therapy in South Africa. *AIDS and Behavior*, *15*(6), 1197–1203. doi:10.1007/s10461-010-9744-6 PMID:20614176

Kaisler, S., Armour, F., Espinosa, J. A., & Money, W. (2013). Big data: Issues and challenges moving forward. In *System Sciences (HICSS), 2013 46th Hawaii International Conference on* (pp. 995-1004). IEEE.

Kale, D. C., Gong, D., Che, Z., Liu, Y., Medioni, G., Wetzel, R., & Ross, P. (2014). An examination of multivariate time series hashing with applications to health care. In *Data Mining (ICDM), 2014 IEEE International Conference on* (pp. 260-269). IEEE. doi:10.1109/ICDM.2014.153

Kang, U., Tsourakakis, C. E., & Faloutsos, C. (2009).Pegasus: A peta-scale graph mining system implementation and observations. In *Data Mining, 2009.ICDM'09. Ninth IEEE International Conference on* (pp. 229-238). IEEE. doi:10.1109/ICDM.2009.14

Kashyap, H., Ahmed, H. A., Hoque, N., Roy, S., & Bhattacharyya, D. K. (2015). *Big data analytics in bioinformatics: A machine learning perspective*. arXiv preprint arXiv:1506.05101

Katal, A., Wazid, M., & Goudar, R. H. (2013). Big Data: Issues, Challenges, Tools and Good Practices. *IEEE Spectrum*, 404–409.

Kempf, M. C., McLeod, J., Boehme, A. K., Walcott, M. W., Wright, L., Seal, P., ... Moneyham, L. (2010). A qualitative study of the barriers and facilitators to retention-in-care among HIV-positive women in the rural southeastern United States: Implications for targeted interventions. *AIDS Patient Care and STDs*, *24*(8), 515–520. doi:10.1089/apc.2010.0065 PMID:20672971

Khalid, Z., & Sezerman, O. U. (2016). Prediction of HIV Drug Resistance by combining Sequence and Structural Properties. *IEEE/ACM Transactions on Computational Biology and Bioinformatics*, 1. doi:10.1109/TCBB.2016.2638821 PMID:27992346

Kim, J., Yoon, J.-H., & Kim, Y.-S. (2013). HIV-1 Tat interacts with and regulates the localization and processing of amyloid precursor protein. *PLoS One*, *8*(11), e77972. doi:10.1371/journal.pone.0077972 PMID:24312169

Kimmel, H. L., Oconnor, J. A. A., Carroll, F. I., & Howell, L. L. (2007). Faster onset and dopamine transporter selectivity predict stimulant and reinforcing effects of cocaine analogs in squirrel monkeys. *Pharmacology, Biochemistry, and Behavior*, *86*(1), 45–54. doi:10.1016/j.pbb.2006.12.006 PMID:17258302

Kleiner, A., Talwalkar, A., Sarkar, P., & Jordan, M. I. (2014). A scalable bootstrap for massive data. *Journal of the Royal Statistical Society. Series B, Statistical Methodology*, *76*(4), 795–816. doi:10.1111/rssb.12050

Koçak, Y., Özyer, T., & Alhajj, R. (2016, August). Classification of HIV data by constructing a social network with frequent itemsets. In *Advances in Social Networks Analysis and Mining (ASONAM), 2016 IEEE/ACM International Conference on* (pp. 949-953). IEEE. doi:10.1109/ASONAM.2016.7752354

Koldsø, H., Christiansen, A. B., Sinning, S., & Schiøtt, B. (2012). Comparative modeling of the human monoamine transporters: Similarities in substrate binding. *ACS Chemical Neuroscience*, *4*(2), 295–309. doi:10.1021/cn300148r PMID:23421681

Koldsø, H., Grouleff, J., & Schiøtt, B. (2015). Insights to ligand binding to the monoamine transporters – from homology modeling to LeuBAT and dDAT. *Frontiers in Pharmacology*, *6*, 208. doi:10.3389/fphar.2015.00208 PMID:26441663

Koldsø, H., Noer, P., Grouleff, J., Autzen, H. E., Sinning, S., & Schiøtt, B. (2011). Unbiased simulations reveal the inward-facing conformation of the human serotonin transporter and Na+ ion release. *PLoS Computational Biology*, *7*(10), e1002246. doi:10.1371/journal.pcbi.1002246 PMID:22046120

Koutsilieri, E., Czub, S., Scheller, C., Sopper, S., Tatschner, T., Stahl-Hennig, C., ... Riederer, P. (2000). Brain choline acetyltransferase reduction in SIV infection. An index of early dementia? *Neuroreport*, *11*(11), 2391–2393. doi:10.1097/00001756-200008030-00011 PMID:10943691

Koutsilieri, E., Meulen, V., & Riederer, P. (2001). Neurotransmission in HIV associated dementia: A short review. *Journal of Neural Transmission (Vienna, Austria)*, *108*(6), 767–775. doi:10.1007/s007020170051 PMID:11478426

Koutsilieri, E., Sopper, S., Scheller, C., ter Meulen, V., & Riederer, P. (2002). Involvement of dopamine in the progression of AIDS Dementia Complex. *Journal of Neural Transmission (Vienna, Austria)*, *109*(3), 399–410. doi:10.1007/s007020200032 PMID:11956960

Krishnamurthy, H., & Gouaux, E. (2012). X-ray structures of LeuT in substrate-free outward-open and apo inward-open states. *Nature*, *481*(7382), 469–474. doi:10.1038/nature10737 PMID:22230955

Krishnamurthy, H., Piscitelli, C. L., & Gouaux, E. (2009). Unlocking the molecular secrets of sodium-coupled transporters. *Nature*, *459*(7245), 347–355. doi:10.1038/nature08143 PMID:19458710

Krissinel, E., & Henrick, K. (2003). Protein structure comparison in 3D based on secondary structure matching (PDBeFold) followed by Cα alignment, scored by a new structural similarity function. *Proceedings of the 5th International Conference on Molecular Structural Biology*, 88.

Kristensen, A. S., Andersen, J., Jørgensen, T. N., Sørensen, L., Eriksen, J., Loland, C. J., ... Gether, U. (2011). SLC6 neurotransmitter transporters: Structure, function, and regulation. *Pharmacological Reviews*, *63*(3), 585–640. doi:10.1124/pr.108.000869 PMID:21752877

Kshetri, N. (2014). Big data′ s impact on privacy, security and consumer welfare. *Telecommunications Policy*, *38*(11), 1134–1145. doi:10.1016/j.telpol.2014.10.002

Kumar, A. M., Fernandez, J. B., Singer, E. J., Commins, D., Waldrop-Valverde, D., Ownby, R. L., & Kumar, M. (2009). Human immunodeficiency virus type 1 in the central nervous system leads to decreased dopamine in different regions of postmortem human brains. *Journal of Neurovirology*, *15*(3), 257–274. doi:10.1080/13550280902973952 PMID:19499455

Kumar, A. M., Ownby, R. L., Waldrop-Valverde, D., Fernandez, B., & Kumar, M. (2011). Human immunodeficiency virus infection in the CNS and decreased dopamine availability: Relationship with neuropsychological performance. *Journal of Neurovirology*, *17*(1), 26–40. doi:10.1007/s13365-010-0003-4 PMID:21165787

Kum, H. C., Krishnamurthy, A., Machanavajjhala, A., Reiter, M. K., & Ahalt, S. (2014). Privacy preserving interactive record linkage (PPIRL). *Journal of the American Medical Informatics Association*, *21*(2), 212–220. doi:10.1136/amiajnl-2013-002165 PMID:24201028

Lamers, S. L., Salemi, M., Galligan, D. C., Morris, A., Gray, R., Fogel, G., ... McGrath, M. S. (2010). Human immunodeficiency virus-1 evolutionary patterns associated with pathogenic processes in the brain. *Journal of Neurovirology*, *16*(3), 230–241. doi:10.3109/13550281003735709 PMID:20367240

J. Lane, V. Stodden, S. Bender, & H. Nissenbaum (Eds.). (2014). *Privacy, big data, and the public good: Frameworks for engagement*. Cambridge University Press. doi:10.1017/CBO9781107590205

Laney, D. (2001). *3-d data management: Controlling data volume, velocity and variety*. META Group, Research Note, February 2001.

Lansdon, E. B., Brendza, K. M., Hung, M., Wang, R., Mukund, S., Jin, D., ... Liu, X. (2010). Crystal structures of HIV-1 reverse transcriptase with etravirine (TMC125) and rilpivirine (TMC278): Implications for drug design. *Journal of Medicinal Chemistry*, *53*(10), 4295–4299. doi:10.1021/jm1002233 PMID:20438081

Larder, B. A., & Stammers, D. K. (1999). Closing in on HIV drug resistance. *Nature Structural Biology*, *6*(2), 103–106. doi:10.1038/5787 PMID:10048915

Lark. (2017). Available from: http://lark.com/

LaValle, S., Lesser, E., Shockley, R., Hopkins, M. S., & Kruschwitz, N. (2011). Big data, analytics and the path from insights to value. *MIT Sloan Management Review*, *52*(2), 21.

Lazer, D., Kennedy, R., King, G., & Vespignani, A. (2014). The parable of Google Flu: Traps in big data analysis. *Science*, *343*(6176), 1203–1205. doi:10.1126/science.1248506 PMID:24626916

Lee, C. H., & Yoon, H. J. (2017). Medical big data: Promise and challenges. *Kidney Research and Clinical Practice*, *36*(1), 3–11. doi:10.23876/j.krcp.2017.36.1.3 PMID:28392994

Lengauer, T., Pfeifer, N., & Kaiser, R. (2014). Personalized HIV therapy to control drug resistance. *Drug Discovery Today. Technologies*, *11*, 57–64. doi:10.1016/j.ddtec.2014.02.004 PMID:24847654

Liang, F., & Kim J., (2013). *A bootstrap Metropolis–Hastings algorithm for Bayesian analysis of big data*. Tech. rep., Department of Statistics, Texas A & M University.

Liang, F., Cheng, Y., Song, Q., Park, J., & Yang, P. (2013). A resampling-based stochastic approximation method for analysis of large geostatistical data. *Journal of the American Statistical Association*, *108*(501), 325–339. doi:10.1080/01621459.2012.746061

Lin, J., & Ryaboy, D. (2013). Scaling big data mining infrastructure: The twitter experience. *ACM SIGKDD Explorations Newsletter*, *14*(2), 6–19. doi:10.1145/2481244.2481247

Lin, N., & Xi, R. (2011). Aggregated estimating equation estimation. *Statistics and Its Interface*, *4*(1), 73–83. doi:10.4310/SII.2011.v4.n1.a8

Liu, S., & Molino, B. F. (2007). Recent developments in monoamine reuptake inhibitors. *Annual Reports in Medicinal Chemistry*, *42*, 13–26. doi:10.1016/S0065-7743(07)42002-4

Loland, C. J. (2014). The use of LeuT as a model in elucidating binding sites for substrates and inhibitors in neurotransmitter transporters. *Biochimica et Biophysica Acta*, *1850*(3), 500–510. doi:10.1016/j.bbagen.2014.04.011 PMID:24769398

Loland, C. J., Norgaard-Nielsen, K., & Gether, U. (2003). Probing dopamine transporter structure and function by Zn2+-site engineering. *European Journal of Pharmacology*, *479*(1–3), 187–197. doi:10.1016/j.ejphar.2003.08.068 PMID:14612149

Lomotey, R. K., & Deters, R. (2014). Towards knowledge discovery in big data. In *Service Oriented System Engineering (SOSE), 2014 IEEE 8th International Symposium on* (pp. 181-191). IEEE. doi:10.1109/SOSE.2014.25

Lovell, S. C., Davis, I. W., Arendall, W. B. III, de Bakker, P. I., Word, J. M., Prisant, M. G., ... Richardson, D. C. (2003). Structure validation by Cα geometry: Φ, ψ and Cβ deviation. *Proteins*, *50*(3), 437–450. doi:10.1002/prot.10286 PMID:12557186

Low, Y., Bickson, D., Gonzalez, J., Guestrin, C., Kyrola, A., & Hellerstein, J. M. (2012). Distributed GraphLab: A framework for machine learning and data mining in the cloud. *Proceedings of the VLDB Endowment International Conference on Very Large Data Bases*, *5*(8), 716–727. doi:10.14778/2212351.2212354

Lu, X., Liu, Y., Jiao, J., & Wang, R. (2016, December). Dynamic evolutions of HIV infection on treatment with combinatorial drugs. In *Bioinformatics and Biomedicine (BIBM), 2016 IEEE International Conference on* (pp. 1856-1863). IEEE.

Lüdemann, S. K., Lounnas, V., & Wade, R. C. (2000). How do substrates enter and products exit the buried active site of cytochrome P450cam? 1. Random expulsion molecular dynamics investigation of ligand access channels and mechanisms. *Journal of Molecular Biology, 303*(5), 797–811. doi:10.1006/jmbi.2000.4154 PMID:11061976

Lyles, C. R., López, A., Pasick, R., & Sarkar, U. (2013). "5 mins of uncomfyness is better than dealing with cancer 4 a lifetime": An exploratory qualitative analysis of cervical and breast cancer screening dialogue on Twitter. *Journal of Cancer Education, 28*(1), 127–133. doi:10.1007/s13187-012-0432-2 PMID:23132231

Ma, P., & Sun, X. (2014). *Leveraging for big data regression.* WIREs Computational Statistics.

Mahajan, A. P., Sayles, J. N., Patel, V. A., Remien, R. H., Ortiz, D., Szekeres, G., & Coates, T. J. (2008). Stigma in the HIV/AIDS epidemic: A review of the literature and recommendations for the way forward. *AIDS (London, England), 22*(Suppl 2), S67. doi:10.1097/01.aids.0000327438.13291.62 PMID:18641472

Manepalli, S., Surratt, C. K., Madura, J. D., & Nolan, T. L. (2012). Monoamine transporter structure, function, dynamics, and drug discovery: A computational perspective. *The AAPS Journal, 14*(4), 820–831. doi:10.1208/s12248-012-9391-0 PMID:22918625

Mann, D. (2004). *Hands-on Systematic Innovation for Business.* CREAX Press.

Manyika, J., Chui, M., Brown, B., Buhin, J., Dobbs, R., Roxburgh, C., & Byers, A. H. (2011). *Big Data: The Next Frontier for Innovation, Competition, and Productivity.* McKinsey Global Institute.

Mao, J. J., Chung, A., Benton, A., Hill, S., Ungar, L., Leonard, C. E., & Holmes, J. H. (2013). Online discussion of drug side effects and discontinuation among breast cancer survivors. *Pharmacoepidemiology and Drug Safety, 22*(3), 256–262. doi:10.1002/pds.3365 PMID:23322591

Marquine, M. J., Umlauf, A., Rooney, A. S., Fazeli, P. L., Gouaux, B. D., Paul Woods, S., ... Moore, D. J. (2014). The veterans aging cohort study index is associated with concurrent risk for neurocognitive impairment. *JAIDS Journal of Acquired Immune Deficiency Syndromes, 65*(2), 190–197. doi:10.1097/QAI.0000000000000008 PMID:24442225

Mattson, M. P., Haughey, N. J., & Nath, A. (2005). Cell death in HIV dementia. *Cell Death and Differentiation*, *12*(S1), 893–904. doi:10.1038/sj.cdd.4401577 PMID:15761472

McArthur, J. C., Steiner, J., Sacktor, N., & Nath, A. (2010). Human immunodeficiency virus-associated neurocognitive disorders: Mind the gap. *Annals of Neurology*, *67*, 699–714. PMID:20517932

McCormick, T. (2012). *Video of my healthier information talk*. Available from: http://tjm.org/2012/04/17/videoof my-healthier-information-talk/

McCutchan, J. A., Marquie-Beck, J. A., Fitzsimons, C. A., Letendre, S. L., Ellis, R. J., Heaton, R. K., ... Grant, I. (2012). Role of obesity, metabolic variables, and diabetes in HIV-associated neurocognitive disorder. *Neurology*, *78*(7), 485–492. doi:10.1212/WNL.0b013e3182478d64 PMID:22330412

McInnes, C., & Rushton, S. (2010). HIV, AIDS and security: Where are we now? *International Affairs*, *86*(1), 225–245. doi:10.1111/j.1468-2346.2010.00877.x

McKenzie, J. F., Neiger, B. L., & Thackeray, R. (2016). *Planning, implementing & evaluating health promotion programs: A primer*. Pearson.

McKinsey. (2011). *Internet matters: The Net's sweeping impact on growth, jobs, and prosperity*. Author.

McKinsey. (2013). *Big Data, Analytics and the Future of Marketing and Sales*. New York: McKinsey.

Meade, C. S., Conn, N. A., Skalski, L. M., & Safren, S. A. (2011a). Neurocognitive impairment and medication adherence in HIV patients with and without cocaine dependence. *Journal of Behavioral Medicine*, *34*(2), 128–138. doi:10.1007/s10865-010-9293-5 PMID:20857187

Meade, C. S., Lowen, S. B., MacLean, R. R., Key, M. D., & Lukas, S. E. (2011). MRI brain activation during a delay discounting task in HIV positive adults with and without cocaine dependence. *Psychiatry Research*, *192*(3), 167–175. doi:10.1016/j.pscychresns.2010.12.011 PMID:21546221

Meyer, P. R., Matsuura, S. E., Mian, A. M., So, A. G., & Scott, W. A. (1999). A mechanism of AZT resistance: An increase in nucleotide-dependent primer unblocking by mutant HIV-1 reverse transcriptase. *Molecular Cell*, *4*(1), 35–43. doi:10.1016/S1097-2765(00)80185-9 PMID:10445025

Meyer, P. R., Matsuura, S. E., So, A. G., & Scott, W. A. (1998). Unblocking of chain terminated primer by HIV-1 reverse transcriptase through a nucleotide-dependent mechanism. *Proceedings of the National Academy of Sciences of the United States of America*, *95*(23), 13471–13476. doi:10.1073/pnas.95.23.13471 PMID:9811824

Michael, K., & Miller, K. W. (2013). Big data: New opportunities and new challenges. *Computer*, *46*(6), 22–24. doi:10.1109/MC.2013.196

Midde, N. M., Gomez, A. M., & Zhu, J. (2012). HIV-1 Tat protein decreases dopamine transporter cell surface expression and vesicular monoamine transporter-2 function in Rat striatal synaptosomes. *Journal of Neuroimmune Pharmacology*, *7*(3), 629–639. doi:10.1007/s11481-012-9369-9 PMID:22570010

Midde, N. M., Huang, X., Gomez, A. M., Booze, R. M., Zhan, C. G., & Zhu, J. (2013). Mutation of tyrosine 470 of human dopamine transporter is critical for HIV-1 Tat-induced inhibition of dopamine transport and transporter conformational transitions. *Journal of Neuroimmune Pharmacology*, *8*(4), 975–987. doi:10.1007/s11481-013-9464-6 PMID:23645138

Midde, N. M., Yuan, Y., Quizon, P. M., Sun, W. L., Huang, X., Zhan, C. G., & Zhu, J. (2015). Mutations at tyrosine 88, lysine 92 and tyrosine 470 of human dopamine transporter result in an attenuation of HIV-1 Tat-induced inhibition of dopamine transport. *Journal of Neuroimmune Pharmacology*, *10*(1), 122–135. doi:10.1007/s11481-015-9583-3 PMID:25604666

Miller, J. A., Oldham, M. C., & Geschwind, D. H. (2008). A systems level analysis of transcriptional changes in Alzheimer's disease and normal aging. *The Journal of Neuroscience*, *28*(6), 1410–1420. doi:10.1523/JNEUROSCI.4098-07.2008 PMID:18256261

Miller, M. D., Margot, N., Lu, B., Zhong, L., Chen, S. S., Cheng, A., & Wulfsohn, M. (2004). Genotypic and phenotypic predictors of the magnitude of response to tenofovir disoproxil fumarate treatment in antiretroviral-experienced patients. *The Journal of Infectious Diseases*, *189*(5), 837–846. doi:10.1086/381784 PMID:14976601

Miller, M., Schneider, J., Sathyanarayana, B. K., Toth, M. V., Marshall, G. R., Clawson, L., ... Wlodawer, A. (1989). Structure of complex of synthetic HIV-1 protease with a substrate-based inhibitor at 2.3 A resolution. *Science*, *246*(4934), 1149–1152. doi:10.1126/science.2686029 PMID:2686029

Mitchell, I., & Wilson, M. (2012). *Linked Data: Connecting and exploiting big data*. White paper. Fujitsu UK, 302.

Mitra, S., Pal, S. K., & Mitra, P. (2002). Data mining in soft computing framework: A survey. *IEEE Transactions on Neural Networks*, *13*(1), 3–14. doi:10.1109/72.977258 PMID:18244404

Mukherjee, S., & Shaw, R. (2016). Big Data–Concepts, Applications, Challenges and Future Scope. *International Journal of Advanced Research in Computer and Communication Engineering*, *5*(2).

Murdoch, T. B., & Detsky, A. S. (2013). The inevitable application of big data to health care. *Journal of the American Medical Association*, *309*(13), 1351–1352. doi:10.1001/jama.2013.393 PMID:23549579

Nair, M. P. N., & Samikkannu, T. (2012). Differential regulation of neurotoxin in HIV clades: Role of cocaine and methamphetamine. *Current HIV Research*, *10*, 429–434. doi:10.2174/157016212802138742 PMID:22591367

Narayanan, A., & Shmatikov, V. (2010). Myths and fallacies of personally identifiable information. *Communications of the ACM*, *53*(6), 24–26. doi:10.1145/1743546.1743558

Nass, S. J., Levit, L. A., & Gostin, L. O. (2009). *HIPAA, the Privacy Rule, and Its Application to Health Research*. Academic Press.

Nath, A., Anderson, C., Jones, M., Maragos, W., Booze, R., Mactutus, C., ... Mattson, M. (2000b). Neurotoxicity and dysfunction of dopaminergic systems associated with AIDS dementia. *Journal of Psychopharmacology (Oxford, England)*, *14*(3), 222–227. doi:10.1177/026988110001400305 PMID:11106300

Nath, A., & Clements, J. E. (2011). Eradication of HIV from the brain: Reasons for pause. *AIDS (London, England)*, *25*(5), 577–580. doi:10.1097/QAD.0b013e3283437d2f PMID:21160414

Nath, A., Jankovic, J., & Pettigrew, L. C. (1987). Movement disorders and AIDS. *Neurology*, *37*(1), 37–41. doi:10.1212/WNL.37.1.37 PMID:3796836

Nath, A., Maragos, W. F., Avison, M. J., Schmitt, F. A., & Berger, J. R. (2001). Acceleration of HIV dementia with methamphetamine and cocaine. *Journal of Neurovirology*, *7*(1), 66–71. doi:10.1080/135502801300069737 PMID:11519485

Nayeem, A., Sitkoff, D., & Krystek, S. (2006). A comparative study of available software for high-accuracy homology modeling: From sequence alignments to structural models. *Protein Science*, *15*(4), 808–824. doi:10.1110/ps.051892906 PMID:16600967

Neiswanger, W., Wang, C., & Xing, E. (2013). *Asymptotically exact, embarrassingly parallel MCMC.* arXiv preprint arXiv: 1311-4780

Nguyen, T., Khosravi, A., Creighton, D., & Nahavandi, S. (2015). Classification of healthcare data using genetic fuzzy logic system and wavelets. *Expert Systems with Applications*, *42*(4), 2184–2197. doi:10.1016/j.eswa.2014.10.027

Niakšu, O., &Kurasova, O. (2012). Data mining applications in healthcare: research vs practice. *Databases Inform Syst Baltic DB&IS, 58.*

Nitrd, N. (2016). *The Federal Big Data Research and Development Strategic Plan.* Networking and Information Technology Research and Development.

Norregaard, L., Frederiksen, D., Nielsen, E. Ø., & Gether, U. (1998). Delineation of an endogenous zinc-binding site in the human dopamine transporter. *The EMBO Journal*, *17*(15), 4266–4273. doi:10.1093/emboj/17.15.4266 PMID:9687495

O'Reilly, M. (1995). Use of medical information by computer networks raises major concerns about privacy. *CMAJ: Canadian Medical Association Journal, 153*(2), 212.

Olsen, L., & McGinnis, J. M. (2010). *Evidence Development for Healthcare Decisions: Improving Timeliness.* Reliability, and Efficiency.

Oweis, N. E., Owais, S. S., George, W., Suliman, M. G., & Snášel, V. (2015). A survey on big data, mining:(tools, techniques, applications and notable uses). In *Intelligent Data Analysis and Applications* (pp. 109–119). Cham: Springer. doi:10.1007/978-3-319-21206-7_10

Papakostas, G. I. (2006). Dopaminergic-based pharmacotherapies for depression. *European Neuropsychopharmacology*, *16*(6), 391–402. doi:10.1016/j.euroneuro.2005.12.002 PMID:16413172

Patel, A. B., Birla, M., & Nair, U. (2012, December). Addressing big data problem using Hadoop and Map Reduce. In *Engineering (NUiCONE), 2012 Nirma University International Conference on* (pp. 1-5). IEEE. doi:10.1109/NUICONE.2012.6493198

PatientsLikeMe. (2013). Available from: http://www.patientslikeme.com/

Patil, R. D., & Jadhav, O. S. (2016). Some Contribution of Statistical Techniques in Big Data: A Review. *International Journal on Recent and Innovation Trends in Computing and Communication*, *4*(4), 293–303.

Patty, J., & Penn, E. M. (2015). Analyzing Big Data: Social Choice and Measurement. *PS, Political Science & Politics*, *48*(1), 95–101. doi:10.1017/S1049096514001814

Paul, M. J., & Dredze, M. (2012). A model for mining public health topics from Twitter. *Health*, *11*, 16–6.

Pei, J., Tang, M., & Grishin, N. V. (2008). PROMALS3D web server for accurate multiple protein sequence and structure alignments. *Nucleic Acids Research*, *36*(Web ServerSuppl. 2), W30–W34. doi:10.1093/nar/gkn322 PMID:18503087

Penmatsa, A., Wang, K. H., & Gouaux, E. (2013). X-ray structure of dopamine transporter elucidates antidepressant mechanism. *Nature*, *503*(7474), 85–90. doi:10.1038/nature12533 PMID:24037379

Penmatsa, A., Wang, K. H., & Gouaux, E. (2015). X-ray structures of drosophila dopamine transporter in complex with nisoxetine and reboxetine. *Nature Structural & Molecular Biology*, *22*(6), 506–508. doi:10.1038/nsmb.3029 PMID:25961798

Piegorsch, W. W. (2015). *Statistical Data Analytics*. New York: Wiley.

Politis, D. N., Romano, J. P., & Wolf, M. (1999). Subsampling. New York: Springer.

Pulley, J. M., Denny, J. C., Peterson, J. F., Bernard, G. R., Vnencak-Jones, C. L., Ramirez, A. H., & Crawford, D. C. (2012). Operational implementation of prospective genotyping for personalized medicine: The design of the Vanderbilt PREDICT project. *Clinical Pharmacology and Therapeutics*, *92*(1), 87–95. doi:10.1038/clpt.2011.371 PMID:22588608

Purohit, V., Rapaka, R., & Shurtleff, D. (2011). Drugs of abuse, dopamine, and HIV-associated neurocognitive disorders/HIV-associated dementia. *Molecular Neurobiology*, *44*(1), 102–110. doi:10.1007/s12035-011-8195-z PMID:21717292

Pyne, S., Rao, B. P., & Rao, S. B. (2016). Big Data Analytics: Views from Statistical and Computational Perspectives. In Big Data Analytics (pp. 1-10). Springer India.

Quizon, P. M., Sun, W. L., Yuan, Y., Midde, N. M., Zhan, C. G., & Zhu, J. (2016). Molecular mechanism: The human dopamine transporter histidine 547 regulates basal and HIV-1 Tat protein-inhibited dopamine transport. *Scientific Reports*, *6*(39048), 1–14. PMID:27966610

Radhi, M. S., Ruslinda, A. R., Fatin, M. F., Hashwan, S. S. B., Arshad, M. M., & Hashim, U. (2016, August). Colorimetric assay of HIV-1 Tat protein and peptide. In *Semiconductor Electronics (ICSE), 2016 IEEE International Conference on*(pp. 200-203). IEEE. doi:10.1109/SMELEC.2016.7573626

Raghupathi, W., &Raghupathi, V. (2014). Big data analytics in healthcare: Promise and potential. *Health Information Science and Systems*, *2*(1), 3.

Ragin, A. B., Wu, Y., Gao, Y., Keating, S., Du, H., Sammet, C., ... Epstein, L. G. (2015). Brain alterations within the first 100 days of HIV infection. *Annals of Clinical and Translational Neurology*, *2*(1), 12–21. doi:10.1002/acn3.136 PMID:25642430

Ray, S., Hossain, S. M. M., & Khatun, L. (2016, September). Discovering preservation pattern from co-expression modules in progression of HIV-1 disease: An eigengene based approach. In *Advances in Computing, Communications and Informatics (ICACCI), 2016 International Conference on* (pp. 814-820). IEEE.

Ray, S., & Maulik, U. (2016). Discovering perturbation of modular structure in HIV progression by integrating multiple data sources through non-negative matrix factorization. *IEEE/ACM Transactions on Computational Biology and Bioinformatics*, 1. doi:10.1109/TCBB.2016.2642184 PMID:28029629

Rhee, S. Y., Gonzales, M. J., Kantor, R., Betts, B. J., Ravela, J., & Shafer, R. W. (2003). Human immunodeficiency virus reverse transcriptase and protease sequence database. *Nucleic Acids Research*, *31*(1), 298–303. doi:10.1093/nar/gkg100 PMID:12520007

Rhee, S. Y., Taylor, J., Wadhera, G., Ben-Hur, A., Brutlag, D. L., & Shafer, R. W. (2006). Genotypic predictors of human immunodeficiency virus type 1 drug resistance. *Proceedings of the National Academy of Sciences of the United States of America*, *103*(46), 17355–17360. doi:10.1073/pnas.0607274103 PMID:17065321

Richard, B. R., John, S. P., Saini, S. K. O., Moukha, C. V., Michael, H., & Baumann, S. A. (2015). Identification of novel allosteric dopamine transporter ligands with nanomolar potency. *Drug and Alcohol Dependence*, *156*, e193–e194. doi:10.1016/j.drugalcdep.2015.07.521

Robertson, K. R., Smurzynski, M., Parsons, T. D., Wu, K., Bosch, R. J., Wu, J., ... Ellis, R. J. (2007). The prevalence and incidence of neurocognitive impairment in the HAART era. *AIDS (London, England)*, *21*(14), 1915–1921. doi:10.1097/QAD.0b013e32828e4e27 PMID:17721099

Roney, K. (2012). *If Interoperability is the Future of Healthcare, What's the Delay. Becker's Hospital Review*.

Rubinstein, I. S. (2012). Big Data: The End of Privacy or a New Beginning? *New York University Public Law and Legal Theory Working Papers*. Paper 357.D

Rumsfeld, J. S., Joynt, K. E., & Maddox, T. M. (2016). Big data analytics to improve cardiovascular care: Promise and challenges. *Nature Reviews. Cardiology*, *13*(6), 350–359. doi:10.1038/nrcardio.2016.42 PMID:27009423

Runyon, S. P., & Carroll, F. (2006). Dopamine transporter ligands: Recent developments and therapeutic potential. *Current Topics in Medicinal Chemistry*, *6*(17), 1825–1843. doi:10.2174/156802606778249775 PMID:17017960

Russom, P. (2011). Big data analytics. *TDWI Best Practices Report, 19*, 40.

Rutherford, A. R., Ramadanović, B., Michelow, W., Marshall, B. D., Small, W., Deering, K., ... Vasaihexyi, K. (2016, December). Control of an HIV epidemic among injection drug users: simulation modeling on complex networks. In *Winter Simulation Conference (WSC)*, 2016 (pp. 13-37). IEEE. doi:10.1109/WSC.2016.7822077

Sabia, S. K., & Kalra, S. (2014). Applications of big Data: Current Status and Future Scope. *SSN (Print)*, *3*(5), 2319–2526.

Sagiroglu, S., & Sinanc, D. (2013).Big data: A review. In *Collaboration Technologies and Systems (CTS), 2013 International Conference on* (pp. 42-47). IEEE. doi:10.1109/CTS.2013.6567202

Salathe, M., Bengtsson, L., Bodnar, T. J., Brewer, D. D., Brownstein, J. S., Buckee, C., & Vespignani, A. (2012). Digital epidemiology. *PLoS Computational Biology*, *8*(7), e1002616. doi:10.1371/journal.pcbi.1002616 PMID:22844241

Sali MODELLER. (1995). *Implementing 3D Protein Modeling, mc2, vol. 2:5*. Molecular Simulations Inc.

Sali. (1995). *MODELLER: Implementing 3D Protein Modeling, mc2, vol. 2:5*. Burlington, MA: Molecular Simulations Inc.

Šali, A., Potterton, L., Yuan, F., Van Vlijmen, H., & Karplus, M. (1995). Evaluation of comparative protein modeling by MODELLER. *Proteins*, *23*(3), 318–326. doi:10.1002/prot.340230306 PMID:8710825

Santos, A. F., & Soares, M. A. (2011). The impact of the nelfinavir resistance-conferring mutation D30N on the susceptibility of HIV-1 subtype B to other protease inhibitors. *Memorias do Instituto Oswaldo Cruz*, *106*(2), 177–181. doi:10.1590/S0074-02762011000200010 PMID:21537677

Sarac, F., & Seker, H. (2016, October). An instance selection framework for mining data streams to predict antibody-feature function relationships on RV144 HIV vaccine recipients. In *Systems, Man, and Cybernetics (SMC), 2016 IEEE International Conference on* (pp. 003356-003361). IEEE. doi:10.1109/SMC.2016.7844752

Sarafianos, S. G., Dasi, K., Dingi, J., Boyer, P. L., Hughes, S. H., & Arnold, E. (1999). Touching the heart of HIV-1 drug resistance: The fingers close down on the dNTP at the polymerase active site. *Chemistry & Biology*, *6*(5), R137–R146. doi:10.1016/S1074-5521(99)80071-4 PMID:10322129

Sardar, A. M., Czudek, C., & Reynolds, G. P. (1996). Dopamine deficits in the brain: The neurochemical basis of parkinsonian symptoms in AIDS. *Neuroreport*, *7*(4), 910–912. doi:10.1097/00001756-199603220-00015 PMID:8724671

Savel, T. G., & Foldy, S. (2012). The role of public health informatics in enhancing public health surveillance. *MMWR. Surveillance Summaries*, *61*(Suppl), 20–24. PMID:22832993

Sayers, E. W., Barrett, T., Benson, D. A., Bolton, E., Bryant, S. H., Canese, K., ... Feolo, M. (2011). Database resources of the national center for biotechnology information. *Nucleic Acids Research*, *39*(suppl 1), D38–D51. doi:10.1093/nar/gkq1172 PMID:21097890

Scanfeld, D., Scanfeld, V., & Larson, E. L. (2010). Dissemination of health information through social networks: Twitter and antibiotics. *American Journal of Infection Control*, *38*(3), 182–188. doi:10.1016/j.ajic.2009.11.004 PMID:20347636

Scheller, C., Arendt, G., Nolting, T., Antke, C., Sopper, S., Maschke, M., ... Koutsilieri, E. (2010). Increased dopaminergic neurotransmission in therapy-naive asymptomatic HIV patients is not associated with adaptive changes at the dopaminergic synapses. *Journal of Neural Transmission (Vienna, Austria)*, *117*(6), 699–705. doi:10.1007/s00702-010-0415-6 PMID:20454983

Schifano, E. D., Wu, J., Wang, C., Yan, J., & Chen, M.-H. (2015). Online Updating of Statistical Inference in the Big Data Setting. *Technometrics*. PMID:28018007

Schmitt, K. C., & Reith, M. E. (2011). The atypical stimulant and nootropic modafinil interacts with the dopamine transporter in a different manner than classical cocaine-like inhibitors. *PLoS One*, *6*(10), e25790. doi:10.1371/journal.pone.0025790 PMID:22043293

Scott, S.L., Blocker, A.W., Bonassi, F.V., Chipman, H., George, E., & McCulloch, R. (2013). Bayes and Big Data: The Consensus Monte Carlo Algorithm. *EFaBBayes 250 Conference*, 16.

Scudellari, M. (2016). *Big Data Tamps Down HIV Outbreaks*. Retrieved March 30, 2017, from http://spectrum.ieee.org/the-human-os/biomedical/diagnostics/big-data-tamps-down-hiv-outbreaks

Seddik, A., Holy, M., Weissensteiner, R., Zdrazil, B., Sitte, H. H., & Ecker, G. F. (2013). Probing the selectivity of monoamine transporter substrates by means of molecular modeling. *Molecular Informatics*, *32*(5-6), 409–413. doi:10.1002/minf.201300013 PMID:23956802

Sedkaoui, S. (2017). The Internet, Data Analytics and Big Data. In Internet Economics: Models, Mechanisms and Management (pp. 185-210). Bentham Science.

Sedkaoui, S., & Monino, J. L. (2016). *Big data, Open Data and Data Development*. New York: ISTE-Wiley.

Seifter, A., Schwarzwalder, A., Geis, K., & Aucott, J. (2010). The utility of "Google Trends" for epidemiological research: Lyme disease as an example. *Geospatial Health*, *4*(2), 135–137. doi:10.4081/gh.2010.195 PMID:20503183

Severinsen, K., Kraft, J. F., Koldsø, H., Vinberg, K. A., Rothman, R. B., Partilla, J. S., ... Sinning, S. (2012). Binding of the amphetamine-like 1-phenyl-piperazine to monoamine transporters. *ACS Chemical Neuroscience*, *3*(9), 693–705. doi:10.1021/cn300040f PMID:23019496

Shafer, R. W., Dupnik, K., Winters, M. A., & Eshleman, S. H. (2001). A guide to HIV-1 reverse transcriptase and protease sequencing for drug resistance studies. *HIV Sequence Compendium*, *2001*, 1. PMID:22324021

Shan, J., Javitch, J. A., Shi, L., & Weinstein, H. (2011). The substrate driven transition to an inward-facing conformation in the functional mechanism of the dopamine transporter. *PLoS One*, *6*(1), e16350. doi:10.1371/journal.pone.0016350 PMID:21298009

Sharma, V., Joshi, N. K., & Manisha. (2015). Big Data Introduction, Importance and Current Perspective of Challenges. *International Journal of Advances in Engineering Science and Technology*, *4*(3), 221–225.

Shivade, C., Raghavan, P., Fosler-Lussier, E., Embi, P. J., Elhadad, N., Johnson, S. B., & Lai, A. M. (2013). A review of approaches to identifying patient phenotype cohorts using electronic health records. *Journal of the American Medical Informatics Association*, *21*(2), 221–230. doi:10.1136/amiajnl-2013-001935 PMID:24201027

Shoenbill, K., Fost, N., Tachinardi, U., & Mendonca, E. A. (2013). Genetic data and electronic health records: A discussion of ethical, logistical and technological considerations. *Journal of the American Medical Informatics Association*, *21*(1), 171–180. doi:10.1136/amiajnl-2013-001694 PMID:23771953

Shroff, G. (2013). *The Intelligent Web, Search, Smart Algorithms and Big Data*. Oxford, UK: Oxford Univ. Press.

Siegel, E. (2016). *Predictive Analytics*. New York: Wiley.

Silverstein, P., Shah, A., Weemhoff, J., Kumar, S. P., Singh, D., & Kumar, A. (2012). HIV-1 gp120 and drugs of abuse: Interactions in the central nervous system. *Current HIV Research, 10*, 369–383. doi:10.2174/157016212802138724 PMID:22591361

Singh, S. K., Piscitelli, C. L., Yamashita, A., & Gouaux, E. (2008). A competitive inhibitor traps LeuT in an open-to-out conformation. *Science, 322*(5908), 1655–1661. doi:10.1126/science.1166777 PMID:19074341

C. M. Spicer, & M. A. Ford (Eds.). (2012). *Monitoring HIV care in the United States: indicators and data systems*. National Academies Press.

Stockner, T., Montgomery, T. R., Kudlacek, O., Weissensteiner, R., Ecker, G. F., Freissmuth, M., & Sitte, H. H. (2013). Mutational analysis of the high-affinity Zinc binding site validates a refined human dopamine transporter homology model. *PLoS Computational Biology, 9*(2), e1002909. doi:10.1371/journal.pcbi.1002909 PMID:23436987

Stone, M. L. (2014). *Big data for media. Reuters Institute For The Study Of Journalism*. University of Oxford.

Sucic, S., Dallinger, S., Zdrazil, B., Weissensteiner, R., Jørgensen, T. N., Holy, M., ... Sitte, H. H. (2010). The N terminus of monoamine transporters is a lever required for the action of amphetamines. *The Journal of Biological Chemistry, 285*(14), 10924–10938. doi:10.1074/jbc.M109.083154 PMID:20118234

Sullivan, S. J., Schneiders, A. G., Cheang, C. W., Kitto, E., Lee, H., & Redhead, J. (2011). What's happening? A content analysis of concussion-related traffic on twitter. *Br J Sports Med*. Available from: http://www.academia.edu/1037228/Whats_happening_A_content_analysis_of_concussion-related_traffic_on_Twitter

Sulzer, D. (2011). How addictive drugs disrupt presynaptic dopamine neurotransmission. *Neuron, 69*(4), 628–649. doi:10.1016/j.neuron.2011.02.010 PMID:21338876

Summary of the HIPAA Privacy Rule. (2017). Dep't Of Health & Human Servs. Retrieved from https://www.hhs.gov/sites/default/files/privacysummary.pdf.

Swan, M. (2013). The quantified self: Fundamental disruption in big data science and biological discovery. *Big Data, 1*(2), 85–99. doi:10.1089/big.2012.0002 PMID:27442063

Szlezák, N., Evers, M., Wang, J., & Pérez, L. (2014). The role of big data and advanced analytics in drug discovery, development, and commercialization. *Clinical Pharmacology and Therapeutics*, *95*(5), 492–495. doi:10.1038/clpt.2014.29 PMID:24642713

Talia, D. (2013). Clouds for scalable big data analytics. *Computer*, *46*(5), 98–101. doi:10.1109/MC.2013.162

Tan, P. N., Steinbach, M., & Kumar, V. (2013). Data mining cluster analysis: basic concepts and algorithms. *Introduction to Data Mining*.

Tang, M. W., Liu, T. F., & Shafer, R. W. (2012). The HIVdb system for HIV-1 genotypic resistance interpretation. *Intervirology*, *55*(2), 98–101. doi:10.1159/000331998 PMID:22286876

Tasse, D. (2012). *Quantifiedself 2012: Some cool things. Tales 'n' ideas*. Available from: http://talesnideas.blogspot.com/2012_09_01_archive.html

Tenenbaum, J. D., Sansone, S. A., & Haendel, M. (2013). A sea of standards for omics data: Sink or swim? *Journal of the American Medical Informatics Association*, *21*(2), 200–203. doi:10.1136/amiajnl-2013-002066 PMID:24076747

Torres, G. E., Gainetdinov, R., & Caron, M. G. (2003). Plasma membrane monoamine transporters: structure, regulation and function. *Nat. Rev. ci.*, *4*(1), 13–25.

Toshniwal, R., Dastidar, K. G., &Nath, A. (2015). Big Data Security Issues and Challenges. *International Journal of Innovative Research in Advanced Engineering*, (2).

Tozzi, V., Balestra, P., Bellagamba, R., Corpolongo, A., Salvatori, M. F., Visco-Comandini, U., ... Narciso, P. (2007). Persistence of neuropsychologic deficits despite long-term highly active antiretroviral therapy in patients with HIV-related neurocognitive impairment: Prevalence and risk factors. *JAIDS Journal of Acquired Immune Deficiency Syndromes*, *45*(2), 174–182. doi:10.1097/QAI.0b013e318042e1ee PMID:17356465

Trichopoulos, D., Sparos, L., & Petridou, E. (1998). Homosexual role separation and spread of AIDS. *Lancet*, *2*, 965–966. PMID:2902413

Turban, E. (2011). *Business Intelligence: A Managerial Approach* (2nd ed.). Upper Saddle River, NJ: Prentice Hall.

Turn, R., & Ware, W. H. (1976). *Privacy and security issues in information systems* (Vol. 5684). Rand Corporation. doi:10.7249/P5684

Uddin, M. F., & Gupta, N. (2014, April). Seven V's of Big Data understanding Big Data to extract value. In American Society for Engineering Education (ASEE Zone 1), 2014 Zone 1 Conference of the (pp. 1-5). IEEE.

Uhl, G. R. (2003). Dopamine transporter: Basic science and human variation of a key molecule for dopaminergic function, locomotion, and parkinsonism. *Movement Disorders*, *18*(S7), S71–S80. doi:10.1002/mds.10578 PMID:14531049

Ularu, E. G., Puican, F. C., Apostu, A., & Velicanu, M. (2012). Perspectives on big data and big data analytics. *Database Systems Journal*, *3*(4), 3–14.

UNICEF. (2016). Global report: UNAIDS report on the global AIDS epidemic 2016. Geneva: UNAIDS.

Unit, E. I. (2012). The deciding factor: Big data &decision making. *Capgemini Reports*, 1-24.

Valcour, V., Shikuma, C., Shiramizu, B., Watters, M., Poff, P., Selnes, O., ... Sacktor, N. (2004). Higher frequency of dementia in older HIV-1 individuals: The Hawaii Aging with HIV-1 Cohort. *Neurology*, *63*(5), 822–827. doi:10.1212/01.WNL.0000134665.58343.8D PMID:15365130

Van Druten, H., Van Griensven, F., & Hendriks, J. (1992). Homosexual role separation: Implications for analyzing and modeling the spread of HIV. *Journal of Sex Research*, *29*(4), 477–499. doi:10.1080/00224499209551663

Ventura, A., Koenitzer, M., Stein, P., Tufano, P., & Drummer, D. (2015).The Future of FinTech: A Paradigm Shift in Small Business Finance. *World Economic Forum, Global Agenda Council on the Future of Financing and Capital.*

Vermesan, D., Prejbeanu, R., Laitin, R., Georgianu, V., Haragus, H., & Nitescu, S. (2014). Meniscal tears left in situ during anatomic single bundle anterior cruciate ligament reconstruction. *European Review for Medical and Pharmacological Sciences*, *18*(2), 252–256. PMID:24488916

Vittinghoff, E., Douglas, J., Judson, F., McKirnan, D., & MacQueen, K. (1999). Per-contact risk of human immunodeficiency virus transmission between male sexual partners. *American Journal of Epidemiology*, *150*(3), 306–311. doi:10.1093/oxfordjournals.aje.a010003 PMID:10430236

Vivithanaporn, P., Nelles, K., DeBlock, L., Newman, S. C., Gill, M. J., & Power, C. (2012). Hepatitis C virus co-infection increases neurocognitive impairment severity and risk of death in treated HIV/AIDS. *Journal of the Neurological Sciences*, *312*(1-2), 45–51. doi:10.1016/j.jns.2011.08.025 PMID:21925684

Vo, Q. T., Cox, C., Li, X., Jacobson, L. P., McKaig, R., Sacktor, N., ... Miller, E. N. (2013). Neuropsychological test performance before and after HIV-1 seroconversion: The Multicenter AIDS Cohort Study. *Journal of Neurovirology*, *19*(1), 24–31. doi:10.1007/s13365-012-0136-8 PMID:23229349

Wainberg, M. A., Zaharatos, G. J., & Brenner, B. G. (2011). Development of antiretroviral drug resistance. *The New England Journal of Medicine*, *365*(7), 637–646. doi:10.1056/NEJMra1004180 PMID:21848464

Walker, S. (2014). *Big data: A revolution that will transform how we live, work, and think*. Academic Press.

Wang, X., Guo, F., Heller, K. A., & Dunson, D. B. (2015). *Parallelizing MCMC with Random Partition Trees*. arXiv preprint arXiv: 1506-03164

Wang, C. I., & Lewis, R. J. (2010). Emerging structure–function relationships defining monoamine NSS transporter substrate and ligand affinity. ochem. *Pharmacol.*, *79*(8), 1083–1091. PMID:19954741

Wang, G. J., Chang, L., Volkow, N. D., Telang, F., Logan, J., ... Fowler, J. S. (2004). Decreased brain dopaminergic transporters in HIV-associated dementia patients. *Brain*, *1*(27), 2452–2458. doi:10.1093/brain/awh269 PMID:15319273

Wang, K. H., Penmatsa, A., & Gouaux, E. (2015). Neurotransmitter and psychostimulant recognition by the dopamine transporter. *Nature*, *521*(7552), 322–327. doi:10.1038/nature14431 PMID:25970245

Westendorp, M. O., Frank, R., Ochsenbauer, C., Stricker, K., Dhein, J., Walczak, H., ... Krammer, P. H. (1995). Sensitization of T cells to CD95-mediated apoptosis by HIV-1 Tat and gp120. *Nature*, *375*(6531), 497–500. doi:10.1038/375497a0 PMID:7539892

West, R., White, R. W., & Horvitz, E. (2013). From cookies to cooks: Insights on dietary patterns via analysis of web usage logs. In *Proceedings of the 22nd international conference on World Wide Web* (pp. 1399-1410). ACM. doi:10.1145/2488388.2488510

Whitcomb, J. M., Parkin, N. T., Chappey, C., Hellmann, N. S., & Petropoulos, C. J. (2003). Broad nucleoside reverse-transcriptase inhibitor cross-resistance in human immunodeficiency virus type 1 clinical isolates. *The Journal of Infectious Diseases*, *188*(7), 992–1000. doi:10.1086/378281 PMID:14513419

White, R. W., Tatonetti, N. P., Shah, N. H., Altman, R. B., & Horvitz, E. (2013). Web-scale pharmacovigilance: Listening to signals from the crowd. *Journal of the American Medical Informatics Association*, *20*(3), 404–408. doi:10.1136/amiajnl-2012-001482 PMID:23467469

Wilkes, J. J. (2014). The Creation of HIPAA Culture: Prioritizing Privacy Paranoia over Patient Care. *BYU L. Rev.*, 1213.

Williams, D. W., Calderon, T. M., Lopez, L., Carvallo-Torres, L., Gaskill, P. J., Eugenin, E. A., ... Berman, J. W. (2013). Mechanisms of HIV entry into the CNS: Increased sensitivity of HIV infected CD14+CD16+ monocytes to CCL2 and key roles of CCR2, JAM-A, and ALCAM in diapedesis. *PLoS One*, *8*(7), e69270. doi:10.1371/journal.pone.0069270 PMID:23922698

Wise, R. A., & Bozarth, M. A. (1987). A psychomotor stimulant theory of addiction. *Psychological Review*, *94*(4), 469–492. doi:10.1037/0033-295X.94.4.469 PMID:3317472

Wlodawer, A., & Erickson, J. W. (1993). Structure-based inhibitors of HIV-1 protease. *Annual Review of Biochemistry*, *62*(1), 543–585. doi:10.1146/annurev.bi.62.070193.002551 PMID:8352596

Wolf, G. (2012). The data-driven life. *The New York Times* Available from: http://www.nytimes.com/2010/05/02/magazine/02self-measurement-t.html

World Health Organization, HIV/AIDS, Media Centre-Fact Sheet. (n.d.). Retrieved from http://www.who.int/mediacentre/factsheets/fs360/en/

Wu, C. F. J. (1989). Bootstrap and other resampling methods in regression analysis. *Ann Stat*, *14*, 1261–1295.

Xiao, H., Neuveut, C., Tiffany, H. L., Benkirane, M., Rich, E. A., Murphy, P. M., & Jeang, K. T. (2000). Selective CXCR4 antagonism by Tat: Implications for in vivo expansion of coreceptor use by HIV-1. *Proceedings of the National Academy of Sciences of the United States of America*, *97*(21), 11466–11471. doi:10.1073/pnas.97.21.11466 PMID:11027346

Yamaguchi, K., Hazan, T., McAllester, D., & Urtasun, R. (2013). *Robustmonocular epipolar flow estimation*. CVPR.

Yamashita, A., Singh, S. K., Kawate, T., Jin, Y., & Gouaux, E. (2005). Crystal structure of a bacterial homologue of Na+/Cl-dependent neurotransmitter transporters. *Nature*, *437*(7056), 215–223. doi:10.1038/nature03978 PMID:16041361

Yau, N. (2011). A year of food consumption visualized. *FlowingData*. Available from: http://flowingdata. com/2011/06/29/a-year-of-food-consumption-visualized/

Yohn, S. E., Gogoj, A., Haque, A., Lopez-Cruz, L., Haley, A., Huxley, P., ... Salamone, J. D. (2016). Evaulation of the effortrelated motivational effects of the novel dopamine uptake inhibitor Prx-14040. *Pharmacology, Biochemistry, and Behavior*, *148*, 84–91. doi:10.1016/j.pbb.2016.06.004 PMID:27296079

Yoo, C., Ramirez, L., & Liuzzi, J. (2014). Big data analysis using modern statistical and machine learning methods in medicine. *International Neurourology Journal*, *18*(2), 50. doi:10.5213/inj.2014.18.2.50 PMID:24987556

Young, S. D. (2015). A "big data" approach to HIV epidemiology and prevention. *Preventive Medicine*, *70*, 17–18. doi:10.1016/j.ypmed.2014.11.002 PMID:25449693

Young, S. D., & Jaganath, D. (2013). Online social networking for HIV education and prevention: A mixed methods analysis. *Sexually Transmitted Diseases*, *40*(2), 162–167. doi:10.1097/OLQ.0b013e318278bd12 PMID:23324979

Young, S. D., Rivers, C., & Lewis, B. (2014). Methods of using real-time social media technologies for detection and remote monitoring of HIV outcomes. *Preventive Medicine*, *63*, 112–115. doi:10.1016/j.ypmed.2014.01.024 PMID:24513169

Yuan, Y., Huang, X., Midde, N. M., Quizon, P. M., Sun, W. L., Zhu, J., & Zhan, C. G. (2015). Molecular mechanism of HIV-1 Tat interacting with human dopamine transporter. *ACS Chemical Neuroscience*, *6*(4), 658–665. doi:10.1021/acschemneuro.5b00001 PMID:25695767

Yuan, Y., Quizon, P. M., Sun, W. L., Yao, J., Zhu, J., & Zhan, C. G. (2016). Role of histidine 547 of human dopamine transporter in molecular interaction with HIV-1 Tat and dopamine uptake. *Scientific Reports*, *6*(1), 27314. doi:10.1038/srep27314 PMID:27250920

Yu, L., Zheng, J., Shen, W. C., Wu, B., Wang, B., Qian, L., & Zhang, B. R. (2012). BC-PDM: data mining, social network analysis and text mining system based on cloud computing. In *Proceedings of the 18th ACM SIGKDD international conference on Knowledge discovery and data mining* (pp. 1496-1499). ACM. doi:10.1145/2339530.2339764

Zaccarelli, M., Perno, C. F., Forbici, F., Soldani, F., Bonfigli, S., Gori, C., ... De Longis, P. (2004). Q151M-mediated multinuclcoside resistance: Prevalence, risk factors, and response to salvage therapy. *Clinical Infectious Diseases*, *38*(3), 433–437. doi:10.1086/381097 PMID:14727218

Zeleny, M. (1987). Management Support Systems: Towards Integrated Knowledge Management. *Human Systems Management*, *7*(1), 59–70.

Zhang, A. (2017). *Data analytics: Practical guide to leveraging the power of Algorithms, data science, data mining, statistics, big data, and predictive analysis to improve business, work, and life*. Kindle Edition.

Zhang, B., Gaiteri, C., Bodea, L. G., Wang, Z., McElwee, J., Podtelezhnikov, A. A., & Fluder, E. (2013). Integrated systems approach identifies genetic nodes and networks in late-onset Alzheimer's disease. *Cell*, *153*(3), 707–720. doi:10.1016/j.cell.2013.03.030 PMID:23622250

Zhu, J., Mactutus, C. F., Wallace, D. R., & Booze, R. M. (2009). HIV-1 Tat protein-induced rapid and reversible decrease in [3H]dopamine uptake: Dissociation of [3H] dopamine uptake and [3H]2beta-carbomethoxy-3-beta-(4-fluorophenyl)tropane (WIN 35,428) binding in rat striatal synaptosomes. *The Journal of Pharmacology and Experimental Therapeutics*, *329*(3), 1071–1083. doi:10.1124/jpet.108.150144 PMID:19325033

Zhu, J., & Reith, M. E. (2008). Role of dopamine transporter in the action of psychostimulants, nicotine, and other drugs of abuse. *CNS & Neurological Disorders - Drug Targets*, *7*(5), 393–409. doi:10.2174/187152708786927877 PMID:19128199

Zicari, R. V. (2014). Big data: Challenges and opportunities. *Big Data Computing*, *564*.

About the Contributors

Ali Al Mazari is an Australian Jordanian Scientist, with more than 18 years of Teaching, Training, Research and Consultation experience in Information & Communication Technologies (ICT) applied sciences and multidisciplinary domains, as well as Business Leadership and Management. Dr. Al Mazari earned his PhD in Science (with specialization in Biomedical Informatics) from the School of Information Technologies, Sydney University in Australia, early 2007, Master of Computing (Major in IT) from the School of Computing, Western Sydney University, Australia, 2001, Master of Leadership & Management in Education, Newcastle University, Australia, 2010, and received his Bachelor of Science in Mathematics and Computer Science, Jordan, 1994. Dr. Al Mazari was working as a Post-Doctoral Biomedical Informatics Researcher, at the School of Information Technologies, the University of Sydney, on investigating research issues in Bioinformatics and Biomedical Informatics (2007 to 2009). Dr. Al Mazari research activities were also taken place at the National ICT Australia (Centre of Excellence) (NICTA), produced Technical Reports and Research Seminars with audiences from many disciplines including ICT, bioinformatics, biostatistics, clinical immunology, molecular biology and machine learning (2007 to 2009). Dr. Al Mazari's science-oriented research experience and interests are in the areas of computational biology, Bioinformatics, life sciences and the development of algorithms and models for biomedical applications and problems, and in the area of Information Security and Cybercrime. Dr. Al Mazari's doctorate research focused on the application of computational methods for the analysis of HIV drug resistance dynamics. His contributions focus on developing algorithms, models, data mining and machine learning tools for the understanding of HIV/AIDS evolutionary behaviours and enabling further insights into understanding the trends of immunological and virological changes with reference to HIV viral evolution, genetic mutation and behaviour.

* * *

Biswa Ranjan Acharya, M.Tech from Dhaneswar Ratha Institute of Management & Studies under BPUT, Odisha, India. He obtained MCA from IGNOU in 2009. He has more than 5years industry experience as well as teaching experience. His research interest Data Analytics, Computer Vision and Image processing, parallel computing and Cloud computing.

Md Tarique Jamal Ansari was born and raised in the state, Uttar Pradesh, India. He is a Research Scholar of Information Technology at Babasaheb Bhimrao Ambedkar University, India. He received his M.Sc. in Information Technology from Babasaheb Bhimrao Ambedkar University. He is a University Gold Medalist during his Master's degree programme. His research interest includes Software Engineering, Requirement Engineering, and Big Data.

Andrés J. Cortés completed his BSc and MSc in Biological Sciences at Universidad de los Andes, Colombia, and earned his PhD in genetics from Uppsala University, Sweden. He has worked at the International Center for Agricultural Research (CIAT), the Botanical Gardens of Ireland, the Swiss Federal Institute for Forest, Snow and Landscape Research (WSL), the Swedish Agricultural University, the University of Gothenburg, and more recently at the Colombian Corporation for Agricultural Research (CORPOICA). He is broadly interested in the extent of genetic adaptation. Dr. Cortés has published 19 articles, 2 books, 1 book chapter, and 2 popular science articles, which, all together, have been cited more than 500 times in the last five years.

Ahmed A. El-Rashedy is a part of the Department of Natural and Microbial Product, Research Division of Pharmaceutical and Drug Industries, National Research Centre, Dokki, Cairo 12622, Egypt. Dr. El-Rashedy published fourteen international journals and two paper under submission and he published a book on medicinal chemistry his titled (Selected Topics In Medicinal Chemistry) published in LAP LAMBERT Academic Publishing, Germany and one chapter entitled (RNA as drug target) published in SM group, Academic Publishing, USA .

Luke Elizabeth Hanna obtained Ph.D in the area of basic medical sciences in the year 2000. Her postdoctoral research includes the field of molecular virology in relation to HIV, from Albert Einstein College of Medicine, New York, USA in the year 2007. From research assistant, she promoted as Scientist B, C, and D in the respective years 2002, 2008, and 2015 after completing her doctorate degree, at NIRT, Chennai. She had 20 years of working experience in the broad area of immunology of infectious diseases including tuberculosis, HIV, and lymphatic filariasis. She is the Chief Laboratory Liaison for WHO HIV Drug Resistance Network activities at TRC, supervisor, and coordinator for activities relating to the Virology Quality Assurance Program (NIH) at NIRT, and laboratory resource person for the second-line ART and early infant diagnosis programs of NACO. She is the principal investigator for the ICMR Biomedical Informatics Project at NIRT and a recognized guide for Ph.D. students registered with the Madras University.

Chinmayee Mohapatra has received B.Tech degree in IT from BPUT, Odisha. She is currently an M.Tech, Computer Science and Engineering student in School of Computer Engineering, KIIT University, Bhubaneswar, Odisha, India. Her areas of interests are Data Mining and Data Analytics.

Dhirendra Pandey is an Assistant Professor of Information Technology at Babasaheb Bhimrao Ambedkar University, India. He received his doctorate in Computer Science from Devi Ahilya Vishwavidyalaya, Indore, India. His areas of specializations are Data Mining, Software Engineering, and Requirement Engineering. He has more than 10 years of teaching experience and research experience. He is the reviewer of many national and international journals. In addition, He has also published many research papers as an author and co-author of more than 60 papers in national and international journals. Dr. Dhirendra Pandey also working as Principal Investigator of Research Project funded by CST, UP, India under Young Scientist scheme.

Manjusha Pandey is presently working as an Assistant Professor in the School of Computer Engineering, Kalinga Institute of Industrial Technology, and Bhubaneswar. She is pursuing her PhD from Indian Institute of Information Technology, Allahabad. She has more than 35 research publications to her credit in journals and conferences of repute. Her research interest areas include Wireless Sensor Network, Security and Privacy in Wireless Sensor Network, Data Analytics, Human Computer Interaction and Computer Networks.

Siddhath Swarup Rautaray is presently working as an Assistant Professor in the School of Computer Engineering, Kalinga Institute of Industrial Technology, Bhubaneswar. He obtained his PhD from Indian Institute of Information Technology, Allahabad. He has more than 50 research publications to his credit in journals and conferences of repute. His research interest areas include Human Computer Interaction, Computer Vision, Data Analytics, Security and Privacy in Wireless Sensor Network, and Computer Networks.

Soraya Sedkaoui is a Senior Lecturer at the department of Economics, Khemis Miliana University in Algeria and Researcher at TRIS laboratory in the University of Montpellier, France. Ph.D In Economic analysis and HDR in Economic and Applied statistics. Her research fields include econometrics, statistics, Big data analytics and data mining, data science, and IT acceptance and uses. Her prior books and research has been published in several refereed editions and journals. She is also Manager of "S.R.Y - Consulting " at Montpellier, France.

A. Nusrath Unissa completed her Ph.D in the interdisciplinary area of Biotechnology-Microbiology - 2010. She worked as lecturer for Biotechnology in couple of colleges from 2001 to 2003. She obtained the GATE award in 2003. She also qualified Indian council of medical research (ICMR)-JRF award in the year 2003, then as ICMR-SRF during 2007, at National Institute for Research in Tuberculosis, (NIRT) Chennai. She was awarded as ICMR -Post Doctoral Fellowship (PDF) in 2013. She has undertaken numerous research studies in the field of TB drug resistance and published several articles being the first and corresponding author in peer reviewed international journals. Currently, she is working in the in silico analysis aspects of HIV drug resistance.

Index

I

K

L

M

N

P

R

S

T

W

www.ingramcontent.com/pod-product-compliance
Lightning Source LLC
LaVergne TN
LVHW081527300926
849161LV00006B/1330